INFECTION AND HEARING IMPAIRMENT

Edited by

V.E. Newton
Human Communication and Deafness,
The University of Manchester

P.J. Vallely
The Virology Unit, Division of Laboratory and Regenerative Medicine,
The University of Manchester

John Wiley & Sons, Ltd

Other Wiley Editorial Offices

John Wiley & Sons Inc., 111 River Street, Hoboken, NJ 07030, USA

Jossey-Bass, 989 Market Street, San Francisco, CA 94103-1741, USA

Wiley-VCH Verlag GmbH, Boschstr. 12, D-69469 Weinheim, Germany

John Wiley & Sons Australia Ltd, 42 McDougall Street, Milton, Queensland 4064, Australia

John Wiley & Sons (Asia) Pte Ltd, 2 Clementi Loop #02-01, Jin Xing Distripark, Singapore
129809

John Wiley & Sons Canada Ltd, 22 Worcester Road, Etobicoke, Ontario, Canada M9W 1L1

Wiley also publishes its books in a variety of electronic formats. Some content that appears in
print may not be available in electronic books.

Library of Congress Cataloging-in-Publication Data
Infection and Hearing Impairment / edited by Valerie E. Newton, Pamela J. Vallely.
    p. ; cm.
Includes bibliographical references and index.
ISBN-13: 978-1-86156-507-5 (pbk. : alk. paper)
ISBN-10: 1-86156-507-0 (pbk. : alk. paper)
1. Deafness. 2. Deafness–Etiology. 3. Infection–Complications.
I. Newton, Valerie E. II. Vallely, Pamela J.
[DNLM: 1. Hearing Loss–etiology. 2. Hearing Loss–microbiology.
3. Hearing Loss–prevention & control. 4. Infection–complications.
WV 270 I43 2006]
RF290.I54 2006
617.8–dc22
                                                                2005025592

British Library Cataloguing in Publication Data
A catalogue record for this book is available from the British Library

ISBN-13   978-1-86156–507-5
ISBN –10   1-86156-507-0

Typeset by SNP Best-set Typesetter Ltd, Hong Kong
Printed and bound in Great Britain by TJ International Ltd, Padstow, Cornwall
This book is printed on acid-free paper responsibly manufactured from sustainable forestry
in which at least two trees are planted for each one used for paper production.

CONTENTS

Contributors   vii

Preface   xiii

1   Basic Anatomy and Physiology of the Ear   1
    J. Irwin

2   Development of the Ear and of Hearing   17
    V.E. Newton

3   Epidemiology of Infection as a Cause of Hearing Loss   31
    A. Smith and C. Mathers

4   Cytomegalovirus   67
    S.B. Boppana and W.J. Britt

5   Rubella   93
    P.A. Tookey

6   Mumps   109
    K.E. Wright

7   Measles   127
    B. Rima

8   Toxoplasma Infection and the Ear   143
    B. Stray-Pedersen

9   Sexually Transmitted Infections   153
    P. Turner

10   Otitis Media   171
    J.J. Gröte and P.J. Vallely

11   Meningitis and Hearing Loss   183
    K.J. Mutton and E.B. Kaczmarski

12   Infectious Diseases and Hearing in the Tropics   217
    R. Hinchcliffe and S. Prasansuk

13   Ototoxic Drugs   239
     R. Taylor and A. Forge

14   Laboratory Diagnosis, Treatment and Prevention of Infection
     Leading to Hearing Loss   257
     P.E. Klapper and P.J. Vallely

15   The Experience of Deafness – Psychosocial Effects   279
     A. Young

References   287

Index   365

CONTRIBUTORS

Chapter 1
Basic Anatomy and Physiology of the Ear

Dr John Irwin
Department of Audiology
School of Medicine
University of Dundee
Dundee DD1 4HN
Scotland, UK

Chapter 2
Development of the Ear and of Hearing

Professor Valerie E. Newton
Emeritus Professor in Audiological Medicine
Human Communication and Deafness
The University of Manchester
Oxford Rd
Manchester M13 9PT, UK

Chapter 3
Epidemiology of Infection as a Cause of Hearing Loss

Dr Andrew Smith
Prevention of Deafness and Hearing Impairment
World Health Organization
20 Avenue Appia CH-1211
Geneva 27
Switzerland

Dr Colin Mathers
Prevention of Deafness and Hearing Impairment
World Health Organization
20 Avenue Appia CH-1211
Geneva 27
Switzerland

Chapter 4
Cytomegalovirus

Professor Suresh B. Boppana M.D.
Associate Professor of Paediatrics
Department of Paediatrics
The University of Alabama at Birmingham
CHB 114
1600 7ᵗʰ Ave. S.
Birmingham, AL 35233-1711
USA

Professor William J. Britt M.D.
Charles A. Alford Professor of Paediatrics
Department of Paediatrics
The University of Alabama at Birmingham
CHB 114
1600 7ᵗʰ Ave. S.
Birmingham, AL 35233-1711
USA

Chapter 5
Rubella

Dr Pat A. Tookey
Senior Lecturer
Centre for Paediatric Epidemiology and Biostatistics
Institute of Child Health
30 Guilford St
London WC1N 1EH, UK

Chapter 6
Mumps

Dr Kathryn E. Wright
Department of Biochemistry, Microbiology and Immunology
Faculty of Medicine
University of Ottawa
451 Smyth Rd
Ottawa
Ontario
Canada K1H 8MD

Chapter 7
Measles

Dr Bertus Rima
Deputy Director, Centre for Cancer Research and Cell Biology

School of Biology and Biochemistry
Medical Biological Centre
97 Lisburn Rd
Belfast BT9 7BL
N. Ireland, UK

Chapter 8
Toxoplasma Infection and the Ear

Professor Babill Stray-Pedersen
Department of Gynaecology and Obstetrics
Rikshospitalet
University of Oslo
0027 Oslo
Norway

Chapter 9
Sexually Transmitted Infections

Dr Paul Turner
Consultant in Public Health
Ashton, Leigh and Wigan Primary Care Trust
Bryan House
61 Standishgate
Wigan WN1 1AH, UK

Chapter 10
Otitis Media

Professor Jan Gröte
Ear Nose and Throat Department
Leiden University Medical Center
PO Box 9600
2300 RC Leiden
The Netherlands

Dr Pamela J. Vallely
Senior Lecturer in Medical Virology
The Virology Unit, Division of Laboratory and Regenerative Medicine
School of Medicine
University of Manchester
3rd Floor Clinical Sciences Building
Manchester Royal Infirmary
Oxford Rd
Manchester M13 9WL, UK

Chapter 11
Meningitis and Hearing Loss

Dr Kenneth J. Mutton
Consultant Virologist/Microbiologist
Health Protection Agency Laboratory
Manchester Medical Microbiology Partnership
3rd Floor, Clinical Sciences Building
Manchester Royal Infirmary
Oxford Road
Manchester M13 9WL, UK

Dr Edward B. Kaczmarski
Consultant Microbiologist
Health Protection Agency Laboratory
Manchester Medical Microbiology Partnership
2nd Floor, Clinical Sciences Building
Manchester Royal Infirmary
Oxford Road
Manchester M13 9WL, UK

Chapter 12
Infectious Diseases and Hearing in the Tropics

Professor Ronald Hinchcliffe
Division of Audiological Medicine
Institute of Laryngology and Otology
University College London Medical School
Gower St
London WC1E 6BT, UK

Professor Suchitra Prasansuk
Bangkok Otological Center
Faculty of Medicine,
15th Floor, Sayarmin Building
Siriraj Hospital
Bangkok 10700
Thailand

Chapter 13
Ototoxic Drugs

Dr Ruth Taylor
University College London Ear Institute Centre for Auditory Research
332 Gray's Inn Road
London WC 1X 8EE, UK

Professor Andrew Forge
University College London Ear Institute Centre for Auditory Research
332 Gray's Inn Road
London WC 1X 8EE, UK

Chapter 14
Laboratory Diagnosis, Treatment and Prevention of Infection Leading to Hearing Loss

Dr Paul E. Klapper
Consultant Clinical Virologist
Clinical Virology
Central Manchester Healthcare Trust
3rd Floor, Clinical Sciences Building
Manchester Royal Infirmary
Oxford Rd
Manchester M13 9WL, UK

Dr Pamela J. Vallely
Senior Lecturer in Medical Virology
The Virology Unit, Division of Laboratory and Regenerative Medicine
School of Medicine
University of Manchester
3rd Floor, Clinical Sciences Building
Manchester Royal Infirmary
Oxford Rd
Manchester M13 9WL, UK

Chapter 15
The Experience of Deafness–Psychosocial Effects

Professor Alys Young
Professor of Social Work
Education and Research
University of Manchester
Coupland III
Oxford Rd
Manchester M13 9PL, UK

PREFACE

Our aim with this book is to provide a text that brings together the expertise from two separate disciplines applied to a shared problem: that of hearing impairment resulting from an infectious cause. We, the Editors, come from each side of these disciplines, one from audiological medicine and the other from medical virology. Our early discussions led us to believe that there is a need for such a volume as the potential exists to make a difference in the prevalence of hearing impairment resulting from infection. Raising awareness within each discipline will be a good first step towards achieving this.

Current World Health Organization (WHO) data, as described in detail in the chapter on epidemiology, suggests that the global burden of hearing loss resulting from infection is probably far greater than was previously recognised and that much of this burden is felt in the developing nations. However, the good epidemiological data that would clearly demonstrate this and show what and where the key problems are remains to be collected. We strongly believe that the first step towards making a difference will be to introduce audiologists to infection and infectious disease specialists to the ear. This is our principal purpose in putting together this book.

We have drawn together contributors with a professional background in audiological medicine, infection or epidemiology from various countries within Europe and North America and Asia. The early chapters provide the anatomical and physiological information needed to understand the ear, how it is formed and how it functions. Chapter 3, on epidemiology, details the current global picture of the impact of infection as a cause of hearing loss and demonstrates how much we still need to know. The major part of the book deals with individual infectious causes of hearing loss. For those organisms known, or thought, to contribute significantly to hearing impairment we have devoted an individual chapter. As well as reporting on the role of the organism in hearing loss, these chapters provide general information on the agent, its clinical significance, epidemiology and pathogenesis. This allows the reader to understand the context of the infection and consider the evidence for, and importance of, its contribution to the problem.

Most notable among these is cytomegalovirus, a common and usually harmless virus that typically causes no symptoms in a healthy individual, yet, as described in Chapter 4, congenital infection with this virus is the leading cause of nongenetic, sensorineural hearing loss in developed countries. Chapters are also devoted to other important viral causes, such as measles, mumps and rubella, all of which are still prevalent in the developing world and have seen a resurgence in recent years in some parts of the developed world. Toxoplasmosis is included as this organism is historically associated with hearing loss in the congenitally affected infant although recent data described in Chapter 8 suggests that it may be less important in this context. In the current era of AIDS and with the recent increase in sexually transmitted diseases, the importance of syphilis, with or without HIV infection, as a cause of congenital and postnatal hearing impairment is highlighted in Chapter 9. Meningitis and otitis media are leading causes of hearing impairment, with meningitis contributing 1.2% and otitis media 0.83% of the total burden of child- and adult-onset hearing loss (WHO), and these proportions are greatly amplified in the developing world. In these chapters the authors have considered the numerous infectious organisms that can contribute to the conditions and attempted to explain how hearing loss results. Although it is clear that the main infectious causes of hearing loss in developing countries are similar to those in the developed world, there are some causes that are specific to particular regions and geographies and for this reason we have also included a chapter that looks at the role of tropical infections in this context.

Finally, in considering causes we have included a chapter (Chapter 13) on the effect of drug treatments that can be toxic to the ear and cause damage to hearing. Such ototoxic treatments are often used as therapy against infection and it is important to consider their effects alongside those of the organism.

Chapter 14 provides an overview of current methods of diagnosis for the organisms identified throughout the book, and where methods for treatment and prevention are available these are described. This chapter highlights the need for greater awareness and cooperation between audiologists, virologists, microbiologists and infectious disease physicians to improve diagnosis, investigation and prevention of audiological problems.

It should not be forgotten that deafness and hearing impairment have profound effects on individuals and the book finishes with a chapter that focuses on the patient and the impact that hearing loss will have on his or her life and the lives of the family. Hearing impairment affects the development of speech, language and cognitive skills in children, slows progress in school, may lead to difficulties later in life when obtaining employment and performing effectively in an occupation and can produce significant social isolation and stigmatisation. All these difficulties are much magnified in developing countries where there are generally very few services or trained staff and little awareness about how to deal with these difficulties. Thus we hope the book will serve as a timely reminder of the potential to make a difference to the individual by concentrating our efforts on these potentially preventable forms of hearing loss.

We hope that the volume is equally accessible to those with a background in either audiology or infection and will be of interest to paediatricians, physicians, researchers, academics, students and others on either side of the infection/hearing spectrum.

1 BASIC ANATOMY AND PHYSIOLOGY OF THE EAR

J. Irwin

Introduction

The ear is a small, complex series of interlinked structures that are involved in both maintenance of normal balance and the sense of hearing. In order to hear, the ear collects the sound waves that arrive as pressure changes in air and converts these into neurochemical impulses that travel along the cochlear-vestibular nerve to the brain. There are both active and passive mechanisms involved in this process. The prime function of the vestibular system is to detect and compensate for movement. This includes the ability to maintain optic fixation despite movement and to initiate muscle reflexes to maintain balance.

For the purposes of describing structure and function the ear is usually split into four distinct parts. These are the outer ear, the middle ear and the auditory and vestibular parts of the inner ear (Figure 1.1).

The outer ear

This is sometimes known as the external ear and consists of the ear that is visible on the side of the head (the pinna), the external auditory meatus (ear hole) and the ear canal (external auditory canal) that leads to the eardrum (or tympanic membrane). The tympanic membrane has three layers and the outer layer is usually included as part of the outer ear.

THE PINNA

This is, for the most part, a piece of cartilage covered by skin (Figure 1.2). There is also a fatty earlobe in most people. The skin covering the cartilage is

Infection and Hearing Impairment. Edited by V.E. Newton and P.J. Vallely
© 2006 John Wiley & Sons, Ltd

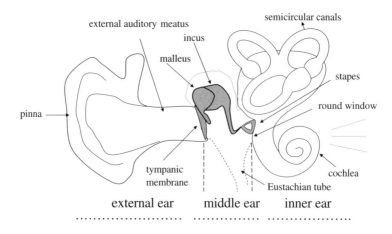

Figure 1.1. Diagrammatic representation of a cross-section through the ear

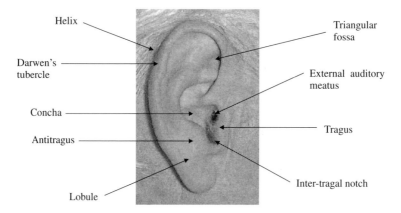

Figure 1.2. The pinna (auricle) and the external auditory meatus of an adult male

very thin with little subcutaneous structure. Any injury or infection can easily lead to deformity – cauliflower ear.

The pinna's shape enables it to funnel sound waves into the external auditory meatus. The various folds in the pinna's structure amplify some high-frequency components of the sound. They also help in the localisation of sound in the vertical plane. As sounds hit the pinna from above and below, their paths to the external auditory meatus vary in length. This means that they take different times to reach the meatus. Again, this is a feature of high-frequency sounds. The difference in time of arrival of the low-frequency and high-frequency components of the sounds allows for localisation.

The pinna is also involved in localisation of sound from in front and behind. As sound waves pass the pinna from behind they are diffracted around the pinna to the meatus whereas sounds from in front do not do this. The slight distortion produced allows for localisation.

Localisation of sound in the lateral plane, i.e. left/right, is a function of the pinnas being on different sides of the head. A sound directly from the left reaches the left ear before the right. The sound is also quieter at the right ear because the head is between the sound and the ear – the head shadow effect. These two factors combine to allow localisation in this plane.

THE EXTERNAL AUDITORY CANAL

Because the middle ear structures are delicate the ear has evolved a mechanism to protect it. This is a tube leading from the external auditory meatus to the tympanic membrane. The middle ear is inside the temporal bone of the skull. This part of the bone is called the petrous temporal bone because of its stone-like density.

The external auditory canal is approximately 25 mm long and is tortuous in its path from the meatus to the eardrum. The canal has bends in both the vertical and horizontal planes. This means that it is difficult for anything poked into the meatus to hit the drum. Any trauma is likely to be to the walls of the canal.

The canal is lined by skin throughout its length – it is the only skin-lined cul-de-sac in the body. The outer one-third is a cartilaginous tube and the skin here has ceruminous glands that secrete wax (cerumen), sweat glands and hairs. The skin of the inner two-thirds is closely adherent to the underlying bone and there is again very little subcutaneous structure.

Skin is a living, growing tissue that is constantly renewed. On the rest of the body, skin grows vertically to the surface, and as it does so the skin cells flatten and die. Dead cells are constantly shed. These dead skin cells form the basis of house dust and sustain the house dust mites, which trigger allergies in some people. The skin of the external canal starts growing from a point near the centre of the eardrum called the umbo. As the skin cells are replaced by new ones they migrate out along the eardrum to the canal wall and then along the canal to the meatus.

The wax and hairs have some protective properties by trapping air-borne particles before they get too deep into the canal. The wax also has some mild antibacterial properties and helps with moisture regulation in the canal: fresh wax is moisture giving and old wax absorbs water. As the skin cells migrate along the canal walls they carry the wax, and anything trapped therein, out of the ear. The outer ear is thus a self-cleaning system.

The external ear canal has one other function. As a cylinder closed at one end it has a resonant frequency whose wavelength is four times the length of the canal or approximately 100 mm. This equates to a sound of approximately

3 kHz and the canal does contribute some amplification of sounds around this frequency.

The middle ear

This is an air-filled space within the petrous part of the temporal bone (Figure 1.3). The prime function of the middle ear is to transmit the vibrations of sound in air gathered at the tympanic membrane to the fluid of the inner ear at the oval window. It is easier to vibrate air than it is to vibrate fluid. There is greater impedance to vibration in fluid. It is difficult to transmit sound between areas of differing impedance – there is usually an echo. The middle ear functions as an impedance matching device to prevent such echoes. If it were not for the middle ear so much sound would be reflected at the air/fluid interface that there would be a hearing loss of 50–60 dB.

The tympanic membrane is the outer (or lateral) border of the middle ear and the air-filled space contains three small bones (ossicles) and the facial nerve and its chorda tympani branch. There are also two muscles and the openings of both the Eustachian tube and the mastoid air cells.

The temporal lobe of the brain, surrounded by its meningeal lining, lies immediately above the roof (superior) of the middle ear and the jugular vein and internal carotid artery are below the floor (inferior). The mastoid air cells in the mastoid part of the temporal bone lie behind (posterior) and the inner ear is the inner (medial) wall.

The middle ear space is lined with respiratory mucous epithelium. Most of the middle ear lies above the level of the external auditory canal and cannot be seen on otoscopy. This is the epitympanic or attic region.

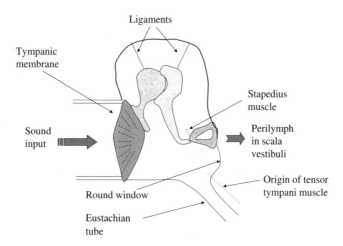

Figure 1.3. Diagram of the middle ear showing the ossicles, muscles and Eustachian tube

THE TYMPANIC MEMBRANE

This is a three-layered structure, the outer layer is skin, the middle layer is supporting connective tissue and the inner layer is respiratory epithelium. It is anchored into the external auditory canal by a thickened rim – the annulus (Figure 1.4). The annulus fits into a groove in the bony wall of the ear canal. A part of the first of the ossicles, the long process of the malleus, is embedded in the lower part of the tympanic membrane. This ends at a point known as the umbo. This is the point of origin of the skin that lines the external canal.

The anterior (front) and posterior (back) malleolar folds divide the tympanic membrane into two distinct parts: the upper pars flaccida and the lower pars tensa. It is the pars tensa that is involved in the transmission of sound. The vibrations are passed on to the ossicular chain via the malleus.

THE OSSICLES

These are the three smallest bones in the body (Figure 1.5). Their function is to transmit vibration into the inner ear at the oval window of the cochlea. The

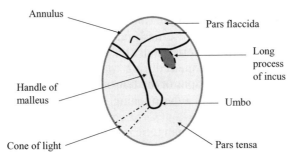

Figure 1.4. A diagrammatic representation of the left tympanic membrane in lateral view

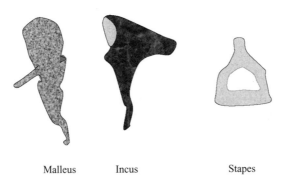

Figure 1.5. The three ossicles of the middle ear

long process of the malleus (hammer) is attached to the tympanic membrane and the footplate of the stapes (stirrup) sits in the oval window. Between these two bones is the incus (anvil). The bulk of the ossicular chain lies in the attic of the middle ear.

THE EUSTACHIAN TUBE

The middle ear is an air-filled space. The air is constantly being absorbed by the mucosal lining and there must therefore be a mechanism whereby this air is replaced: this is the Eustachian tube. This runs from the middle ear to the naso-pharynx behind the nose. It is in two parts and is lined with ciliated respiratory epithelium. The cilia beat and move mucus towards the naso-pharynx and away from the middle ear.

The first part is a bony tube continuous with the middle ear cavity. This tube is approximately 10 mm long and runs between the carotid artery and the mandible of the jaw. The bony canal of the tensor tympani muscle runs immediately above the Eustachian tube at this point. The bony portion is oval in cross-section and is narrowest where it meets the cartilaginous part.

The inner part of the tube is approximately 25 mm long and is angled down at about 45 degrees towards the naso-pharynx in adults. In children this portion of the tube is more horizontal, at a 10 degree angle. This portion of the tube is closed at rest and opens during swallowing and yawning. This is an active process due to contractions of the tensor veli Palatini muscle. There may be minor roles in Eustachian tube opening for the tensor tympani and the levator veli Palatini muscles.

The classic role of the Eustachian tube is to allow air from the naso-pharynx to enter the middle ear to replace air absorbed. The middle ear needs to be filled with air at, or near, ambient atmospheric pressure to allow the tympanic membrane to vibrate efficiently in response to sound. The Eustachian tube also has a protective role in preventing passage from the naso-pharynx to the middle ear and allowing drainage of mucus and fluids from the middle ear. This latter is an active process.

THE MASTOID AIR CELLS

These lie behind the middle ear in the mastoid part of the temporal bone. They act as a reservoir of air for the middle ear. The mastoid bone develops these air cells between the ages of one and six years. The mastoid air cells are contiguous with each other and have the same epithelial lining as the rest of the middle ear. The air cell system opens into the attic of the middle ear via the aditus ad antrum.

THE MIDDLE EAR MUSCLES

There are two muscles in the middle ear: the tensor tympani and the stapedius muscle. The tensor tympani runs in a canal along the roof of the Eustachian tube and its tendon emerges into the middle ear at the cochleariform process. The tendon attaches to the handle of the malleus. The muscle is supplied by a branch of the mandibular branch of the trigeminal (fifth cranial) nerve. Contraction of the muscle is a reflex triggered by loud sounds or a puff of air on the eyeball. Contraction pulls the tympanic membrane inwards and restricts its freedom of movement. This serves to protect the ear from loud noise or trauma.

The stapedius is the smallest muscle in the body. It arises from the pyramidal eminence on the posterior wall of the middle ear, inserts into the neck of the stapes bone and is supplied by a branch of the facial (seventh cranial) nerve. Contractions are reflex, initiated by loud sounds, and when it contracts it pulls the stapes posteriorly, so tilting its footplate. This has the effect of damping the ossicular chain vibration and hence limits the potential damage caused by loud noise.

THE FACIAL NERVE

This travels along the internal auditory canal with the eighth cranial nerve. It then enters the facial canal and travels between the cochlea and the vestibule and runs just above the oval window on the medial wall of the middle ear. It reaches the posterior wall near the aditus ad antrum and then turns downwards to leave the middle ear. Within the facial canal it gives off two branches: the nerve to the stapedius, which reaches the muscle in the pyramid, and the chorda tympani.

The chorda tympani runs over the upper part of the inner surface of the tympanic membrane across the root of the handle of the malleus. The nerve supplies parasympathetic and secretomotor fibres to the submandibular and sublingual salivary glands and carries fibres from the anterior two-thirds of the tongue and floor of the mouth concerned with taste.

IMPEDANCE MATCHING

As stated above, the main function of the middle ear is to overcome the impedance mismatch between the air in the outer ear and the fluid of the inner ear. The largest contribution to this is the difference in surface area between the tympanic membrane and the stapes footplate. This means that vibrations are collected from a large area and transmitted to a much smaller area, increasing the force/mm^2. There is also a small lever effect due to the way the ossicles vibrate (Figure 1.6).

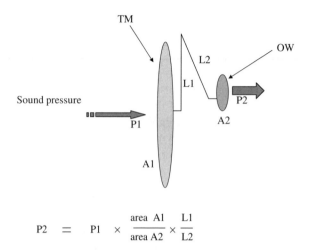

$$P2 \quad = \quad P1 \quad \times \quad \frac{\text{area } A1}{\text{area } A2} \times \frac{L1}{L2}$$

Figure 1.6. A diagram to illustrate the impedance matching mechanism (or trans-former mechanism) of the middle ear. P1 = pressure at the tympanic membrane; P2 = pressure at the oval window (OW); A1 = area of the tympanic membrane; A2 = area of the oval window; L1 = manubrium lever of the malleus; L2 = long process of the incus lever

The inner ear

The inner ear is an intricately shaped membranous tube suspended within a bony tube – the labyrinth. The inner ear has two functions. The first is the trans-duction of sound pressure into neurochemical impulses in the auditory (eighth cranial) nerve. This takes place in the cochlea. The second function is to main-tain optic fixation in the presence of movement and to help to maintain upright posture. This occurs in the vestibular system.

THE COCHLEA

This comprises $2\frac{3}{4}$ turns of a spiral. The base of the spiral protrudes into the middle ear as the promontory of the medial wall. The bony wall of the cochlea has two defects, each covered by a thin membrane. These are the round window and the oval window. The latter contains the footplate of the stapes, which is held in place by the annular ligament.

A cross-section of one turn of the cochlea (Figure 1.7) shows that the cochlea is divided into three segments. From above down these are the scala vestibuli, the scala media and the scala tympani. Each scala is fluid-filled. The scala media contains endolymph and the other two contain perilymph. There is communication between the perilymph of the scala vestibuli and the scala tympani at the apex of the cochlea at a point known as the helicotrema (Figure 1.8).

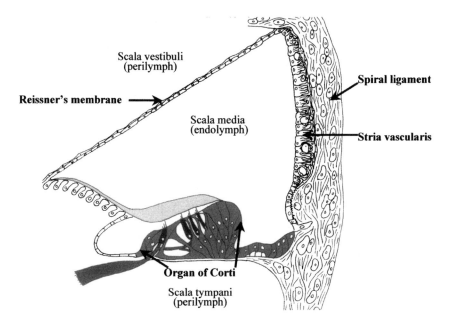

Figure 1.7. A cross-section of the cochlea showing the organ of Corti and the stria vascularis. (Reproduced with permission, Taylor and Forge, 2005)

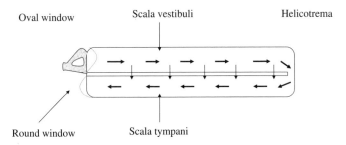

Figure 1.8. A diagram illustrating the movements of the fluid in the inner ear as a result of the inward movement of the stapes

The scala media is a closed, triangular cavity bounded above by Reissner's membrane and below by the basilar membrane. The stria vascularis forms the base of the triangle lying against the bony wall of the cochlea. The organ of Corti sits on the basilar membrane and it is here that the transduction of sound happens.

THE ORGAN OF CORTI

The basilar membrane runs between the inner and outer bony spiral laminae. It is narrower and more taut at the base of the cochlea and wider and floppier at its apical end. At its inner end sits the organ of Corti. This comprises the limbus, the tectorial membrane, the inner and outer rods (or pillars) of Corti with the tunnel of Corti between them, one row of inner hair cells, three rows of outer hair cells and supporting cells of Claudius, Deiter and Hensen.

There are approximately 12 000 outer hair cells and 3500 inner hair cells (Figure 1.9) in humans. The auditory branch of the eighth cranial nerve (the cochlear-vestibular nerve) contains fibres that run from the cochlea to the brain stem – afferent fibres – and efferent fibres that run in the opposite direction. Around 90% of the afferent fibres come from the inner hair cells. Each fibre comes from only one cell but each cell may have up to 10 fibres. The remaining 10% of the afferent fibres and all of the efferent ones are associated with the outer hair cells. Each of the nerves associated with the outer hair cells is connected with many cells.

Each hair cell has many hairs (cilia). The cilia of each outer hair cell are arranged in a 'W' shape (with a very shallow central notch) and those of the inner hair cells in a gentle curve. The hairs of the outer hair cells are embedded into the tectorial membrane whereas at rest the hairs of the inner hair cells are not. The cilia of each hair cell are connected by tip links. The outer hair cells contain contractile actin and myosin fibres which allow for the cells to alter their length.

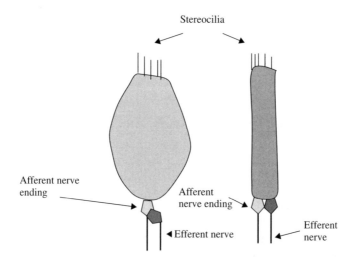

Figure 1.9. An outer hair cell (left) and an inner hair cell (right)

THE COCHLEAR FLUIDS

Perilymph is a fluid that is similar in character to extracellular fluid. Endolymph is chemically and electrically different. It has a high concentration of potassium and low concentrations of sodium and calcium similar to cerebrospinal fluid (CSF). The resting potential of endolymph is approximately +80 mV. The inner and outer hair cells have resting potentials of approximately −45 and −70 mV respectively. There is therefore a resting potential difference across between the endolymph and the hair cell of between 125 and 150 mV.

The scala media has an endolymph-containing duct that joins with a similar duct from the vestibular system to form the endolymphatic duct. This ends in the endolymphatic sac, which lies close to the meningeal lining of the brain.

There are two possible sources of endolymph. One theory is that the endolymph is produced directly from CSF at the endolymphatic sac and is actively reabsorbed by the stria vascularis. The other main theory is that the cochlear fluids are produced by effusion from the outer walls of the perilymphatic spaces. The perilymph passes across the semi-permeable Reissner membrane and is again actively reabsorbed by the stria vascularis. Small molecular weight markers introduced into the perilymph do pass into the endolymph and on into the stria vascularis.

THE STRIA VASCULARIS

This is a metabolically very active structure with a rich blood supply. It is responsible for the maintenance of the chemical and electrical composition of the endolymphatic space. It is a convoluted structure with many folds and indentations to increase the surface area. There are three types of cells arranged in three layers. The inner basal are cells in one continuous layer. These cells may be of neural crest or possibly mesodermal in origin. The outer layer lines the lumen of the cochlear duct and consists of epithelial cells. Between these two layers are intermediate cells. These are a type of migratory melanocyte. It is likely that these cells are responsible for the endocochlear potential and high potassium content of endolymph that are necessary for transduction of sound. The intermediate and basal cells are joined by gap junctions. Gap junction proteins such as Connexin probably also have a role in maintaining the high potassium concentration within the endolymph.

TRANSDUCTION OF SOUND

When the stapes footplate moves in response to incoming sound pressure waves the vibrations are transmitted into the scala vestibuli. This is possible because of the helicotrema and the round window. As the stapes footplate moves in, the round window membrane moves out.

The pressure waves make the organ of Corti move. Because of the hinge action of the limbus, the basilar membrane and the tectorial membrane do not move exactly in unison. This means that the cilia of the outer hair cells that are embedded in the tectorial membrane are displaced laterally. The tip links mean that more of the cilia are deflected. As the cilia move, potassium and calcium channels on the upper surface of the hair cells are exposed. This allows for equalisation of the chemical and electrical differences between the endolymph and the hair cell. It is this depolarisation that triggers the action potential in the cochlear-vestibular nerve. The cells have other ion exchange pumps in their walls that restore the original balance by removing the potassium (repolarisation).

INTENSITY RESOLUTION

It is the afferent nerve fibres from the inner hair cells that carry the information about hearing to the brain. The outer hair cells act as controlling and fine-tuning mechanisms.

When the organ of Corti moves in response to sounds of low intensity the cilia of the inner hair cells do not contact the tectorial membrane. The brain receives impulses from the afferent fibres of the outer hair cells and is, therefore, aware that there is a sound. However, there is no perception of sound as there are no impulses from the inner hair cells. Signals are sent along the efferent nerve fibres to the outer hair cells, causing them to shorten in length. This pulls the tectorial membrane closer to the basilar membrane, allowing the cilia of the inner hair cells to impact the tectorial membrane. Deflection of the cilia leads to depolarisation and action potentials from the inner hair cells and perception of sound.

High-intensity sounds lead to more movement of the organ of Corti. In order to protect the cilia, efferent impulses cause the outer hair cells to lengthen and push the tectorial membrane away from the basilar membrane.

FREQUENCY RESOLUTION

The anatomy of the basilar membrane allows for resolution of frequencies in sound. The membrane is stiffer and narrower at the base of the cochlea and more floppy and narrower at the apex. The fibres that comprise the basilar membrane run in parallel across the width of the basilar membrane and are necessarily shorter at the base and longer at the apex. The basilar membrane therefore has different resonant frequencies along its length with high frequencies at the base and low frequencies at the apex. This leads to a point of maximum displacement for pure tones that varies along the length of the cochlea for different frequencies.

There is thus a point where more impulses are transmitted from the inner hair cells. The vibration envelope of the basilar membrane is such that there is very little movement further along the basilar membrane than the point of maximum displacement. This, and the control mechanisms of the outer hair cells, inhibit afferent impulses at adjacent areas.

The vestibular system

This comprises the three semicircular canals and the saccule and utricle (Figure 1.1). The semicircular canals are concerned with the rotation and the saccule and utricle with gravitation.

THE SEMICIRCULAR CANALS

There are three semicircular canals on each side of the head. They are arranged in three planes at right angles to each other. They are the anterior (or superior) canal, the posterior (or inferior) canal and the lateral (or horizontal) canal. Each end of the canals opens into the utricle but there are only five openings as the anterior and posterior canals unite. The opposite end of these two canals is swollen into the ampulla and the lateral canal has an ampulla close to that of the anterior canal.

The endolymph of the vestibular system is continuous with that of the cochlea and is surrounded by perilymph. The endolymphatic space within the ampullae contains the sensory organ – the crista ampullaris. This is a crest of hair cells. The cilia are of different lengths and are arranged in order of height to the kinocilium. The hairs are embedded in a gelatinous structure – the cupola. There are about 23 000 hair cells divided between the three cristae on each side of the head and there are both afferent and efferent nerve fibres to each hair cell.

Any change in rotation speed of the head results in motion in the endolymph. This causes the cupola to move and brings about a shearing movement of the cilia. There is the same depolarisation process as within the cochlea, resulting in action potentials in the vestibular branch of the eighth nerve. As with other sensory systems in the body there is a resting firing rate of neurons within the vestibular nerve. Deflection of the vestibular hair cells towards the kinocilium results in an increase in this firing rate and deflection away from the kinocilium reduces the rate. Because of the orientation of the semicircular canals rotation will produce an increase in firing rate in the vestibular nerve on one side of the head and a reduction on the other side.

The prime function of this system is to allow the individual to maintain optic fixation in the presence of movement. This is through the vestibulo-ocular reflex at the brainstem level. Thus as the head moves in one direction the eyes are moved in the opposite direction so they can remain focused on the same point.

The semicircular canals also form one of the inputs into the body's mechanism for the maintenance of upright posture in the face of movement via the vestibulo-spinal reflex.

THE UTRICLE AND SACCULE

The utricle and saccule both contain endolymph. Within each structure is a gravitational sense organ – the macula. There are hair cells in each macula and the cilia project into the otolithic membrane. This is a gelatinous structure containing small crystals of calcium carbonate – the otoliths. Any linear motion displaces this membrane in the opposite direction. This again produces deflection of the cilia and depolarisation of the hair cells.

The macula of the utricle is situated on the floor, while in the saccule it extends on to the medial wall. The macula of the utricle is thought to respond to lateral, side-to-side motion whereas that of the saccule responds to movement in the vertical plane. The hair cells within these structures are orientated with reference to a central plane – the striola. In the utricle the cilia are arranged so that the kinocillium is towards the striola whereas in the saccule the kinocilia are arranged away from the striola.

There is again both an afferent and an efferent nerve supply to the hair cells of the maculae.

THE EIGHTH CRANIAL NERVE
(COCHLEAR-VESTIBULAR NERVE)

The eighth cranial nerve is, in effect, three distinct nerves. There are two vestibular nerves (superior and inferior) and the cochlear nerve. They run together through the skull in the internal auditory canal. This canal also contains the seventh cranial nerve (the facial nerve) and the blood supply to the inner ear – the internal auditory artery. The nerves pass through the meninges to the brainstem. The vestibular nerves go to the vestibular nuclei and the cochlear nerve to the cochlear nuclei.

THE CENTRAL AUDITORY CONNECTIONS

The afferent fibres travelling from the cochlear hair cells have their first synapse in the spiral ganglion within the cochlea. Thus the cochlear nerve consists of second-order neurones. The cochlear nerve runs via the internal auditory meatus, through the skull and meninges to the cochlear nuclei in the brainstem. This is at the level of the medulla oblongata. There is another synapse at this level.

The auditory pathway then crosses to the superior olivary nucleus on the other side of the medulla and then up towards the auditory cortex via a bundle of fibres called the lateral lemniscus. Some fibres in the lateral lemniscus cross back to the original side of the cochlear nerve. The lateral lemniscus runs to the inferior colliculus in the mid brain and then the pathway goes to the medial geniculate body of the thalamus.

The auditory cortex is located in the temporal lobes of the brain in an area called the superior temporal gyrus. This is just behind and below the lateral sulcus.

The frequency-specific anatomy of the cochlea is mirrored in the central auditory pathway. Neurones carrying high-frequency information travel towards the outside of the cochlear nerves and specific parts of each part of the pathway up to and including the cortex have different places for different frequencies. At the level of the primary auditory cortex high frequencies are coded posterior to the low frequencies.

2 DEVELOPMENT OF THE EAR AND OF HEARING

V.E. Newton

Introduction

Development is a serial process that may be identifiable over time but is not defined by time (Michel and Tyler, 2005). Certain processes have to occur before others can develop; some structures need to be present before others are formed. Organisms are particularly sensitive to damaging agents during development and especially during the period of organ differentiation. Those organs that are particularly affected are those undergoing the most rapid cellular growth at the time when the teratogen is introduced. This is the period of organ differentiation which, in humans, is from 18 to 55 days after fertilisation. At this time the ear is undergoing maximum development although the process of development of the auditory system continues into postnatal life.

Development of the ear

The ear starts to develop early in the embryonic period and is derived from all three primary germ layers – ectoderm, mesoderm and endoderm. It consists of the external ear, the middle ear and the inner ear. The external ear includes the pinna (auricle) and the external auditory meatus. The middle ear is separated from the external auditory meatus by the tympanic membrane (eardrum). The inner ear consists of the cochlea and the vestibular apparatus (see Chapter 1).

THE EXTERNAL EAR

The external auditory meatus develops around the fourth to fifth week from the first pharyngeal groove, which deepens to form a funnel-shaped opening

Infection and Hearing Impairment. Edited by V.E. Newton and P.J. Vallely
© 2006 John Wiley & Sons, Ltd

that is separated from the tubo-tympanic recess by a plate of mesoderm. The external auditory canal is filled with ectoderm which, around the eighth week of gestation, canalises to form the external auditory canal. The tympanic membrane forms at the point where the external auditory canal meets the middle ear cleft. It is formed as a result of a thinning out of the intervening mesoderm and is a layer of fibrous tissue lined on the external surface by an ectodermal layer and internally by a layer of entoderm, which also lines the middle ear cavity.

Three pairs of auditory hillocks start to develop around the first pharyngeal groove about the sixth week after fertilisation and are clearly visible by the eighth week, which marks the end of the embryonic period. These hillocks arise from the mesoderm overlying the first and second branchial arches, and coalesce to form the pinna. In the process they extend over the top of the groove to form the helix (Figure 2.1). The rudimentary pinna is formed by 60 days and in the fourth month the adult form can be seen (Wright, 1997). The pinna continues to grow throughout intrauterine life and postnatally. Initially the position of the external ear is at neck level but it becomes progressively higher in fetal life. By 13–16 weeks the ears move to their final position at the side of the head. Low-set ears are seen in infants where development is arrested at an early stage.

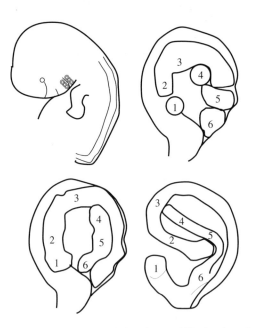

Figure 2.1. Stages in the development of the pinna. Hillocks that develop around the first pharyngeal cleft become: (1) the tragus, (2) and (3) the helix, (4) and (5) the antihelix and (6) the antitragus

Further development of the external ear takes place after birth with growth of the temporal bone. The direction of the external auditory canal alters and, as a result, the tympanic membrane, which is almost horizontal in the neonate, comes to lie at an angle to the horizontal plane.

THE MIDDLE EAR

The development of the middle ear starts during the third week of embryonic life. The pouch of the first arch gives rise to the tubo-tympanic recess which, later in intrauterine life, embraces the ossicles and forms the tympanum (middle ear cavity). The middle ear cleft, lined with endoderm, lies in close proximity to the ectoderm of the first pharyngeal groove. The growth of mesenchyme between the ectoderm and endoderm results eventually in a tympanic membrane with three layers (Figure 2.2).

There are three ossicles in the middle ear – the malleus, the incus and the stapes. These arise from the first and second branchial arches. They can be identified from the fourth week, begin to ossify at 4 months and are adult sized by 25 weeks (Wright, 1997). The head of the malleus is believed to be of first arch origin whereas the origin of the handle of the malleus is the second arch. The incus also has a dual origin, the body of the incus arising from the first arch and the long process from the second arch. The stapes is derived from the second arch. The footplate of the stapes, while derived from second arch cartilage has contributions from the otic capsule (Fritsch and Sommer, 1991). In late pregnancy, the middle ear cavity expands by means of programmed cell death and resorption into the loose mesenchyme of the pharyngeal arches, resulting in the middle ear ossicles becoming suspended within the cavity (McLaughlin, 2002).

There are two muscles in the middle ear, the tensor tympani and the stapedius muscles. These arise from the first and second arches respectively. The nerve of the first arch is the mandibular division of the fifth cranial nerve and this nerve supplies the tensor tympani muscle. The seventh cranial nerve, which is the nerve of the second arch, supplies the stapedius muscle.

The Eustachian tube arises from the tubo-tympanic recess and has the same lining. Its initial direction is more horizontal than that adopted in the adult.

The mastoid antrum starts to develop in the middle of the fetal period but the mastoid air cells develop postnatally in infancy and childhood (Wright, 1997).

THE INNER EAR

The inner ear consists of a bony vestibule containing perilymph with an inner membranous compartment filled with endolymph. The 20th day after fertili-

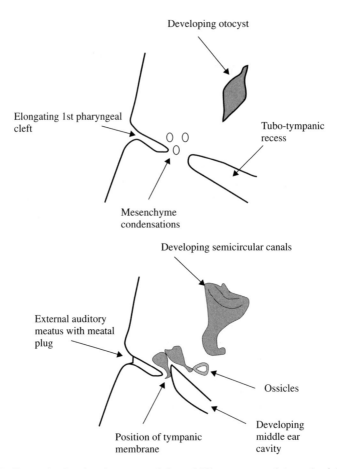

Figure 2.2. Stages in the development of the middle ear around 4 weeks (above) and by the 6th week (below)

sation sees the otic placode forming as a thickening in the surface ectoderm (Figure 2.3). This invaginates and loses its connection with the surface to form the otic vesicle or otocyst, which is closely linked with cells of the neural crest.

A fold developing in the otocyst differentiates to form the membranous labyrinth and this process is complete by the 10th week. The otocyst divides into cochlea and vestibular sections and gives rise to the appendage that later becomes the endolymphatic sac and duct. The dorsal or vestibular section becomes the semicircular canals and the utricle (Figure 2.3). The sensory organs of the utricle and saccule, the maculae, have developed into their adult form by 14–16 weeks whereas the cristae, the sensory organs of the semicircular canals, reach their adult size by 23 weeks (Lim, 1984; Wright, 1997).

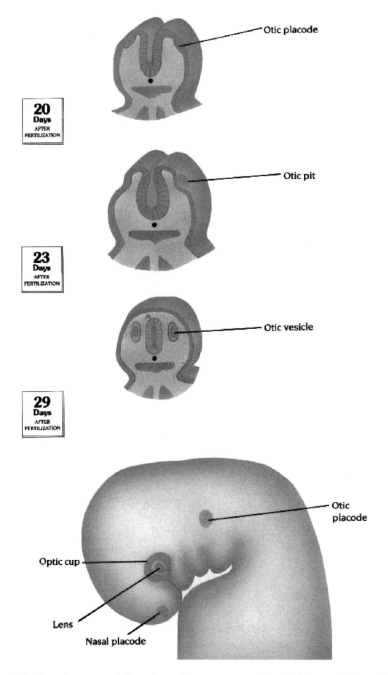

Figure 2.3. Development of the otic vesicle or otocyst. (Used with permission of John C. McLachlan from McLachlan, 1994)

The cochlear section gives rise to the cochlea and the saccule, the latter becoming separated from the cochlea by the formation of a constriction known as the ductus reuniens. The developing cochlea elongates as the cochlear duct and coils into a spiral (Figure 2.4). By the eighth week it has developed two turns and later will expand to 2.5 turns. The cochlea duct becomes the scala media. The epithelium of the outer wall develops into the stria vascularis. The first signs of differentiation of the stria vascularis appears at the 11th week and by the 17–18th week the three layers can be identified (Bibas *et al.*, 2000). By the 21st week the appearance of the stria vascularis resembles the adult structure (Bibas *et al.*, 2000).

The epithelium of the roof of the cochlea duct becomes the lining of the future Reissner membrane (Wright, 1997). The scala vestibuli and scala tympani are formed from adjacent tissues and, 16 weeks after fertilisation, the scala tympani communicates with the scala vestibuli at the helicotrema.

The sensory organ of the cochlea, the organ of Corti, develops from the epithelium of the floor of the cochlear duct. It begins to differentiate by the seventh week of gestation (Pearson *et al.*, 1973). By the beginning of the third month the tectorial membrane overlies a thickening in the epithelium that gives rise to the hair cells of the organ of Corti. Hair cells begin to differenti-

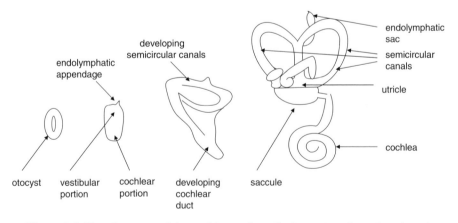

Figure 2.4. Development of the cochlea and vestibular system from the otocyst

ate at 11–12 weeks gestation and their appearance is preceded by nerve fibres entering the epithelium (Pujol and Lavigne-Rebillard, 2004). The three outer rows of this thickened area give rise to the three rows of outer hair cells whereas the single row of inner hair cells develop from the inner layer. The rows are visible by 14 weeks along the length of the cochlea, with the exception of the apical extremity (Lavigne-Rebillard and Pujol, 1990) (Figure 2.5). Stereocilia develop on the surface of the hair cells with a single kinocilium. The kinocilium later degenerates. The tunnel of Corti forms between the rows of inner and outer hair cells.

The cochlea starts functioning at 18–20 weeks and at 30–36 weeks is mature (Pujol and Lavigne-Rebillard, 2004). The inner ear is relatively hypoxic compared to that of the neonate and this leads to a reduced endocochlear potential and to a reduction in cochlear transduction and amplification, giving the fetus a slight sensorineural hearing loss (Sohmer and Freeman, 2001).

The bony labyrinth forms from the mesoderm around the membranous labyrinth and begins to ossify in the fifth or sixth month (McLaughlin, 2002). It becomes filled with perilymph. Jeffrey and Spoor (2004) examined 41 postmortem human fetuses using high-resolution magnetic resonance imaging and stated that the prenatal labyrinth reaches adult size between the 17th and 19th week of gestation.

Development of the cochlear branch of the auditory nerve was investigated by Ray et al. (2005) using light and electron microscopy. Fetuses between 12 and 38 weeks gestation were examined and nerve fasicles were revealed as early as 12 weeks and were compacted by 18 weeks. They observed Schwann cells in between unmyelinated axons at 12 weeks and myelinated fibres were readily distinguishable at 28 weeks. Development of the right cochlear nerve was in advance of that of the left cochlear nerve.

The spiral ganglia are complete by 25 weeks (Wright, 1997). Experimental and comparative animal data indicate that otic ganglion cells are derived from the otic placode (Fritzsch, Barald and Lomax, 1998). Cells from the neural crest, an early and transitory developmental structure, give rise to some of the neurones in the vestibular ganglion and to cells that are the precursors of the melanocytes found in the intermediate layer of the stria vascularis of the inner ear.

The central auditory system is not mature at the time of birth and continues to develop anatomically and functionally in the following few years, not being complete until 4–8 years (Pujol and Lavigne-Rebillard, 2004). Others have indicated a longer period of maturation (Illing, 2004). The direction of maturation is from the peripheral ear towards the auditory cortex. Like the cochlea, cochlear nuclei, superior olives and inferior colliculi, the auditory cortex is tonotopically ordered with neurones responding to particular frequencies orderly represented. Evidence has accumulated to show that tonotopic organisation of these structures is dependent upon sensory input.

First signs of hair
cell differentiation
(i, inner hair cells;
o, outer hair cells;
scale bar, 10 µm)

Surface of a 14 week
human fetus cochlea
just prior to the onset
of function
(i, inner hair cells;
o, outer hair cells;
scale bar, 10 µm)

At the end of its
development (30
weeks' gestation) the
human organ of Corti
looks like this
(photograph from
a month-old rat)

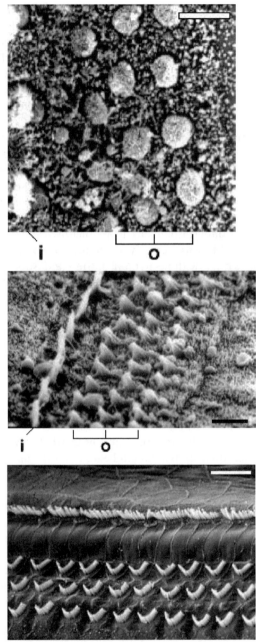

Figure 2.5. The two developmental stages (human cochleas) are by Mireille Lavigne-Rebillard, reproduced with permission from 'Promenade around the cochlea' EDU website by Rémy Pujol *et al.* INSERM and University Montpellier 1. The mature cochlea is by Marc Lenoir, reproduced with permission from 'Promenade around the cochlea' EDU website by Rémy Pujol *et al.* INSERM and University Montpellier 1

Fetal responses to sound

Responses to sound have been investigated by monitoring fetal movements and heart rate and it has been demonstrated that the fetus hears and discriminates sounds. Some recent investigations have explored the electrical activity of the fetal brain to sound and recorded the results using magnetoencephalography (MEG), enabling the temporal processing of short-term auditory memory to be examined.

The fetus is able to respond to sounds after 20 weeks' gestation (Sohmer et al., 2001). Development of hearing begins in fetal life with low- to middle-frequency discrimination (Lippe and Rubel, 1985). Animal experiments have indicated that the basal end of the cochlea is first to mature and that initially this region responds to low-frequency sounds. With increasing maturity there is a shift in frequency coding along the basilar membrane and low-frequency sounds are coded at the apex in the mature animal (Hyson and Rudy, 1987).

Environmental sounds can penetrate maternal tissues and fluids and stimulate the ear through bone conduction (Sohmer and Freeman, 2001; Sohmer et al., 2001). The sounds are mainly low frequency as sounds above 0.5 kHz are attenuated by 40–50 dB (Gerhardt and Abrams, 2000). Gerhardt and Abrams reported that the fetus could detect vowel sounds easily but not consonants, as these were quieter and of higher frequency.

Pitch changes, rhythm and stress, which are the prosodic features of speech, are available to the fetus (Moon and Fifer, 2000). It has been shown that the term fetus is capable of differentiating between its mother's voice and that of a stranger. Kisilevsky et al. (2003) observed that fetal heart rate increased when the mother's voice was heard but not when the voice heard was that of a stranger. Therien et al. (2004) examined the recognition ability of preterm infants of less than 32 weeks gestation who had normal cranial ultrasound on examination. They used event-related cortical potentials to investigate whether or not the infants could (a) detect and discriminate speech sounds and (b) recognise their mother's voice compared to that of a stranger. They were unable to demonstrate recognition of maternal voice in the preterm infants compared to full-term controls. Patterns of speech discrimination in the preterm infants also differed from those of infants born at term. It is possible that auditory recognition memory had not been established at the low rate of gestation at which the preterm infants were born.

The short-term auditory memory of 17 fetuses of gestational age 35–40 weeks has been examined using an odd-ball paradigm, and recording MMNn. This is the magnetic counterpart of MMN (magnetic mismatch negativity) which is a cortical evoked response to stimulation (Huotilainen et al., 2005). The standard had a fundamental frequency of 500 Hz and the deviant a fundamental frequency of 750 Hz. Recording was performed using a magnetoencephalographic approach. An MMN was recorded in 12 out of the 17 fetuses, indicating that the fetuses were able to detect the change in frequencies.

Responses to music have been explored and Kisilevsky *et al.* (2004) investigated responses in fetuses with gestational ages from 28 weeks to term. They used a five-minute recording of Brahms' lullaby and monitored heart rate and body movement. They showed that the youngest fetuses increased their heart rate when the music was loud and that, with increased gestation age, responses were obtained at lower intensities. At 35 weeks the increased heart rate was sustained and body movement was recorded at 38 weeks gestation. Fetuses near term showed an ability to discriminate the tempo of the music.

The ability of the fetus to hear and to differentiate sounds may be an important stimulus towards furthering the development of the auditory system as well as postnatal stimulation.

Effect of auditory input on central auditory system development: plasticity

Animal studies and clinical research with patients fitted with hearing aids or cochlear implants have shown that early exposure to sound is important for the development of the central auditory system. There is a limited time during which this auditory input is crucial. This has been called the 'critical period' or 'sensitive period'.

ANIMAL STUDIES

An early experiment by Levi-Montalcini (1949), in which a chick otocyst was removed or suffered damage, showed that this resulted in anatomical changes in the chick auditory pathways. Nakahara, Zhang and Merzenich (2004), using rats, were able to show that, during the 'sensitive' period of development, the temporal order and rate of repetitive auditory stimuli affected the organisation of the auditory cortex and that this representation persisted into adulthood.

In contrast, a hearing loss is believed to deprive the brain of the stimulation needed for its normal development. Neural connections, which are functional, can be established in the central auditory system without the need for auditory stimulation (Hartmann *et al.*, 1997). Research, however, indicates that sound deprivation has an effect upon dendritic branching in the auditory cortex. Pujol and Lavigne-Rebillard (2004) showed the influence of early stimulation in experiments on the auditory cortex of cats. In deaf white cats the dendritic branching seen in the adult was much less extensive than that found in cats receiving normal stimulation. Lack of auditory input can result in a more rudimentary auditory pathway than would otherwise exist (Shepherd and Hardie, 2001).

Reorganisation of the role of different cortical areas takes place when there is sound deprivation. Mount *et al.* (1991) discovered loss or damage of hair cells in the lower frequency areas of the cochleae of cats correlated with a significant reorganisation of the lower frequency area in the cortex. In a high-frequency loss there was normal low-frequency representation in the cortex but the high-frequency area was remapped to a common low frequency. They concluded that the pattern of cochleotopic organisation of the cortex is dependent on the pattern of activity in the ascending auditory pathway during early developmental stages. Harrison *et al.* (1991), also investigating neonatal high-frequency hearing loss, found that areas of the cortex devoted to high frequencies contained neurones, almost all of which were tuned to a common low frequency corresponding to the border between normal and damaged hair cell regions.

Hemodynamic and electromagnetic studies have shown that a modality specific area deprived of its normal sensory input can respond to other sensory modalities (Kujala, Alho and Naatanen, 2000). The loss of auditory stimulation has been shown to result in cells of the auditory cortex taking on a non-auditory function. Lee *et al.* (2001a) were able to demonstrate that in the absence of auditory stimulation some of the auditory cortex took over a visual function.

Other areas within the auditory system are affected by the lack of sound stimulation. Wu *et al.* (2003), working with rats deafened neonatally, found that prolonged auditory deprivation dramatically alters the organisation of the inferior colliculus.

Electrical stimulation after a period of sound deprivation has resulted in metabolic changes demonstrable in animals. Wong-Riley *et al.* (1981) was able to show a partial reversal of low cytochrome oxidase levels in animals given chronic electrical stimulation following a hearing loss of long duration. Electrical stimulation of the auditory nerve of cats deafened for a long time has also resulted in neuronal change (Matshushima *et al.*, 1991).

The period of plasticity of the central auditory system is limited. Harrison *et al.* (1991) found that, at the level of the inferior colliculus, tonotopic plasticity was evident in chinchillas only in the three-week period following birth, but not in the adult animal. Others, e.g. Kral *et al.* (2001), have demonstrated that, in deaf cats, plasticity at the level of the auditory cortex was only evident if electrical stimulation was given prior to the age of six months.

CLINICAL STUDIES

Studies with children with a congenital or early onset hearing impairment fitted with hearing aids or given cochlear implants have supported the presence of plasticity within the auditory system and a period of sensitivity for introduction of a stimulus. Children with sensorineural hearing impairment habilitated with hearing aids before the age of six months have been shown to have significantly better language scores when examined at an older age than children whose hearing impairment was habilitated after this age (Yoshinaga-Itano, Coulter and Thomson, 2000).

Children given cochlear implants early have better language abilities than those im-planted at a later age. Harrison, Gordon and Mount (2005) analysed speech perception performance in children with severe prelingual hearing impairment implanted at 1–15 years. Their results showed that after long implant use children implanted at young ages performed better than those implanted when older.

Some researchers have reported that the period of plasticity of the auditory system is limited. Sharma, Dorman and Spahr (2002), using evoked potentials to examine the sensitive period for development of the central auditory system, concluded that the period during which the auditory system retains maximum plasticity after development is about 3.5 years, but can remain in some until the age of about seven years. There is evidence, however, that some plasticity extends beyond this age (Pantev *et al.*, 2003).

The presence of plasticity in the auditory system has implications for effective auditory rehabilitation. The evidence for a critical period during which stimulation must be introduced to be maximally effective makes it essential that a hearing impairment is detected as early as possible in children.

Development of auditory behaviour

The ability of infants to hear and discriminate sounds has been explored by examining behavioural responses. These in turn are influenced by nonsensory stimuli such as an ability to attend to a stimulus and auditory memory as well as the stage of the infant's motor development. The neonate's psychoacoustic thresholds are better than the behavioural response to sound. A response to a loud sound in the neonatal period elicits a general body response with increased respirations and an increase in heart rate. As the infant develops, behavioural responses are elicited to quieter sounds and the response is more specific. The six–seven month infant has developed good head control and can turn and locate the source of a sound introduced in the horizontal plane. This ability is the basis of the 'distraction test' used to examine hearing in infants (Hickson, 2002). The ability to localise in the vertical plane is acquired at around 15 months. Werner and Gray (1998) pointed out that poor localisation ability at a very young age may be because of the changes in head size that are occurring at this time. This could mean that interaural clues that specify particular spacial locations on the cortical map of auditory space are also changing.

Intensity discrimination is poorer in children than in adults, who have the ability to discriminate differences in the intensity of a pure tone of 1 dB (Maxon and Hochberg, 1982). The intensity difference limen approaches adult values at about the age of six years (Werner and Gray, 1998). Frequency discrimination in neonates is initially poor, particularly in the higher frequencies, but this improves in the high frequencies until, at the age of six months, the frequency limen is similar to that of adults (Olsho, Koch and Halpin, 1987).

Discrimination of low frequencies improves over a longer period (Werner and Gray, 1998).

Pitch perception and spectral shape that indicate sound quality are important in speech perception. There are indications that infants have these abilities within the adult range by seven months of age (Clarkson and Clifton, 1985; Trehub, Endman and Thorpe, 1990). The limitations of behavioural testing for exploring psychoacoustic abilities in infants and young children may account for the apparent maturation of responses in some instances.

Factors affecting the developing ear and hearing

There are many genes that influence the development of the ear and increasingly these are being identified and their functions explored (Read, 2000; Hawkins and Lovett, 2004). Mutations in these genes cause syndromal or nonsyndromal hearing impairment.

Infections and various teratogens such as ototoxic drugs can affect the developing ear, the type and degree of the effect depending upon the gestational stage at which the damaging agent is introduced. If exposed to infections or other teratogens at a sensitive period in development there may be marked structural and functional damage affecting the auditory and the vestibular system which are demonstrable radiologically by a CT (computed tomography) scan or MRI (magnetic resonance imaging). These may be defects of the outer, middle or inner ear. An absent or vestigial vestibulo-cochlear nerve is rarely found. Intrauterine infections tend to damage the membranous cochlea, in which case a CT scan or MRI would not show any abnormality. At a later developmental stage the damaging effect of a teratogen may be absent or minimal.

During the development stage the fetus is more susceptible to aminoglycosides than after birth. This means that the preterm neonate has a greater susceptibility to develop ototoxic damage than the full-term infant at similar dosage of aminoglycosides (Pujol, 1986).

HEARING IMPAIRMENT

Other causes of a hearing impairment in the perinatal period and postnatally can influence the development of the central auditory system through auditory deprivation, as described earlier. The result of prenatal or postnatal damage may be a conductive, sensorineural or mixed hearing impairment. A conductive hearing loss is where the cause lies in the outer ear or middle ear. It may be the result of defects in the development of the external ear such as congenital atresia. Congenital defects of the middle ear include an absent middle ear, ossicular abnormalities and ossicular fixation.

In a sensorineural hearing loss the cause lies in the cochlea, vestibulo-cochlear nerve or auditory pathways; in a mixed hearing loss the cause is both conductive and sensorineural. Congenital abnormalities of the cochlea such as aplasia or various degrees of dysplasia have been described, e.g. the Michel defect or Mondini defect of the cochlea (Fritsch and Sommer, 1991). Intrauterine infections such as congenital rubella result in a sensorineural hearing loss, but usually as a result of damage to structures forming part of the membranous rather than the bony cochlea.

Hearing loss resulting from infections is, with the exception of mumps, usually bilateral but may be unilateral. A bilateral hearing loss is particularly disabling for the infant and young child who is developing speech and language if it is congenital or of early onset. It can also be very disabling for an adult, especially if of sudden onset. Hearing aids can amplify sounds but do not restore normal hearing and cochlear implants, which are useful if the hearing loss is very severe/profound, again do not render hearing normal.

A unilateral hearing loss can also be disadvantageous. There is an intensity advantage when two ears are listening and it is easier to concentrate on a speaker in reverberant conditions. It is also possible to localise the source of a sound signal more accurately. A person with hearing in only one ear is particularly disadvantaged in a noisy environment but is helped by turning the head and by using visual clues.

Summary

The ear is a complex structure. It starts to develop early in intrauterine life and further development continues postnatally. Auditory experience is one of the factors affecting development. Infections are a potentially preventable cause of auditory deprivation and, if not prevented, are a known risk factor, a fact that should alert clinicians and facilitate early detection and rehabilitation of any hearing loss present.

3 EPIDEMIOLOGY OF INFECTION AS A CAUSE OF HEARING LOSS

A. Smith and C. Mathers

Outline

This chapter reviews current knowledge on the global and regional burden of hearing impairment and its infectious causes. The perspective is that of the World Health Organization (WHO).

It discusses the levels of hearing impairment in current use by WHO, and recent estimates of the global and regional numbers of child- and adult-onset hearing loss in 2000 and their increase over the last two decades. This is followed by a detailed discussion of the use of child and adult prevalence data and the methodology for calculation of global and regional burdens of hearing loss, and their contributions to the global burden of the disease project being carried out by WHO. The key measure of burden, the disability-adjusted life year (DALY), and its components, the years of health life lost (YLL) and the years lived with disability (YLD), are described. These measures show that hearing loss makes a substantially greater contribution to the overall burden of disease than was previously thought.

A review of data currently available by WHO regions[1] on infectious causes of hearing loss demonstrates their much greater burden in developing countries, but also that there is a massive shortage of epidemiologically acceptable data that would quantify these burdens accurately. Such information is needed to enhance the credibility of infection as a cause of hearing loss in comparison to other contributors to the global burden of hearing loss.

---

[1] WHO regions: AMR, Region of the Americas; AFR, African Region; EMR, Eastern Mediterranean Region; EUR, European Region; SEAR, South-East Asian Region; WPR, Western Pacific Region. The constituent countries of the regions are shown in the Appendix.

Infection and Hearing Impairment. Edited by V.E. Newton and P.J. Vallely
© 2006 John Wiley & Sons, Ltd

For the global burden of disease estimates, WHO measures the total burden of all sequelae of those infections that can cause hearing impairment, but so far it has disaggregated the burden of hearing loss separately for only two infectious causes, meningitis and chronic otitis media (COM). The second half of the chapter reviews the incidence, prevalence and DALY burden estimates for hearing impairment from these infections. It shows that these burdens of hearing loss from meningitis and COM contribute 7.1 and 18.8% respectively to the burden of all sequelae of these infections, and 1.2 and 0.83% respectively of the total burden of child- and adult-onset hearing loss. The largest burden by a WHO region for hearing loss overall and for hearing loss caused by meningitis and by COM occurs in South-East Asia. Africa ranks second for the burden of hearing loss caused by meningitis.

In the future, further epidemiologically appropriate surveys of the occurrence and causes of hearing impairment are needed in key regions of the world. WHO needs to quantify further the burden of hearing loss, especially by disaggregating hearing loss data from those for all sequelae of other major infections.

Global and regional burden of hearing loss and its contribution to the global and regional burden of disease

WHO GRADES AND DEFINITIONS

During the last decade, WHO has been involved in setting levels of assessment of hearing impairment and in developing tools for their measurement in populations. Figure 3.1 shows the grades of hearing impairment, currently used by WHO (1991), from none, slight, moderate, severe to profound. It also shows

Grade 0 None	**25 dB or less**	No/slight problems Hears whispers	
Grade 1 Slight	**26 - 40 dB**	Hears/repeats words in normal voice at 1m	
Grade 2 Moderate	**Child 31 - 60 dB** **Adult 41 - 60 dB**	Hears/repeats words in raised voice at 1m	**Disabling hearing impairment**
Grade 3 Severe	**61 - 80 dB**	Hears words shouted into better ear	**Disabling hearing impairment**
Grade 4 Profound	**81 dB or more**	Cannot hear/understand shouted voice	**Disabling hearing impairment**

[Average 0.5, 1, 2, 4 kHz in better ear]

Figure 3.1. WHO grades of hearing impairment

that moderate, severe and profound hearing impairment in the better ear define the group of people having disabling hearing impairment[2]. This table was originally developed for a performance test when audiometry was not available; the ISO dB equivalents were included later. These definitions of hearing impairment are currently used in WHO surveys[3] and disabling hearing impairment is used in the estimation of global deafness and hearing impairment for the global burden of disease rankings.

GLOBAL NUMBERS WITH DISABLING HEARING IMPAIRMENT (PAST AND CURRENT)

WHO estimates of the global number with disabling hearing impairment have increased substantially in the last 15 years. This number was originally estimated at 42 million in 1985 and then increased to 120 million in 1995 at the time of the last World Health Assembly Resolution on Prevention of Hearing Impairment (WHO, 1995); the most recent figure is 250 million in the year 2001, which is approximately 4.2% of the world's population (WHO, 2001d). Three-quarters of these people have adult-onset hearing loss[4]; 340 million persons have mild hearing loss, of adult- and child-onset (see Table 3.1 which shows year 2000 estimates).

At least two-thirds of the burden of hearing loss is found in developing countries (WHO, 2001d). This is proportionally slightly less than the proportion of the population in the developing world and is probably accounted for by the larger numbers of elderly people in the developed world having deafness and hearing impairment.

The increase in the WHO estimates since 1985 is most likely due to a combination of better identification of cases through improved diagnosis and earlier detection of hearing loss, longer survival of elderly people who have the highest prevalences of deafness and hearing impairment, and the proba-

---

[2] WHO definition of disabling hearing impairment:
The permanent unaided hearing threshold level for the better ear of 41 or 31 dB or greater in age over 14 or under 15 years respectively; for this purpose the 'hearing threshold level' is to be taken as the better ear average hearing threshold level for the four frequencies 0.5, 1, 2, and 4 kHz.
(From WHO, 1991, with adaptations from WHO, 1997a.)
[3] In some surveys in the field and as recommended by the WHO Ear and Hearing Disorders Survey Protocol, testing was only done at 1, 2 and 4 kHz but not at 0.5 kHz, because of the likelihood of false positive results when 0.5 kHz is included.
[4] The prevalence of adult-onset hearing loss was estimated by subtracting from prevalences at ages 20 and over, the estimated prevalence of hearing loss for teenage children (15–19 years) or the nearest similar age group for which prevalences were available. It is assumed that the incidence of adult-onset hearing loss associated with otitis media and other infectious and noninfectious causes included elsewhere in the GBD 2000 cause list is negligible compared to the incidence of adult-onset hearing loss associated with age-related hearing degeneration or noise-induced loss.

Table 3.1. Estimated global prevalence of hearing loss, Global Burden of Disease (GBD) 2000, Version 2. (From Mathers, Smith and Concha, 2005)

Severity (dB HTL)	Males	Females	Persons
Mild or greater (26+)			
Adult-onset	215	197	413
Child-onset	89	86	175
Total	304	284	588
Moderate or greater (41+)			
Adult-onset	94	93	187
Child-onset	31	31	61
Total	125	123	248
Severe or greater (61+)			
Adult-onset	21	25	46
Child-onset	3	3	7
Total	24	29	53
Profound (81+)			
Adult-onset	3	5	8
Child-onset	3	3	6
Total	6	8	14

ble increased incidence due to causes such as noise-induced hearing loss and ototoxic drugs.

PREVALENCE OF CHILD- AND ADULT-ONSET HEARING LOSS

Estimates of the prevalence of childhood hearing loss up to age 15 years and adult-onset hearing loss from age 20 years (Mathers, Smith and Concha, 2005) have recently been used to estimate the burden of this disability in adults, according to the 17 WHO subregions used in all WHO work on the global burden of disease (see the Appendix, Tables 3.11 and 3.12). The sources of data on which these estimates are based are shown in Tables 3.2 (children) and 3.3 (adults). All the surveys in these tables were population-based and used audiometric measurements (there are relatively few surveys that fulfil these two criteria) generally using the WHO definition. Where non-WHO thresholds were used, the prevalence of hearing impairment at the WHO thresholds was interpolated assuming that the log of the cumulative prevalence is linear with threshold. This relationship holds reasonably well in most studies. Prevalence rates of disabling hearing impairment were obtained for the 17 WHO subregions by means of a model based on the data from the countries listed in Tables 3.2 and 3.3. Standardised prevalence rates from a country level were used to calculate the subregional prevalence rates. The prevalence rates from countries in the same WHO subregion were taken as representative data of the subregion. When there were several available data sources, average prevalence

Table 3.2. Prevalence studies for hearing impairment: children

Country	Study population	Reference	Years	Definition used	Sample size	Age range	Prevalence (%)
Developed	Review	Davidson, Hyde and Alberti, 1988	Review	41+ dB HL better ear		Childhood	0.05–0.23
UK	Trent region	Fortnum and Davis, 1997	1985–93	40+ dB HL better ear at 0.5, 1, 2, 4 kHz	552 558	0–9	0.133 birth prevalence[a]
USA	Atlanta	Van Naarden, Decouflé and Caldwell, 1999	1991–3	40+ dB HL better ear at 0.5, 1, 2 kHz	255 742	3–10	0.11
USA	NHANES II and Hispanic HANES	Lee, Gomez-Marin and Lee, 1996	1982–4	31+ dB HL better ear	7888	6–19 African-American Cuban American Mexican American White, non-Hispanic	0.78 1.21 0.60 0.38
USA	NHANES III	Niskar et al., 1998	1988–94	16+, 26+ dB HL at 0.5, 1, 2 kHz better ear	6166	6–19	0.7 (16+) 0.4 (26+)
Developing	Review	Davidson, Hyde and Alberti, 1988	Review	41+ dB HL better ear		Childhood	0.2–0.42
Thailand	Bangkok schools Rural schools	Prasansuk, 2000	?	41+ dB HL better ear	10242 2153	School age children	3.9 6.1
Sierra Leone	Panguma	Seely et al., 1995	1992	26+, 41+, 61+ dB HL better ear	2015	5–15	2.58 (26–40) 0.65 (41–60) 0.50 (61+)
Angola	Luanda	Bastos, Reimer and Lundegren, 1993	1981–2	31+ dB HL better ear at 0.5, 1, 2 kHz	1030	School children	2.0

Table 3.2. *Continued*

Country	Study population	Reference	Years	Definition used	Sample size	Age range	Prevalence (%)
Zimbabwe	Primary schools, SE highlands	Jones, 1974	1972	31+ dB HL better ear	885	School children	3.2
Kenya	Kiambu district	Hatcher et al., 1995	1992	31+ dB HL better ear at 2, 4 kHz	5368	Primary school age	2.2
Tanzania	Northern inland district	Bastos et al., 1995	1995	31+ dB HL either ear at 0.5, 1, 2 kHz Severe/profound	854	Primary school age	3.0 0.35
South Africa	Poor rural district in Western Cape	Prescott and Kibel, 1991	1990?	21+, 31+, 41+ dB HL better ear	401	6–13	2.0 (31+) 0.5 (41+)
Swaziland	First year school children	McPherson and Swart, 1997					
Saudi Arabia	Riyadh	Zakzouk, 2003	1997	20+ dB HL, air conduction at 0.25–0.8 kHz and 0.5–4 kHz bone conduction, unilateral or better ear bilateral	6421	2 months–12 years	7.7

[a]This figure refers to what the authors call 'permanent childhood hearing impairment', i.e. mainly sensorineural hearing loss, and includes 16% who had postnatally acquired loss. The prevalence rate for congenital hearing impairments was 0.112%. The figures are not directly comparable with data from the WHO studies which include all conductive loss.

Table 3.3. Data sources for prevalence estimates of adult-onset hearing loss (Mathers, Smith and Concha, 2005)

Country	Study population	Reference	Years	Definition used	Sample size	Age range	Prevalences available by
UK	Four cities	Davis, 1989, 1994	1980–6	25+, 45+, 65+ dB HL in the better ear	2910	17–80	Age, sex
Italy	Milan, Padua, Florence, Bari, Palermo	Quaranta 1996	1989	25+, 45+, 65+, 90+ dB HL in the better ear	2170	18+	Age
Denmark	Copenhagen males	Parving et al., 1997	1976	25+ dB HL in the better ear (0.5, 1, 2, 4)	300	49–69	Age
Denmark	Jutland (rural)	Karlsmose, Lauritzen and Parving, 1999	Early 1990s	25+ dB HL; 35+ dB HL; 45+ dB HL	1397	31–50	Age × sex
Finland	Northern Ostrobothnia	Uimonen et al., 1999	1997	21+, 40+, 70+, 95+ dB HL in the better ear (0.5, 1, 2, 4)	5400	5–75	Age
USA	Framingham	Moscicki et al., 1985	1979	25+ dB HL (0.5, 1, 2, 4 kHz) in the better ear	2293	57–89	
USA	Beaver Dam, Wisconsin	Cruickshanks et al., 1998a, 1998b; Dalton et al., 1998	1993–5	26+, 41+, >60 in the worse ear (0.5, 1, 2, 4 kHz); >25 dB HL in the better ear (0.5, 1, 2, 4)	3753	48–92	Age × sex (26+ only)
USA	Beaver Dam, Wisconsin	Popelka et al., 1998, 2000	1987–8	26+, 41+, >60 in the worse ear (0.5, 1, 2, 4 kHz)		48–92	
USA	NHANES 1 national	Reuben, 1998, 1999	1971–5	25+ dB HL in the better ear (HFPTA scale 1, 2, 4 kHz)	2506	55–74	Age × sex

Table 3.3. *Continued*

Country	Study population	Reference	Years	Definition used	Sample size	Age range	Prevalences available by
USA	HHANES Hispanic Americans	Lee *et al.*, 1991	1982–4	26+, 41+ in the worse ear (0.5, 1, 2 kHz)	2751	20–74	Age × sex
Brazil	Residents of Canoas	Beria, 2003	2003	26+, 41+, 61+, 81+ dB HL in the better ear	3858	All ages	Age, sex
Australia	South Australia	Wilson *et al.*, 1999	1996	25+, 35+, 45+, 65+ dB HL in the better ear (0.5, 1, 2, 4 kHz)	9027	15+	Age × sex
Oman	National	Al-Khabori *et al.*, 1996	1996–7	26+, 41+ dB HL in the bilateral/better ear (1, 2, 3 kHz)	11 402	All ages	Age
India	Vellore, Taluk, Tamil Nadu	WHO, 1997b; Mackenzie, 2002	1997–8	26+, 41+, 61+, 81+ dB HL in the better ear	5432	All ages	Age
India	Lucknow rural	Singh *et al.*, 1980	1975–6	15+, 30+, 60+ dB HL, bilateral deafness, unilateral deafness	904	All ages	Age × sex (15+) Age (30+, 60+)
India	Lucknow urban	Jitendra *et al.*, 1974	1970	15+, 30+, 60+ dB HL, bilateral deafness, unilateral deafness	904	All ages	Age × sex (15+) Age (30+, 60+)
Sri Lanka	Kandy district	WHO, 1997b; Mackenzie, 2002	1998–2000?	26+, 41+, 61+, 81+ dB HL, better ear (1, 2, 4 kHz bilateral/better ear)	4858	All ages	Age (41+ only)

Country	Location	Reference	Year	Definition	N	Age range	Breakdown
Nepal	Two regions	Little et al., 1993	1990?	31, 51+, 81+ dB HL, better ear (1, 2, 4kHz bilateral/better ear)	15845	5+ years	Age
China	Sichuan	Liu et al., 1993; Bu, 2002	1986-7	27+, 56+, 91+ dB HL, better ear	126876	All ages	Age, sex (27+ only)
Korea	Community-based and health clinics	Kim et al., 2000	1994-7	27+, 41+, 56+, 71+ dB HL, both ears; presbycusis only	39004	25+	Age × sex Age (56, 71)
Thailand	17 provinces	Prasansuk, 2000	1988-90	41 dB HL, better ear	7499	All ages	Total only
Thailand	Bangkok +5 provinces	Prasansuk, 2000	1986-7	41+, 61+, 81+ dB HL, better ear (0.5, 1, 2kHz bilateral/better ear)	1797	All ages	Age
Indonesia	Bandung municipality & district	WHO, 1997b; Mackenzie, 2002	1997-8	26+, 41+, 61+, 81+ dB HL (1, 2, 4kHz bilateral/better ear)	5604	All ages	Age (41+ only)
Myanmar	Yangon	WHO, 1997b; Mackenzie, 2002	1997-8	26+, 41+, 61+, 81+ dB HL (1, 2, 4kHz bilateral/better ear)	5604	All ages	Age (41+ only)
Vietnam	Six selected provinces (3 north, 3 south)	Dung, Cio and Thuy, 2003		26+, 41+, 61+, 81+ dB HL (1, 2, 4kHz bilateral/better ear)	13120	Six months and older	Age × sex
Nigeria	Three states: Akua Ibom, Benue, Katsina	Nwawolo, 2003	2000-2001	26+, 41+, 61+, 81+ dB HL (1, 2, 4kHz bilateral/better ear)	8975	All ages	Age (41+ only)

rates weighted on sample size were calculated and then used for the subregional estimates. For subregions where there were no population-based surveys available, the prevalence rates were estimated to be the same as for other subregions with similar health level indices. The prevalence of adult-onset hearing loss was estimated by subtracting from prevalences at ages 20 and over the estimated prevalence of hearing loss for teenage children (15–19 years) or the nearest similar age group for which prevalence values were available.

This prevalence data for adults is shown in Figure 3.2 and Table 3.4. It should be noted that this work is still in an interim phase. As more accurate data become available especially from developing countries, the estimates will be refined and updated.

DALYs, YLL AND YLD: DESCRIPTION AND TYPE OF DATA NEEDED, AND RANKINGS

Since 2001, WHO has included adult-onset hearing loss in the tables of the global burden of disease (GBD) in the World Health Report (WHO, 2001c). The causes of the GBD are assessed according to the percentage of total disability adjusted life years (DALYs) in the world attributable to each cause. DALYs are a measure of the years of healthy life lost due to premature mortality (YLL), and the years lived with disability (YLD), hence taking much more account of the burden of chronic conditions than was the case with previous indicators that focused only on mortality. One DALY can be thought of as one lost year of 'healthy' life and the burden of disease as a measurement of the gap between the current situation and an ideal situation where everyone lives up to the age of the standard life expectancy, free of disease and disability. YLL for hearing loss is assumed to be zero so all the DALY burden comes from YLD. The data required to estimate YLD are disability incidence, disability duration, age of onset and distribution by severity class, all of which must be disaggregated by age and sex. These in turn require estimates of incidence, remission, case fatality rates or relative risks, by age and sex. A specific software tool, DisMod, has been produced to assist in the development of internally consistent estimates. The basic calculation for YLD is the product of the number of incident cases in the reference period, the disability weight and the average duration of disability in years. The disability weight reflects the severity of the disease or condition on a scale from 0 (perfect health) to 1 (death). It is planned to use results from the new World Health Survey, currently being conducted, to comprehensively revise the disability weights.

In general, the results of measurement surveys contribute more to YLD calculations than self-reported interview surveys, and population-based epidemiological studies provide the most useful information (Mathers *et al.*, 2004). The WHO Ear and Hearing Disorder Survey Protocol (WHO, 1999) was developed to encourage countries to fulfil these needs by conducting

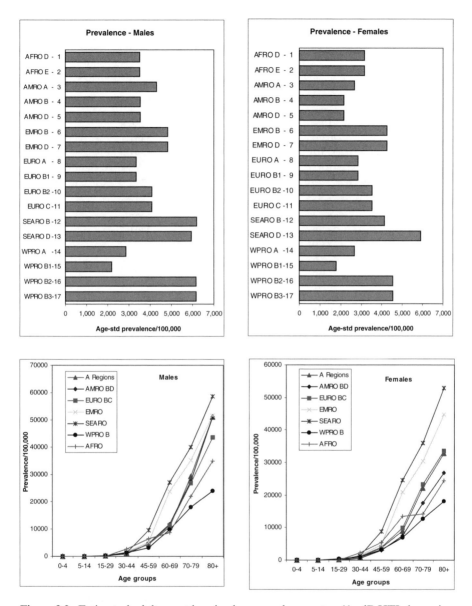

Figure 3.2. Estimated adult-onset hearing loss prevalence rates, 41+ dB HTL, by region and sex, GBD 2000, Version 2

population-based, random cluster sample surveys (see the next section for further details). In the majority of cases, routine data on consultations by diagnosis are not helpful in estimating burden since these are almost always based on samples of the disability present in the community and does not give a true

Table 3.4. Adult-onset hearing loss (41+ dB HTL): age-standardised incidence and prevalence estimates for WHO epidemiological subregions, 2000

Subregion	Age-standardised incidence/100 000		Age-standardised prevalence/100 000	
	Males	Females	Males	Females
AFRO D	213.8	167.8	3466.8	2919.3
AFRO E	203.9	169.2	3451.1	2976.7
AMRO A	323.1	189.0	4351.5	2643.0
AMRO B	264.7	150.1	3500.9	2119.8
AMRO D	260.3	150.8	3498.1	2107.9
EMRO B	324.2	281.3	4829.5	4200.5
EMRO D	322.8	279.1	4829.0	4241.4
EURO A	234.9	190.0	3337.6	2795.5
EURO B1	233.8	189.7	3301.7	2803.7
EURO B2	273.0	228.9	4037.9	3557.5
EURO C	274.8	235.0	4078.6	3561.7
SEARO B	421.8	336.7	6390.3	4901.9
SEARO D	363.2	360.0	5870.1	5827.1
WPRO A	243.1	187.7	2859.6	2685.9
WPRO B1	159.5	127.4	2567.5	2056.6
WPRO B2	430.7	346.4	6352.3	4506.2
WPRO B3	326.8	278.1	5081.0	4163.0
World	271.5	220.1	4036.3	3326.7

picture of the situation in the whole population. However it may be possible to use hospital data to measure some conditions where the coverage is good; those relevant to hearing loss may include perinatal conditions and meningitis (Mathers *et al.*, 2004).

Adult-onset hearing loss ranks 15th among the leading causes of the DALY burden in the year 2002, coming after perinatal conditions, respiratory infections, HIV/AIDS, depression, diarrhoea, heart disease, strokes, malaria, road accidents, tuberculosis, maternal conditions, chronic lung disease, congenital anomalies and measles in that order of ranking (Mathers *et al.*, 2004). However, on a regional basis these rankings vary considerably; thus adult-onset hearing loss ranks 6th, 10th and 11th in the WHO European, Western Pacific and South-East Asian regions respectively. It does not rank at all in the first 15 places in the African region, which includes most sub-Saharan African countries where infectious diseases and trauma dominate. If mortality is excluded and disability considered alone using the assessment of years lived with disability (YLD), adult-onset hearing loss ranked second in 2002 at 4.2% of the total YLD. Unipolar depressive disorders ranked first with 12.1% of the total (see Table 3.5 (Mathers *et al.*, 2004)).

Table 3.5. Ten leading causes of YLD: global estimates for 2002

		% of total YLD
All countries		
1	Unipolar depressive disorders	11.8
2	Hearing loss, adult onset	4.6
3	Cataracts	4.5
4	Alcohol use disorders	3.3
5	Maternal conditions	3.3
6	Schizophrenia	2.8
7	Perinatal conditions	2.7
8	Osteoarthritis	2.6
9	Vision loss, age-related and other	2.5
10	Bipolar affective disorder	2.5

Preliminary estimates have recently been made to show the burden of childhood and adult onset combined for the 17 subregions and the proportions in the 6 regions (see Table 3.6). These show that the total global burden is 33.344 million DALYs, with the largest proportions of this burden in the South-East Asian and Western Pacific regions. These figures will be updated as more recent, accurate data become available and are assessed for inclusion.

NEED FOR DATA AND DEVELOPMENT OF THE WHO SURVEY PROTOCOL

Despite the improvements in estimation of the burden of deafness and hearing impairment, there remains a widespread scarcity of appropriate data, particularly from developing countries (Pascolini and Smith, 2005). More, and more accurate, data are urgently needed in order to raise awareness, prioritise interventions, predict needs, monitor outcomes and underpin credible economic analyses, such as in cost-of-illness and cost-effectiveness studies. The latter could be included in the menu of estimates of cost-effectiveness of a wide range of health interventions that WHO is compiling, which are intended to be used by governments to determine good investments for health.

To help to address this need, WHO in 1999 published a protocol (WHO, 1999), developed by an expert group, for conducting population-based surveys on ear and hearing disorders. The protocol includes software for data entry and analysis and comprises a section on survey methods, a questionnaire to record information on demographics, audiometry, ear examination, family history, diagnosis of ear diseases and cause of hearing impairment and actions needed, and a set of coding instructions to go with the questionnaire. The protocol recommends a cluster sampling method which may be multistage and stratified, with a minimum sample size of approximately 6000 individuals. The method can be used at national or district level. The use of this standardised

Table 3.6. Childhood and adult-onset hearing loss: YLD, YLL and DALY estimates by subregion and region, 2000

	YLD/100000 Males	YLD/100000 Females	YLL/100000 Males	YLL/100000 Females	Total YLD ('000)	Total YLL ('000)	Total DALYs ('000)	% of total DALYs	WHO region	% of total DALYs by WHO region
AFRO D	807.7	847.9	0.0	0.0	2764	0.0	2764	8.3	AFR	16.8
AFRO E	825.9	858.5	0.0	0.0	2843	0.0	2843	8.5		
AMRO A	499.1	379.7	0.0	0.0	1357	0.0	1357	4.1	AMR	8.9
AMRO B	346.5	288.7	0.0	0.0	1404	0.0	1404	4.2		
AMRO D	303.8	251.5	0.0	0.0	198	0.0	198	0.6		
EMRO B	507.0	459.2	0.0	0.0	675	0.0	675	2.0	EMR	4.1
EMRO D	482.4	498.0	0.0	0.0	677	0.0	677	2.0		
EURO A	470.0	451.7	0.0	0.0	1893	0.0	1893	5.7	EUR	12.1
EURO B1	354.6	358.9	0.0	0.0	592	0.0	592	1.8		
EURO B2	421.1	448.5	0.0	0.0	221	0.0	221	0.7		
EURO B3	509.8	576.8	0.0	0.0	1340	0.0	1340	4.0		
SEARO B	735.3	598.9	0.0	0.0	2631	0.0	2631	7.9	SEA	37.0
SEARO D	700.5	738.5	0.0	0.0	9694	0.0	9694	29.1		
WPRO A	354.7	467.9	0.0	0.0	616	0.0	616	1.8	WPR	21.2
WPRO B1	418.6	379.0	0.0	0.0	5423	0.0	5423	16.3		
WPRO B2	725.1	644.3	0.0	0.0	972	0.0	972	2.9		
WPRO B3	667.7	604.3	0.0	0.0	44	0.0	44	0.1		
Total	559.2	543.9	0.0	0.0	33344	0.0	33344	100.0		100

methodology in surveys will enable comparison between surveys conducted in different places or surveys conducted in the same place at different times.

Surveys using the protocol have so far been conducted in a part or all of the following countries (with the prevalence of disabling hearing impairment in parentheses). Oman (2.1%), Indonesia (4.6%), Myanmar (8.4%), Sri Lanka (8.8%), India (6.3%), Nigeria (three states 4.4–7.6%), Vietnam (three Northern provinces 7.8%, three Southern provinces 4.7%), Southern Brazil (6.8%) and a pilot study in Jiangsu Province China (6.4%). A full study is underway in Madagascar and is about to start in Jiangsu. It is planned that other provinces in China will start in future. Data obtained using the protocol will be incorporated in a global review of available data on deafness and hearing impairment to be published soon (Pascolini and Smith, 2005), and will be used in updates of regional and GBD calculations, as well as in forthcoming economic analyses. A new edition of the protocol and software will be ready later this year.

AWARENESS

A major problem in addressing this field is the general lack of awareness about issues related to deafness and hearing impairment in all parts of society. The population as a whole is generally not aware of the specific effects this problem has on individuals. They may not know about its huge cost to society or that there are good opportunities for intervention for prevention and management. Since the true size of the problem is not accurately known, there is a lack of political will to deal with it, which leads to a lack of resources for programmes. Hence, the collection of accurate data will help to raise awareness both among the general public and among health planners and decision makers.

EFFECTS ON INDIVIDUALS

In dealing with populations, it should never be forgotten that deafness and hearing impairment have profound effects on individuals. In particular, they damage the development of speech, language and cognitive skills in children, especially if commencing prelingually; they slow progress in school, they lead to difficulties in obtaining and keeping and performing effectively in an occupation; for all ages and for both sexes, they produce significant social isolation and stigmatisation. All these difficulties are much magnified in developing countries where there are generally very few services or trained staff and little awareness about how to deal with these difficulties.

THE NEED FOR A PUBLIC HEALTH APPROACH

However, in order to prevent deafness and hearing impairment on a large scale and help hard of hearing people around the world, it is essential to develop a public health approach to this problem. Health professionals and health planners need to reorientate their thinking and activities along a public health route to address the situation. We need to find ways to make a difference in the population in addition to treating people on an individual basis. Conditions should be selected for targeting on a massive scale according to whether they have, at the same time, high prevalence in the population, together with cost-effective means of prevention or control. Unfortunately, there is a shortage of appropriate and effective interventions in this field, not only at the basic, scientific level but also in terms of programme implementation. Good data will be essential in determining the conditions that should be targeted and assessing the cost-effectiveness of new interventions.

Contribution of major infectious causes of hearing loss to the global and regional burden of hearing loss

OVERVIEW OF AVAILABLE DATA

An attempt has been made to review available epidemiological data on infectious causes of hearing loss according to the 17 subregions of WHO. This would add credibility to current estimates and also show where gaps exist for future data gathering. Published and unpublished surveys were sought that complied with the following criteria (these are similar to those employed in the collection of surveys for a forthcoming global database of deafness and hearing impairment):

- The surveys reported prevalence of hearing impairment, preferably from cross-sectional surveys on representative populations of a country or area of a country, and if by sample preferably using a random sampling method. If no population-based surveys were available, random sample surveys from normal schools were accepted but, because of the likelihood of bias, clinical studies from hospitals, surveys from schools for the deaf and data from neonatal screening surveys were excluded.
- The definitions of hearing impairment were clearly stated and threshold hearing levels and frequencies tested were reported.
- The methods of the studies were described: design, sampling, sample size, preferably sampling and nonsampling errors were reported and discussed. The sample size should have been at least 500 subjects.
- The response rate was adequate.
- The type of audiometric testing, the otological examination, the background noise and the location of the examination were described.
- The studies reported results for 'persons' and not only for 'number of ears' but preferably of bilateral hearing impairment.
- The surveys should have assessed infectious causes of hearing loss and have been performed in the last 20 years.

- Surveys covered 'nonpermanent' as well as 'permanent' childhood hearing impairment (PCHI) since an assessment should be made of the DALY burden from nonpermanent hearing loss, such as that caused by chronic otitis media, which in developing countries may be long-lasting if not permanent. The concept of PCHI is more relevant in a clinical or service development context in developed countries, but less so in a public health context for developing countries.

It was already known from data searches for the available data (Pascolini and Smith, 2005) that there is a scarcity of epidemiologically sound surveys for prevalence; studies that include accurate information on cause are even rarer, probably mainly because of the difficulties determining cause of hearing loss, especially in field surveys in developing countries. Thus the results expressed here are necessarily tentative and await the conduct of better surveys and more accurate and portable methods of determining causation. A more detailed discussion of the limitations of surveys of deafness and hearing impairment is given in Pascolini and Smith (2005).

ESTIMATES OF PROPORTION DUE TO INFECTION AND REGIONAL PREVALENCE

When the criteria given in the previous section for selection of studies (which are essential for collecting accurate and credible epidemiological data) are applied, it is clear that there is a severe dearth of such surveys around the world and not just in developing countries. Indeed, for several sub-regions, no suitable survey was available (see Table 3.7). A large number of surveys had to be excluded because of non-adherence to these basic epidemiological principles, and the relatively few acceptable epidemiological studies that report causes of hearing impairment probably reflect the difficulty of determining cause in field surveys, especially in developing countries. In addition the surveys often use different definitions of hearing impairment or have determined causes in different ways, thus limiting the scope and accuracy of comparison between them.

In terms of the importance of infection as a cause of hearing loss, there are some indications that in certain regions it is much more important than in others. Thus in the African region (sub-Saharan African countries) both available population-based surveys report infection as contributing 48 and 54% respectively to the overall prevalence of hearing loss. However, the third study from the African region (Seely et al., 1995), although not assessing the total proportion of infections in this way, showed that matched cases and controls with and without hearing loss had very similar rates of measles and mumps. Thus, data from field surveys showing these infections as causing hearing loss should be interpreted with caution. Studies from other regions and subregions containing mainly developing countries (EMRO B, SEARO B & D, WPRO

Table 3.7. Burden of infectious causes of hearing loss by WHO regions and subregions

Subregion (17)	Country	Reference	Date of study	Type of study[c]	Population from which sample is selected
African region					
R01 AFRO D	Nigeria	Nwawolo, 2003	January 2000	WHO pbrss	3 states from whole country
R01 AFRO D	Sierra Leone	Seely et al., 1995	1992	pbrss	Eastern province around the town of Panguma, rural
R02 AFRO E	Zimbabwe	Stewart et al., 1998	1998	sbs	All primary schools in Manicaland province
Americas region					
R03 AMRO A	USA	Van Naarden, Decouflé and Caldwell, 1999	1991–2	rds	Atlanta city
R04 AMRO B	NA				
R05 AMRO D	Brazil	Beria et al., 2005[g]	2003	WHO pbrss	Canoas city
Eastern Mediterranean region					
R06 EMRO B	Saudi Arabia	Al-Muhaimeed, 1996[h]	1988–90	pbrss	Riyadh city
R06 EMRO B	Oman	Al-Khabori and Khandekar, 2004	1997	WHO pbrss	Whole country
R07 EMRO D	NA				
European region					
R8 EURO A	UK	Fortnum and Davis, 1997	1994–5	rch	Trent Health region

Sample description	Ages	Sample size	Definition of hearing impairment[d]	Number[a] of sample subjects (prevalence %)[b]	
				Any level of hearing impairment (as defined in study)	Disabling hearing impairment, (WHO defn[e])
30 clusters of people from 3 states	≥6 months	8975	WHO defn	1691 (18.8%)	510 (6.6%)
All children in study area (estimate 20% nonattenders)	5–15 years	2015	>25 dB HL average 0.5, 1, 2 kHz in either ear	184 (9.1%)	23
Random selection of schools (weighting for larger schools); all pupils in a school tested	4–20 years	5528	>30 dB HL at 1, 2, 4 kHz in either ear	135 (2.4%)	NA
Children ascertained from special needs programme testing	3–10 years	324327	40 dB or more HL averaged at 0.5, 1, 2 kHz	nd	250
Random cluster sample of whole population	≥6 months	2427	WHO defn	685 (28.2)	183 (7.5%)
Stratified three-stage random; children had audiometry if 'at risk' or positive history	2 months –12 years	6421	Mild or greater hearing loss	494 (7.7)	NA
Cluster sampling; 2-stage: screen/full test	≥6 months	11400	WHO defn	511 (4.5) (age/sex adjusted: 5.5)	223 (2.0) (adjusted: 2.1)
Children born 1985–93	1–10 years	552558	PCHI[j] ≥40 dB HL BEA at 0.5, 1, 2, 4 kHz	653 (0.12)	ND

Table 3.7. *Continued*

Subregion (17)	Country	Reference	Date of study	Type of study[c]	Population from which sample is selected
R9 EURO B1	NA				
R10 EURO B2	NA				
R11 EURO C	Estonia	Uus and Davis, 2000[i]	1985–90	rch	Whole country
South-East Asian region					
R12 SEARO B	Indonesia	Mackenzie, 2002		WHO pbrss	Bandung municipality
R13 SEARO D	India	Mackenzie, 2002		WHO pbrss	Vellore district
Western Pacific region					
R14 WPRO A	NA				
R15 WPRO B1	China	Liu *et al.*, 2001	2000	pbrss	Sichuan Province
R16 WPRO B2	Vietnam	Dung, 2003	2001	WHO pbrss	Six provinces (3 in North, 3 in South)
R17 WPRO B3	NA				

[a] Numbers are numbers of cases, not ears.
[b] Prevalences and %ages are calculated using all hearing impaired not just those with 'disabling hearing impairment', unless otherwise stated.
[c] pbrss = population-based random sample survey, WHO pbrss = population-based random sample survey using the WHO protocol, rch = retrospective cohort study, sbs = school-based survey, rds = routine data surveillance.
[d] Hearing impairment means any level of hearing loss including deafness.
[e] WHO defn = WHO definition of hearing impairment and disabling hearing impairment (see text).

Sample description	Ages	Sample size	Definition of hearing impairment[d]	Number[a] of sample subjects (prevalence %)[b]	
				Any level of hearing impairment (as defined in study)	Disabling hearing impairment, (WHO defn[e])
Children born 1985–90		144 186 births	PCHI ≥40 dB HL BEA	NA	248 (172 per 100 000 births)
Random cluster	6 months+	5 604	WHO defn	670 (12.0)	230 (4.1)
Random cluster	6 months+	5 428	WHO defn	1 130 (20.8)	319 (5.9)
Stratified sample from whole province	All ages	126 876	≥26 dB BEA	4 164 (3.3)	NA
Random cluster	6 months+	13 120	WHO defn	2 675 (20.4)	786 (5.99)

[f] 'High fever' is grouped under unknown causes.

[g] Data unadjusted; causes %ages of disabling hearing impairment.

[h] Zakzouk (1997) reported 48 of these children had laboratory confirmation of HSV-1 (16 children), *Toxoplasma gondii* (11), cytomegalovirus (10), multiple serology (11) (as well as 4 with rubella, listed separately). These 48 are not included in the group of all infections.

[i] Prevalence figures are per 100 000 births. Some meningitis cases had additional causes.

[j] PCHI = permanent childhood hearing impairment (includes permanent conductive causes), BEA = better ear average, NA = not available; ND = not done.

Table 3.7. *Continued*

	Number[a] of sample subjects (% prevalence)/(% of all causes) for:			
Subregion (17)	Sensorineural hearing impairment	All infections	Other causes	Unknown causes[f]
African region				
R01 AFRO D	NA	804 (9.0)/(47.5)	236 (2.6)/(14.0)	651 (7.3)/ (38.5)
R01 AFRO D	NA	NA	NA	NA
R02 AFRO E	56 (1.0)	73 (1.3)/(54.1)	35 (0.63)/(26.0)	27 (0.49)/ (20.0)
Americas region				
R03 AMRO A	NA	25 (0.008)/(10.0)	30 (0.009)/(12.0)	195 (0.06)/ (78.0)
R04 AMRO B				
R05 AMRO D	NA	28 (1.2)/(15.3)	52 (2.1)/(28.4)	103 (4.2)/ (56.3)
Eastern Mediterranean region				
R06 EMRO B	168 (2.6)	349 (5.4)/(70.6)	130 (2.0)/(26.3)	15 (0.23)/ (3.0)
R06 EMRO B	NA	92 (0.8/18.0)	307 (2.6/60.1)	104 (0.9/20.3)
R07 EMRO D				
European region				
R8 EURO A	NA	56 (0.01)/(8.6)	330 (0.06)/ (50.5)	267 (0.05)/ (40.9)
R9 EURO B1				
R10 EURO B2				

Number[a] (prevalence %)/(% of all causes) / (% of all infectious causes) for:

All COM	OME	CSOM	Meningitis	Congenital rubella	Other congenital infections	Measles	Mumps	Other infections
563 (6.3)/ (33.3)/ (70.0)	203 (2.3)/ (12.0)/ (25.2)	316 (3.5)/ (18.7)/ (39.3)	162 (1.8)/ (9.6)/ (20.1)	0	0	71 (0.8)/ (4.2)/ (8.8)	(0.089)/ (0.47)/ (1.0)	0
NA	NA	124 (6.1)/ (67.4)/ NA	NA	NA	NA	96 (4.8)/ (52.2)/ NA	23 (1.1)/ (12.5)/ NA	4 cases and no controls
56(1.0)/ (41.5)/ (76.7)	28 (0.51)/ (20.7)/ (38.4)	22 (0.4)/ (16.2)/ (30.1)	2 (0.04)/ (1.5)/ (2.7)	1 (0.02)/ (0.7)/(1.4)	0.0	2 (0.04)/ (1.5)/ (2.7)	4 (0.07)/ (3.0)/ (5.4)	1 case 'following flu'
15 (0.005)/ (6.0)/ (60.0)	ND	ND	10 (0.003)/ (4.0)/ (40.0)	0	0	0	0	0
24 (0.1)/ (13.1)/ (85.7)	7 (0.29)/ (3.8)/ (25.0)	0.0	NA	NA	NA	NA	NA	NA
326 (65.7)/ (66.0)/ (93.4)	232 (3.6)/ (47.0)/ (66.5)	94 (1.5)/ (19.0)/ (26.9)	15 (0.23)/ (3.0)/ (4.3)	4 (0.06)/ (0.8)/(1.1)	See footnote		4 (0.06)/ (0.8)/ (1.1)	
79 (0.7)/ (15.5)/ (85.9)	11 (0.1)/ (2.1)/ (12.0)	31 (0.3)/ (6.0)/ (33.7)	NA	NA	NA	NA	NA	NA
ND	ND	ND	35 (0.006)/ (5.3)/ (62.5)	8 (0.001)/ (1.2)/(14.2)	12 (0.002)/ (1.8)/(21.4)	0	0	1

Table 3.7. *Continued*

	Number[a] of sample subjects (% prevalence)/(% of all causes) for:			
Subregion (17)	Sensorineural hearing impairment	All infections	Other causes	Unknown causes[f]
R11 EURO C		28	135	85
South-East Asian region				
R12 SEARO B		23 (0.4)/(10.0)	153	28
R13 SEARO D		125 (2.3)/(39.2)	157	25 (0.46)/ (2.2)
Western Pacific region				
R14 WPRO A				
R15 WPRO B1	3 041 (2.4)/ (73.0)	1 118 (0.88)/ (26.8)	2 390 (1.9)/ (57.4)	656 (0.52)/ (15.8)
R16 WPRO B2	NA	168 (1.3)/(6.3)	(63.5%)	(26%)
R17 WPRO B3				

B1 & B2) generally show infections to be similarly contributing the major proportion of hearing loss. However, studies from Brazil (Beria *et al.*, 2005), Oman (Al-Khabori and Khandekar, 2004), Indonesia (Mackenzie, 2002) and Vietnam (Dung, 2003) show contributions of 15, 18, 10 and 6% respectively, which are more like those from developed world studies, such as 10% in the USA (Van Naarden, Decouflé and Caldwell, 1999) and 8.6% in the UK (Fortnum and Davis, 1997).

Chronic otitis media (COM) is by far the largest infectious cause in those developing country surveys showing a high prevalence of infectious hearing loss. However, it is relatively easy to diagnose in the field and it may be that

			Number[a] (prevalence %)/(% of all causes) / (% of all infectious causes) for:					
All COM	OME	CSOM	Meningitis	Congenital rubella	Other congenital infections	Measles	Mumps	Other infections
ND	ND	ND	21 (14.5)/ (8.5)/ (75.0)	3 (2.1)/ (1.2)/ (10.7)	4 (2.8)/ (1.6)/(14.3)	0	0	
21 (0.37)/ (9.1)/ (91.3)	1 (0.04)/ (0.4)/ (4.3)	12 (0.2)/ (5.2)/ (52.2)	NA	NA	NA	NA	NA	2
123 (2.3)/ (38.6)/ (98.4)	9 (0.17)/ (2.8)/ (7.2)	26 (0.48)/ (8.2)/ (20.8)	NA	NA	NA	NA	NA	2
1 034 (0.81)/ (24.8)/ (92.5)	NA	NA	NA	NA	NA	NA	NA	NA
160 (1.2)/ (5.98)/ (95.2)	81 (0.62)/ (3.0)/ (48.2)	51 (0.39)/ (1.9)/ (30.4)	NA	NA	NA	NA	NA	NA

other causes are underdiagnosed. In addition, as is seen in a later section, the total burden of hearing loss caused by meningitis is almost twice that for COM, presumably due to its greater severity and longer-lasting effect.

The main message from this review of available data is that there is still a considerable shortage of good epidemiological surveys, conducted in a standard way. This is especially so from the developing world, and that, except for COM and meningitis, it is probably premature to extrapolate the available data to regional and global levels to make meaningful assessments of the burden from all causes of infectious hearing loss. More data are urgently needed.

Known epidemiology of specific infectious causes

This section addresses two major infectious causes, meningitis and chronic otitis media, for which WHO has specific burden data on the cause in relation to deafness and hearing impairment. For other infectious causes, such as congenital rubella and other viral or parasitic diseases, their contribution to the burden of disease estimates has not been disaggregated according to the sequelae of deafness and hearing impairment (in fact the only other specific disease in the global burden estimates in which the sequelae of deafness and hearing impairment are disaggregated is iodine deficiency).

MENINGITIS

The definitions of the various types of meningitis used by WHO in the burden estimates are shown in Table 3.8 (Mathers *et al.*, 2004). Even though it does not specifically mention 'better ear average hearing loss', the definition of

Table 3.8. Sequelae and definitions of meningitis

1. *Streptococcus pneumoniae*: episodes	Acute bacterial disease with sudden onset and fever, intense headache, nausea, vomiting and neck stiffness. The disease must be accompanied by laboratory evidence (in cerebrospinal fluid or blood) of *Streptococcus pneumoniae*
2. *Haemophilus influenzae*: episodes	Acute bacterial disease with sudden onset and fever, intense headache, nausea, vomiting and neck stiffness. The disease must be accompanied by laboratory evidence (in cerebrospinal fluid or blood) of *Haemophilus influenzae* type B
3. *Neisseria meningitidis*: episodes	Acute bacterial disease with sudden onset and fever, intense headache, nausea, vomiting and neck stiffness. The disease must be accompanied by laboratory evidence (in cerebrospinal fluid or blood) of *Neisseria meningitidis*
4. Meningococcaemia without meningitis: episodes	Invasion of the bloodstream with *Neisseria meningitidis*
5. Deafness	At least moderate impairment, where the person is able to hear and repeat words using a raised voice at 1 metre; resulting from meningitis
6. Mental retardation	IQ of 70 or below
7. Motor deficit	Spasticity or paresis of one or more limbs; resulting from meningitis
8. Seizure disorder	Seizures of any type that were present at least 6 months after hospitalisation; resulting from meningitis

deafness used here is the same as the definition of 'disabling hearing impairment' given at the start of the chapter, using the same decibel thresholds and frequencies. Meningitis definitions are according to the most recent descriptions in the International Classification of Diseases (ICD9 codes: 036, 320–322; ICD10 codes: A39, G00, G03).

Figure 3.3 shows the estimated incidence rates of deafness and hearing impairment due to meningitis in the 17 WHO subregions (this and subsequent similar data are provided by the WHO global burden of disease project, variously described in papers by Mathers *et al.* and Murray and Lopez in the reference list). The highest rates are seen in regions WPRO B3 (Western Pacific Islands), SEARO B (Brunei Darussalam, Indonesia, Malaysia, Philippines, Singapore, Sri Lanka, Thailand), AFRO D (mainly those in Saharan and sub-Saharan Central and West Africa in the so-called 'meningitis belt', first described by Lapéyssonnie, 1963). SEARO D, AFRO E, AMRO B and D have lower rates but still substantially greater than the rest of the world. This pattern is substantially different from the incidence of all sequelae of meningitis (including death), where the highest rates by far are seen in AFRO D followed by AFRO E. Rates in AMRO B and D still stand out at lower levels but the rest of the world is very much less. The patterns for prevalence rates are very similar to those for incidence rates, both for deafness alone and for all sequelae.

When the data are analysed according to age, the incidence of meningitis-induced deafness and hearing impairment is extremely high only at ages from 0 to 15 years, is lowest at ages 30–44 years and then rises somewhat to reach a plateau from age 60 years and above. The prevalence (see Figure 3.4) increases progressively by age, especially in AFRO and SEARO regions, and again reaches a plateau at age 60 and above. This latter trend would be expected because of the permanent sensorineural hearing loss induced by meningitis.

The total global burden of meningitis-induced hearing loss is 411 000 DALYs (Table 3.9), which is 7.1% of the global burden for all sequelae of meningitis and 1.2% of the total burden of child- and adult-onset hearing loss. This burden for meningitis occurs overwhelmingly in the developing world, with developing countries (i.e. all subregions except those with developed market economies and economies in transition) experiencing 396 000 DALYs, which is almost 25-fold larger than for all non-developing countries (WHO subregions AMRO A, EURO A, B1, B2, C, WPRO A), which experienced 16 000 DALYs in 2000.

By far the largest burden is in SEAR (56.9% of total burden of meningitis-induced deafness), followed by AFR (25.4%), AMR (10.6%) (see Table 3.9 for percentages of this burden for all regions and subregions). This pattern is different from that for all hearing loss (Table 3.6), where WPR has a much greater proportion of the total burden of hearing loss, putting it in second position after SEAR.

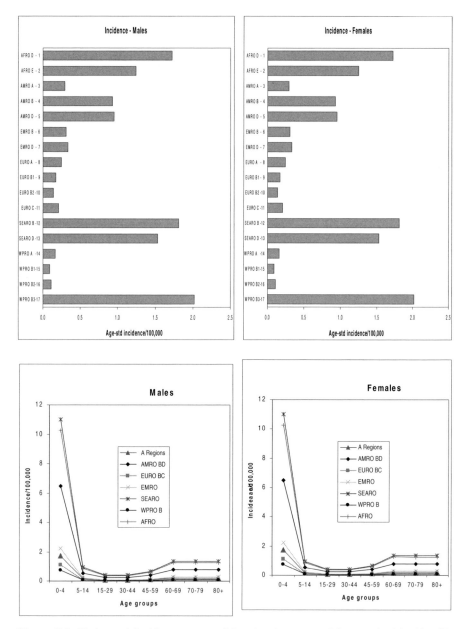

Figure 3.3. Estimated incidence rates of hearing loss caused by meningitis, 41+ dB HTL, by region and sex, GBD 2000, Version 2

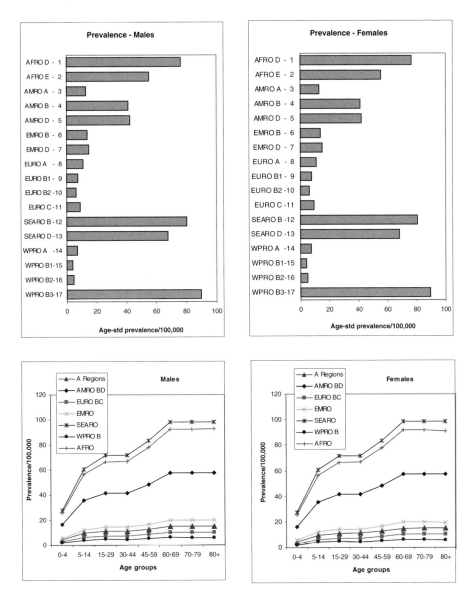

Figure 3.4. Estimated prevalence rates of hearing loss caused by meningitis, 41+ dB HTL, by region and sex, GBD 2000, Version 2

OTITIS MEDIA

Otitis media is the only other major infectious cause of hearing loss in the burden of disease estimates for which WHO has so far attempted to quantify separately its contribution to the burden of hearing impairment. However, the

Table 3.9. Hearing loss caused by meningitis: YLD, YLL and DALY estimates by subregion, 2000

	YLD/100000 Males	YLD/100000 Females	YLL/100000 Males	YLL/100000 Females	Total YLD (000)	Total YLL (000)	Total DALYs (000)	% total DALYs	WHO region	% total DALYs by WHO region
AFRO D	18.4	18.2	0.0	0.0	61	0	61	14.8	AFR	25.4
AFRO E	13.0	12.8	0.0	0.0	44	0	44	10.6		
AMRO A	1.7	1.6	0.0	0.0	5	0	5	1.2	AMR	10.6
AMRO B	7.4	7.2	0.0	0.0	32	0	32	7.8		
AMRO D	9.0	8.8	0.0	0.0	6	0	6	1.5		
EMRO B	2.6	2.7	0.0	0.0	4	0	4	0.9	EMR	2.0
EMRO D	3.2	3.1	0.0	0.0	4	0	4	1.1		
EURO A	1.2	1.1	0.0	0.0	5	0	5	1.2	EUR	2.3
EURO B1	1.0	1.0	0.0	0.0	2	0	2	0.4		
EURO B2	1.2	1.2	0.0	0.0	1	0	1	0.1		
EURO B3	1.0	0.9	0.0	0.0	2	0	2	0.6		
SEARO B	14.4	14.1	0.0	0.0	56	0	56	13.6	SEA	56.9
SEARO D	13.1	13.3	0.0	0.0	178	0	178	43.3		
WPRO A	0.8	0.8	0.0	0.0	1	0	1	0.3	WPR	2.8
WPRO B1	0.6	0.6	0.0	0.0	8	0	8	1.9		
WPRO B2	0.9	0.8	0.0	0.0	1	0	1	0.3		
WPRO B3	19.0	19.2	0.0	0.0	1	0	1	0.3		
Total	6.9	6.8	0.0	0.0	411	0	411			

data are at present less detailed than those for meningitis. The definitions of otitis media used are those in the ICD9 codes: 381–382 and the ICD10 codes: H65–H66, which define episodes of 'inflammation of the middle ear'. No distinction is made between acute and chronic otitis media although the vast preponderance of the burden of deafness and hearing impairment will be from chronic otitis media. The definition of deafness uses the same parameters as for meningitis: at the least moderate impairment resulting from otitis media, a person is able to hear and repeat words using a raised voice at 1 metre.

The most recent estimate for the global burden of moderate or worse hearing loss in the better ear caused by otitis media is 276 900 DALYs in 2000, which is two-thirds of the equivalent burden of deafness and hearing impairment from meningitis, 18.8% of the total burden of otitis media, and 0.83% of the global burden of hearing loss. This burden for otitis media occurs overwhelmingly in the developing world, with developing countries (i.e. all subregions except those for developed countries) experiencing 250 700 DALYs, which is almost ninefold larger than for developed countries (WHO subregions AMRO A, EURO A, EURO C, WPRO A), which experienced 29 000 DALYs in 2000. As with meningitis, the largest burden is in SEAR (34.5% of the total burden of otitis media-induced deafness), followed by WPR (23.7%) and AFR (16.4%) (see Table 3.10 for percentages of this burden for all regions and subregions). These results are generally supported by the prevalence data presented in the preceding section.

The distribution by subregion (see Table 3.10) shows that WPRO B1 (China, Mongolia, Republic of Korea) ranks second after SEARO D, whereas for meningitis it ranked considerably lower. This may be because China has a much larger problem from otitis media-induced hearing loss than from meningitis.

Further information may become available in due course as these data are extended and refined.

Summary and pointers for further research

Although there is a substantial body of published work that addresses the epidemiology of deafness and hearing impairment, the studies that have been performed frequently have deficiencies, usually in methodology, that make the data unsuitable for WHO work on the construction of regional and global databases. Even where such surveys are performed in an epidemiologically sound way, there are still considerable difficulties in determining whether and which type of infection caused the hearing loss. It is vital to improve data-gathering methods because these databases are essential for the assessment of the total burden of hearing loss and its contribution to the burden of disease estimates, as well as to ascertain the contributions that infectious causes of hearing loss make to this burden.

Table 3.10. Hearing loss caused by otitis media: YLD, YLL and DALY estimates by subregion, 2000

	YLD/100000 Males	YLD/100000 Females	YLL/100000 Males	YLL/100000 Females	Total YLD ('000)	Total YLL ('000)	Total DALYs ('000)	% total DALYs	WHO region	% total DALYs by WHO region
AFRO D	6.7	6.6	0.0	0.0	22	0	22	8	AFR	16
AFRO E	6.9	6.9	0.0	0.0	23	0	23	8		
AMRO A	2.4	2.2	0.0	0.0	7	0	7	3	AMR	12
AMRO B	5.1	4.9	0.0	0.0	22	0	22	8		
AMRO D	6.2	6.0	0.0	0.0	4	0	4	2		
EMRO B	5.9	6.2	0.0	0.0	8	0	8	3	EMR	6
EMRO D	6.1	6.1	0.0	0.0	8	0	8	3		
EURO A	1.9	1.8	0.0	0.0	8	0	8	3	EUR	7
EURO B1	2.5	2.4	0.0	0.0	4	0	4	1		
EURO B2	5.9	5.6	0.0	0.0	3	0	3	1		
EURO B3	2.2	1.9	0.0	0.0	5	0	5	2		
SEARO B	5.1	4.9	0.0	0.0	20	0	20	7	SEA	35
SEARO D	5.6	5.6	0.0	0.0	76	0	76	27		
WPRO A	1.8	1.6	0.0	0.0	3	0	3	1	WPR	24
WPRO B1	4.1	4.0	0.0	0.0	55	0	55	20		
WPRO B2	5.4	5.1	0.0	0.0	7	0	7	3		
WPRO B3	6.1	6.2	0.0	0.0	0	0	0	0.2		
Total	4.6	4.5	0.0	0.0	277	0	277	100		100

There is thus a huge need for more acceptable data, especially from developing countries. Data that would be acceptable for incorporation in the WHO data bank should be collected according to the following criteria:

- Data should be population-based and collected by random sampling with adequate sample size and quality control.
- Hearing levels should be measured by audiometric testing or other objective tests of hearing, before removal of wax but without the subject wearing a hearing aid.
- Test instruments should be calibrated and background noise measured and controlled.
- Definitions of hearing impairment should be clearly stated and hearing levels and frequencies should be reported.
- Data should be analysed by hearing loss in the better ear and not by individual ears.
- There should be conformity to the provisions of the WHO Ear and Hearing Disorders Survey Protocol (WHO, 1999), which addresses all the above criteria in more detail.

Research needs to be done on identifying better methods for field testing in remote areas, especially on testing of young children, on eliminating the effects of background noise and on better methods for ascertaining the cause(s) of hearing loss. This last need is a prerequisite for determining the individual burdens of the different infectious causes of hearing loss and other causes.

For WHO, there is a need for the burden of disease estimates on conditions with hearing loss sequelae to be disaggregated so as to indicate the contribution the hearing loss makes to the burden of that condition (e.g. measles, mumps, rubella and other perinatal infections, other infectious causes, other major causes). However, this may not come about until more data are available and collected according to the criteria listed above.

Appendix

For geographic disaggregation of the global burden of disease, the six WHO regions of the world have been further divided into 14 subregions, based on levels of child (under five years) and adult (15–59 years) mortality for WHO member states (see Table 3.12). The classification of WHO member states into the mortality strata were carried out using population estimates for 1999 (UN Population Division 1998) and estimates of $_5q_0$ and $_{45}q_{15}$ based on WHO analyses of mortality rates for 1999 (WHO, 2000).

When these mortality strata are applied to the six WHO regions, they produce 14 mortality subregions. These are listed in Table 3.11, together with the WHO member states in each subregion.

Table 3.11. Regional epidemiological analysis categories for the Global Burden of Disease 2000 Project: GBD regions and 17 subregions

GBD region	Mortality stratum	Region code	WHO member states	Reporting subregion
AFRO	D	1	Algeria, Angola, Benin, Burkina Faso, Cameroon, Cape Verde, Chad, Comoros, Equatorial Guinea, Gabon, Gambia, Ghana, Guinea, Guinea-Bissau, Liberia, Madagascar, Mali, Mauritania, Mauritius, Niger, Nigeria, Sao Tome and Principe, Senegal, Seychelles, Sierra Leone, Togo	AFRO D
			Djibouti, Somalia, Sudan	EMRO D
AFRO	E	2	Botswana, Burundi, Central African Republic, Congo, Côte d'Ivoire, Democratic Republic of the Congo, Eritrea, Ethiopia, Kenya, Lesotho, Malawi, Mozambique, Namibia, Rwanda, South Africa, Swaziland, Uganda, United Republic of Tanzania, Zambia, Zimbabwe	AFRO E
AMRO	A	3	Canada, United States of America	AMRO A
AMRO	B	4	Antigua and Barbuda, Argentina, Bahamas, Barbados, Belize, Brazil, Chile, Colombia, Costa Rica, Dominica, Dominican Republic, El Salvador, Grenada, Guyana, Honduras, Jamaica, Mexico, Panama, Paraguay, Saint Kitts and Nevis, Saint Lucia, Saint Vincent and the Grenadines, Suriname, Trinidad and Tobago, Uruguay, Venezuela	AMRO B
			Cuba	AMRO A
AMRO	D	5	Bolivia, Ecuador, Guatemala, Haiti, Nicaragua, Peru	AMRO D
EMRO	B	6	Bahrain, Cyprus, Iran (Islamic Republic of), Jordan, Kuwait, Lebanon, Libyan Arab Jamahiriya, Oman, Qatar, Saudi Arabia, Syrian Arab Republic, Tunisia, United Arab Emirates	EMRO B

EMRO	D	7	Egypt, Iraq, Morocco, Yemen	EMRO D
EURO	A	8	Andorra, Austria, Belgium, Croatia, Czech Republic, Denmark, Finland, France, Germany, Greece, Iceland, Ireland, Israel, Italy, Luxembourg, Malta, Monaco, Netherlands, Norway, Portugal, San Marino, Slovenia, Spain, Sweden, Switzerland, United Kingdom	EURO A
EURO	B1	9	Albania, Bosnia and Herzegovina, Bulgaria, Georgia, Poland, Romania, Slovakia, the former Yugoslav Republic of Macedonia, Turkey, Yugoslavia	EURO B
EURO	B2	10	Armenia, Azerbaijan, Kyrgyzstan, Tajikistan, Turkmenistan, Uzbekistan	EURO B
EURO	C	11	Belarus, Estonia, Hungary, Kazakhstan, Latvia, Lithuania, Republic of Moldova, Russian Federation, Ukraine	EURO C
SEARO	B	12	Indonesia, Sri Lanka, Thailand	SEARO B
			Malaysia, Philippines	WPRO B
			Brunei Darussalam, Singapore	WPRO A
SEARO	D	13	Bangladesh, Bhutan, India, Maldives, Nepal	SEARO D
			Afghanistan, Pakistan	EMRO D
WPRO	A	14	Australia, Japan, New Zealand	WPRO A
WPRO	B1	15	China, Mongolia, Republic of Korea	WPRO B
			DPR Korea	SEARO D
WPRO	B2	16	Cambodia, Lao People's Democratic Republic, Vietnam	WPRO B
			Myanmar	SEARO D
WPRO	B3	17	Cook Islands, Fiji, Kiribati, Marshall Islands, Micronesia (Federated States of), Nauru, Niue, Palau, Papua New Guinea, Samoa, Solomon Islands, Tonga, Tuvalu, Vanuatu	WPRO B

Table 3.12. Definitions of mortality strata used to define WHO subregions for the GBD 2000

Mortality stratum	Child mortality	Definition	Adult mortality
A	Very low child mortality (first quintile of $_5q_0$)	$_5q_0 < 0.0122$	Low adult mortality
B	Low child mortality (second and third quintile of $_5q_0$)	$0.0122 < {_5q_0} < 0.062$	Low adult mortality
C	Low child mortality (second and third quintile of $_5q_0$)	$0.0122 < {_5q_0} < 0.062$	High adult mortality
D	High child mortality (fourth and fifth quintile of $_5q_0$)	$0.062 < {_5q_0}$	High adult mortality
E	High child mortality (fourth and fifth quintile of $_5q_0$)	$0.062 < {_5q_0}$	Very high adult mortality

For the purposes of burden of disease epidemiological analyses, two of these regions have been further subdivided: EURO B into EURO B1 and EURO B2 – the latter including the central Asian states; and WPRO B into WPRO B1 (mainly China), WPRO B2 (South-East Asian countries) and WPRO B3 (Pacific Islands). Additionally, some member states have been reclassified into subregions with similar epidemiological/geographic/ethnic patterns in order to maximise the epidemiological homogeneity of the subregions for the purposes of epidemiological analysis. These subregions are used for analysis in the GBD 2000, but the resulting estimates are mapped back to the 14 subregions defined in Table 3.11 for all reporting purposes.

4 CYTOMEGALOVIRUS

S.B. Boppana and W.J. Britt

Introduction

Human cytomegalovirus (HCMV) is a ubiquitous cause of human infection. Infection with this virus as measured by serologic reactivity exceeds 80% of most populations in the developing world and in certain populations in North America and northern Europe. The virus was first isolated and identified in the middle of the 20th century, although the human infection that was initially thought to be the single manifestation of HCMV infection, cytomegalic inclusion disease (CID) of the newborn, was described by pathologists early in the 20th century. As tissue culture isolation and serological assays became more widely available, researchers linked HCMV to a variety of illnesses, many that have subsequently been shown to be unrelated to HCMV. Studies in renal transplant patients and patients receiving large amounts of blood definitively linked HCMV to disease in humans, particularly in the immunocompromised patient (Rifkind, 1965; Lang and Hanshaw, 1969; Prince *et al.*, 1971; Bowden, 1995; Rubin, 2002). Suppression of host immune responsiveness was recognised as a common characteristic of patients at risk for invasive HCMV infections and the onset of the AIDS epidemic in the early 1980s was associated with a dramatic increase in the spectrum of disease caused by HCMV. Human cytomegalovirus eventually became the most common opportunistic infection in HIV infected patients with AIDS and remained a major cause of morbidity and mortality in these patients until the introduction of highly active antiretroviral therapy (Jacobson and Mills, 1988; Gallant *et al.*, 1992; SOCA, 1992; Munoz *et al.*, 1993; Spector *et al.*, 1999). Currently, HCMV continues to cause disease in patients with AIDS, but similar to the natural history of other opportunistic infections in AIDS patients responding to antiretroviral therapy, the

Infection and Hearing Impairment. Edited by V.E. Newton and P.J. Vallely
© 2006 John Wiley & Sons, Ltd

incidence of invasive HCMV disease is low, even in patients with minimally reconstituted immune systems (Whitcup et al., 1999; Jacobson et al., 2000). Today, HCMV is primarily a cause of disease in newborn infants and in transplant patients. Perhaps of even greater potential medical importance is the proposed role of chronic HCMV infections in diseases such as coronary atherosclerosis and human cancers.

The spectrum of human disease associated with HCMV infections can be best understood by considering the manifestations of acute infections and those that may arise following chronic persistent infection as separate pathogenic processes. The manifestation of acute infections include end-organ damage and, in the most severe forms of HCMV infection, death (Table 4.1).

This type of infection most commonly occurs in immunocompromised patients, either secondary to AIDS or treatment with cytolytic agents in the post-transplant period. Severe disease can also occur in newborn infants following intrauterine infection (Table 4.1). Although the mechanism of disease during acute infection is not known, the most consistent correlate of disease is an increased virus burden in the blood compartment or in a specific organ. Thus, it appears that the lytic cycle associated with HCMV replication leads to cell death and organ dysfunction. Consistent with this proposed pathogenesis of acute HCMV infection is the response of symptomatic HCMV disease to antiviral agents that prevent virus replication but do not limit expression of virus encoded early genes. Viral tropism for specific organs is poorly understood but at least in solid-organ transplant recipients, the transplanted organ is often the site of virus replication (Pass et al., 1978; Bowden et al., 1986; Gnann et al., 1988; Wreghitt et al., 1988; Dummer, 1990; Goodrich, Boeckh and Bowden, 1994; Evans et al., 1999). In general, active virus replication is limited in these patients, often sparing the central nervous system (Table 4.1) (Rubin, 2002). In contrast, virus replication can be demonstrated in almost every organ following fetal infection (Table 4.1); however, the relationship between the developmental age and the widespread susceptibility of various cell types in the fetus to HCMV infection remains undefined. Most investigators would argue that both the developmental status of cells within individual fetal organs at the time of HCMV infection and the level of maternally derived immune functions influence the extent of disease in these patients.

The spectrum of disease associated with chronic, persistent HCMV infections remains to be determined. Human cytomegalovirus infection results in life-long persistence and community acquired reinfections with new strains of this virus are probably common (Drew et al., 1984; Spector, Hirata and Newman, 1984; Bale et al., 1996; Boppana et al., 2001). Thus, viruses maintained in an individual are likely to represent the cumulative exposure to HCMV and also include strains that arise following recombination between different strains of HCMV in the persistently infected host. In contrast to the correlation between virus replication and disease in patients with acute HCMV syndromes, the level of virus replication does not appear to be directly related to

Table 4.1. Clinical manifestations of CMV infection

Population	Clinical manifestations	
	Acute Infection	Chronic Infection
Immunocompetent	Subclinical infection; mononucleosis syndrome	Persistent infection; recurrent virus shedding; vascular disease?
Immunocompromised		
Fetuses	Hepatitis; encephalitis; retinitis; thrombocytopenia; microcephaly	Persistent virus shedding; progressive hearing loss; developmental delay
Allograft recipients	Fever; hepatitis; pneumonitis; haematological abnormalities; graft dysfunction	Graft dysfunction/loss; transplant vasculopathy; predisposition to fungal superinfection
AIDS	Retinitis; encephalitis; colitis; esophagitis; malabsorption	Vision loss; wasting syndrome; increased mortality; encephalopathy/ encephalitis

disease associated with chronic infection. A variety of common diseases have been suggested to be linked to chronic HCMV infections, including vascular disease such as atherosclerosis and chronic graft rejection in transplant recipients (Table 4.1) (Everett *et al.*, 1992; Epstein *et al.*, 1996; Epstein, Zhou and Zhu, 1999; Hosenpud, 1999; Browne *et al.*, 2001b; Soderberg-Naucler and Emery, 2001; Streblow, Orloff and Nelson, 2001; Libby, 2002). The association between HCMV and vascular disease leading to the loss of transplanted allografts has been noted for solid-organ allografts and is best described for cardiac allograft recipients (Grattan *et al.*, 1989; Koskinen *et al.*, 1999). Evidence linking HCMV infection to vascular disease includes: (a) increased HCMV seroprevalence in patients with vascular disease such as coronary atherosclerotic vascular disease, (b) increased titres of HCMV-specific antibodies in patients with progressive atherosclerotic vascular disease, (c) the demonstration of viral nucleic acids and virus-encoded proteins in the wall of diseased vessels and (d) the development of animal models that recapitulate most characteristics of vascular disease observed in allografts undergoing rejection (Bruning *et al.*, 1994; Speir *et al.*, 1994, 1996; Lemstrom *et al.*, 1995, 1997; Epstein *et al.*, 1996; Zhou *et al.*, 1996, 1999; Berencsi *et al.*, 1998; Martelius *et al.*, 1999; Stals, 1999; Zhu *et al.*, 1999; Sorlie *et al.*, 2000; O'Connor *et al.*, 2001; Orloff *et al.*, 2002; Streblow *et al.*, 2003). Together, these data argue strongly for a role of HCMV in the pathogenesis of vascular disease. The association between chronic HCMV infection and human cancers has been suggested by epidemiologic studies or *in vitro* studies. Past studies have linked the HCMV infection and the development of cervical cancer, but study populations in several of these reports also had evidence of exposure to other infectious agents associated with the development of malignancy, including human papilloma virus (HPV) (Huang et al., 1984; Shen et al., 1993). More recently, HCMV nucleic acids and viral proteins have been demonstrated in CNS (central nervous system) tumours and adenocarcinoma of the colon (Huang and Pagano, 1978; Cobbs et al., 2002; Harkins et al., 2002). Whether this virus participates in the transformation or malignant behaviour of these cell types is unknown. Alternatively, HCMV could be merely a passenger in cells found within human cancers and have no role in the malignant phenotype of these cells. The localisation of HCMV to areas of inflammation together with the association of human cancers with chronic infections and inflammation suggests several possible mechanisms by which HCMV could promote the malignant phenotype. Additional studies will be required to define the relationship between HCMV and human cancers.

Epidemiology of HCMV infection

Human cytomegalovirus is acquired early in life in most populations, with the exception of people in economically well-developed countries of northern Europe and North America. In the developing world, acquisition of HCMV is nearly universal in early childhood (Table 4.2). Although the mode of acquisition is unknown, it is assumed to be through the close physical contacts that result from crowded living conditions. Presumably, exposure to saliva and

Table 4.2. Sources of HCMV exposure and routes of infection in different populations

Sources of CMV infections	
Community acquired	
Age	**Mode of acquisition**
Perinatal	Intrauterine fetal infection (congenital); intrapartum exposure to virus; breast milk acquired
Infancy and childhood	Exposure to saliva and other body fluids
Adolescence and adulthood	Sexually transmitted; exposure to young children
Hospital acquired	
Source	**Risks associated with virus transmission**
Blood products	Blood products from seropositive donors; multiple transfusions; white blood cell containing blood products
Allograft recipients	Allograft from seropositive donors; graft rejection

other body fluids containing infectious virus is a primary mode of spread and because infants infected with HCMV characteristically excrete significant amounts of virus for months to years following infection, virus spread is relatively efficient. Similar routes of exposure of HCMV have been proposed for children from countries with more developed economies that are infected as a result of attending group child care facilities (Adler, 1985, 1988, 1989; Murph *et al.*, 1986; Pass and Hutto, 1986; Dobbins *et al.*, 1993). Perinatal acquisition, including congenital infection, also contributes to the spread of HCMV into a population by introduction of infected infants who persistently excrete several logs of virus (Table 4.2). An additional and less well appreciated mode of virus spread is through breast milk. It is estimated that over 80% of breast-fed infants of persistently infected mothers will be exposed to HCMV as a result of breast feeding (Stagno *et al.*, 1980; Dworsky *et al.*, 1983; Ahlfors and Ivarsson, 1985; Minamishima *et al.*, 1994; Asanuma *et al.*, 1996; Vochem *et al.*, 1998; Hamprecht *et al.*, 2001). Infants infected through breast feeding excrete virus for prolonged periods of time, making them ideal vectors for the spread of virus. Children are infected throughout childhood, but during adolescence and early adulthood the rate of infection increases significantly secondary to sexual exposure. Significant titres of infectious HCMV can be found in semen and cervical secretions, suggesting that exposure to these body fluids could result in HCMV infection (Lang and Kummer, 1975; Stagno *et al.*, 1975a; Waner *et al.*, 1977; Drew and Mintz, 1984; Collier *et al.*, 1995). The natural history of HCMV infection in adolescents and adults has been shown to parallel STI (sexually transmitted infection). Homosexual men and women attending STI clinics have an increased incidence of HCMV infection (Drew and Mintz, 1984; Chandler, Handsfield and McDougall, 1987; Sohn *et al.*, 1991). Thus, HCMV should be considered an STI in adults that can effectively spread through a sexually active population (Table 4.2).

EPIDEMIOLOGY OF MATERNAL AND CONGENITAL HCMV INFECTION

Numerous cross-sectional, serological studies, dating back from the 1960s, have demonstrated that HCMV infection is ubiquitous in humans. Increased rates of HCMV serological reactivity have been demonstrated in nonwhite and low-income populations in both developed and developing countries (Alford, Stagno and Pass, 1980; Alford *et al.*, 1981). The prevalence of maternal HCMV infection is an important determinant of the frequency and significance of vertical transmission of HCMV in a population. The rates of congenital HCMV infection are directly proportional to the rates of maternal seropositivity in the population (Alford and Pass, 1981; Alford *et al.*, 1981).

The natural history of HCMV infection during pregnancy is complex and has not been defined completely. Unlike rubella and toxoplasmosis, where intrauterine transmission is thought to occur as a result of primary infection acquired during pregnancy, congenital HCMV infection has been shown to occur in children born to mothers who have had HCMV infection prior to pregnancy (nonprimary infection) (Stagno et al., 1977b; Peckham et al., 1983; Ahlfors et al., 1984; Morris et al., 1994). In fact, congenital HCMV infection following a nonprimary maternal infection has been shown to be common, especially in highly seroimmune populations (Table 4.3) (Stagno et al., 1977b; Schopfer, Lauber and Krech, 1978; Peckham et al., 1983; Ahlfors et al., 1984). Studies of risk factors for congenital HCMV infection have documented the association between young maternal age and increased rates of congenital HCMV infection (White et al., 1989; Pass et al., 1991; Fowler et al., 1993, 1996). In addition, nonwhite race and single marital status were independently associated with an increased risk of congenital HCMV infection (Preece et al., 1986; Walmus et al., 1988; White et al., 1989; Fowler, Stagno and Pass, 1993). An increased risk of congenital HCMV infection in offspring of women with sexually transmitted diseases, single mothers and those less than 20 years of age has been reported (Fowler et al., 1991).

Although the mechanisms of intrauterine transmission of HCMV have not been clearly defined, the maternal immune response has been shown to be a crucial determinant of the transplacental transmission of HCMV. The importance of maternal immune responses is evident from the substantial protection that preconceptional seroimmunity to HCMV provides against intrauterine transmission. Although this protection is not complete, transmission rates decrease by about 25-fold in mothers with preconceptional seroimmunity compared to those with primary infection (Medearis, 1982; Griffiths and Baboonian, 1984; Stagno et al., 1986). Primary maternal infection is defined as an initial acquisition of HCMV during pregnancy and is identified by conversion from serum antibody negative to antibody positive or by the detection of circulating IgM antibody to HCMV. However, one should be cautious with the latter definition because of the low sensitivity of commercial

Table 4.3. Classification of maternal HCMV infection and outcome of infants infected in utero

	Primary[a]	Nonprimary
Rate of congenital infection	13%[b]	87%
	40%[b]	60%
Rate of symptomatic congenital infection	60%[b]	40%
Rate of infected infants with long-term sequelae	25%[c]	8%

[a] Classification of maternal infection based on serological reactivity as initially described by Stagno (Stagno et al., 1982). Primary infection is defined as the acquisition of serologic reactivity during pregnancy. Nonprimary infection is defined as preconception serologic reactivity.
[b] Results from an ongoing screening programme in the authors' institution. Less than half of enrolled women can be definitively classified as primary or nonprimary.
[c] Results from an analysis of the nonscreened population (Fowler et al., 1992).

IgM assay (~70%) and the demonstration of HCMV IgM antibodies in women with evidence of past infection (Griffiths *et al.*, 1982; McVoy and Adler, 1989). Although the occurrence of congenital HCMV infection in children born to immune mothers (nonprimary maternal infection) was documented more than 25 years ago, it was thought that congenitally infected children who were born to mothers with a nonprimary maternal infection rarely if ever develop long-term sequelae (Stagno *et al.*, 1977b, 1982, 1986; Fowler *et al.*, 1992). However, more recent data from the natural history studies of congenital HCMV infection in the Europe and the US suggested that a significant proportion of these children are also at risk for an adverse outcome (Ahlfors, Ivarsson and Harris, 1999; Boppana *et al.*, 1999; Casteels *et al.*, 1999).

The mechanisms of transplacental transmission of HCMV in immune women are not clearly defined. A nonprimary maternal infection could be due to reactivation of endogenous latent HCMV or reinfection with a new virus strain. The results of a recent study demonstrated that acquisition of a new CMV strain between pregnancies in women who were previously HCMV seropositive was associated with an increased risk of intrauterine transmission and severe fetal infection (Boppana *et al.*, 2001). The results of that study also showed that the virus isolated from the infected infants was similar to an HCMV strain acquired most recently by the mother. These women also had serologic evidence of reinfection between pregnancies.

Clinical manifestations of intrauterine HCMV infection

Of the estimated 40000 children born each year in the US with congenital cytomegalovirus (CMV) infection, only about 10–15% exhibit clinical findings suggestive of congenital infection at birth (symptomatic infection) (Fowler *et al.*, 1992). It was thought that clinically apparent or symptomatic congenital CMV occurs almost exclusively following a primary CMV infection; however, more recent data from natural history studies of congenital CMV infection have documented that symptomatic infection occurs in children born to immune mothers more frequently than has previously been recognised (Boppana *et al.*, 1999). The typical findings that have been associated with generalised cytomegalic inclusion disease are characterised by multiorgan disease with prominent involvement of the reticuloendothelial and central nervous systems (McCracken *et al.*, 1969; Becroft, 1981; Ho, 1982; Boppana *et al.*, 1992a, 1997). About 10% of infants with symptomatic congenital CMV infection die during early infancy due to multiorgan disease with severe hepatic dysfunction, bleeding diathesis and secondary bacterial infections (Boppana *et al.*, 1992a). The frequency of various clinical and laboratory findings in 106 neonates with symptomatic congenital HCMV infection is shown in Table 4.4. Petechiae, jaundice and hepatosplenomegaly are the most frequently noted abnormalities and are present in approximately 75% of symptomatic neonates (Boppana *et al.*, 1992a). In addition, approximately 50% of infants were micro-

Table 4.4. Clinical and laboratory findings in children with symptomatic congenital HCMV infection[a]

Finding	% positive
Prematurity	34
Small for gestational age	50
Petechiae	76
Jaundice	67
Hepatosplenomegaly	60
Purpura	13
Microcephaly	53
Seizures	7
Elevated alanine aminotransferase (ALT) (>80 IU/mL)	83
Thrombocytopenia (platelet count <100 × 10³/mm³)	77
Conjugated hyperbilirubinemia (direct bilirubin >2 mg/dL)	81

[a] Modified from a report of symptomatic congenital HCMV infection (Boppana et al., 1992b).

cephalic and small for gestational age and about a third were born prematurely, suggestive of significant prenatal insult. About two-thirds of symptomatic infants have clinical neurological abnormalities such as microcephaly, lethargy/hypotonia, poor suck and/or seizures. Of the neonates who had ophthalmologic and audiologic assessments, chorioretinitis and/or optic atrophy were noted in 20% and an abnormal hearing screen in about half the children (Boppana et al., 1992). Other less frequent findings include hydrocephalus, pneumonitis and haemolytic anaemia. The presence or absence of clinical abnormalities in congenitally infected children is an important prognostic determinant of outcome. Between 40 and 60% of infants with clinically apparent or symptomatic congenital HCMV infection will develop hearing loss compared with about 7–10% of infants with subclinical or asymptomatic infection (Dahle et al., 2000).

The virus

Human cytomegalovirus is the largest and most complex member of the family of human herpesviruses. Its genome of double-stranded linear DNA consists of over 230 kilobase pairs that encode somewhere between 170 and 260 open reading frames (ORFs) (Mocarski and Tan Courcelle, 2001). The genome organisation differs from other CMVs (with the possible exception of chimpanzee CMV) and other β-herpesviruses in that it contains both internal and terminal repeated sequences, thus permitting it to isomerise into four different forms; however, the biological consequences of isomerisation of the genome is unknown (Mocarski and Tan Courcelle, 2001). The genome can be divided into a unique long sequence (U_L) and a unique short sequence (U_S)

that are separated by repeat sequences. In general, gene blocks encoding essential viral replicative functions such as the viral DNA polymerase and structural proteins are in the U_L sequences and often colinear with other herpesviruses. Viral genes that encode functions such as chemokine receptors, cytokine analogues and regulatory enzymes that could influence the tropism of HCMV growth in different cell types are typically found in the U_S regions. These regions contain the greatest sequence variation between different mammalian CMVs (Mocarski and Tan Courcelle, 2001).

The replicative cycle of HCMV is typical of other members of the herpesvirus family in that it is temporally coordinated and viral genes are expressed in a sequential fashion, described as immediate-early, early and late (Mocarski and Tan Courcelle, 2001). Viral genes expressed at various times often modulate expression of viral genes in the subsequent temporal class, thereby providing further regulation of the production of infectious progeny and the lytic replicative cycle. Immediate-early gene products have a common function, modification of both viral and host cell functions, and facilitate early viral gene expression. HCMV early genes include viral proteins that are important for viral DNA replication, including the viral DNA polymerase, alkaline exonuclease, ribonucleotide reductase and other replicative enzymes. Virion structural proteins are thought to be expressed late in the replicative cycle, but numerous virion structural proteins including one of the major envelope glycoproteins have also been shown to be expressed at both early and late times following infection. The replicative cycle of HCMV is the longest of members of the β-herpesvirus family and requires approximately 48 hours for generation of progeny virus. Viral DNA replication takes place in the nucleus of infected cells and concatameric DNA is cleaved during packaging into the procapsid by mechanisms that closely resemble the pathway of bacteriophage assembly. Recent studies in the assembly of α-herpesviruses have provided a much greater understanding of the mechanisms and pathways of viral capsid assembly and DNA packaging and the interested reader is referred to these studies (Newcomb et al., 1999). The viral capsid leaves the nucleus by as yet undetermined mechanisms and enters the cytoplasm as a partially tegumented, subviral particle. Assembly of the mature particle takes place in the cytoplasm of the infected cell in a specialised compartment that has been termed the assembly compartment (Sanchez et al., 2000). It is believed that this is a modified secretory compartment in close proximity to the trans-Golgi (Sanchez et al., 2000; Homman-Loudiyi et al., 2003). Virion structural proteins are transported to this compartment and, presumably through a series of protein interactions, the virus is assembled and finally enveloped. This latter step is of considerable complexity because of the large number of virion glycoproteins that comprise the envelope of infectious virions (Chee et al., 1990). Virus is presumably released by cell lysis in cells such as fibroblasts and by as yet poorly defined exocytic pathways in certain other cell types (Fish et al., 1998).

Human cytomegalovirus is highly species specific, as are other β-herpesviruses, and productive replication takes place *in vitro* only in cells of human origin. Biopsy and autopsy specimens have indicated that HCMV can infect and induce cellular pathology in a wide variety of tissue and cell types (Borisch *et al.*, 1988; Sinzger *et al.*, 1993, 1995; Plachter, Sinzger and Jahn, 1996; Sinzger and Jahn, 1996; Halwachs-Baumann *et al.*, 1998; Bissinger *et al.*, 2002). Virus has been detected in fibroblast, epithelial, neuronal and glial cells, and in some hematopoietic cells. Although most investigators view HCMV as a chronic persistent infection characterised by low-level virus replication, recent studies have clearly demonstrated latent infection (Soderberg-Naucler, Fish and Nelson, 1997). Studies in other mammalian species have demonstrated that CMV infections can persist as a latent infection (Balthesen, Messerle and Reddehase, 1993; Reddehase *et al.*, 1994; Grzimek *et al.*, 2001). Studies carried out *in vitro* have relied almost exclusively on primary human fibroblasts for virus propagation. Rapidly growing transformed cell lines are rarely susceptible to productive infection with HCMV, emphasising the importance of terminal differentiation in permissive targets of HCMV infection. Rarely, malignant cells derived from human tumours will support HCMV replication and interestingly enough these cells often maintain some characteristics of differentiated cells such as motility in glial derived tumour cells that support productive HCMV infection.

The explanation for the restricted growth of HCMV in different cell types is unknown. As examples, HCMV undergoes a lytic replicative cycle in primary fibroblasts while in primary aortic endothelial cells, productive infection has been reported to take place in the absence of cell lysis (Fish *et al.*, 1998). Other cell types, such as macrophages and some epithelial cells, do not exhibit the typical cytopathic effects (CPE) observed in human fibroblasts infected with HCMV (Fish *et al.*, 1995; Fish, Britt and Nelson, 1996; Jarvis *et al.*, 1999). The role of viral genes in cellular tropism is well appreciated but not well understood. Laboratory adapted viruses, such as the commonly used strains AD169 and Towne, appear to lack viral genes that confer growth in nonfibroblast derived cells such as primary endothelium, epithelium and monocyte derived macrophages (Sinzger and Jahn, 1996; Jahn *et al.*, 1999; Sinzger *et al.*, 1999; Kahl *et al.*, 2000; Grazia Revello *et al.*, 2001; Gerna *et al.*, 2002). Intense current study is aimed at defining these viral functions as it is believed that such genes not only confer tissue tropism but also may contribute to the pathogenesis of certain HCMV associated disease states.

Pathogenesis

The pathogenesis of HCMV infections remains poorly understood and thus far has only been directly associated with virus replication. Levels of virus replication, the so-called virus burden, have been related to disease manifestation in both immunocompetent and immunocompromised HCMV infected hosts (Stagno *et al.*, 1975a; Fox *et al.*, 1995; Cope *et al.*, 1997a, 1997b; Zaia *et al.*, 1997; Zanghellini *et al.*, 1998; Emery, 1999; Hassan-Walker *et al.*, 1999; Spector *et al.*, 1999; Emery *et al.*, 2000). It is important to consider that these correlations have been made for disease states that can be described as acute following HCMV infection or reactivation. In acute disease states, HCMV replicates in a wide variety of cells and disease presumably results from cellular damage, organ dysfunction and end-organ failure. This mechanism of HCMV disease is best illustrated in immunocompromised allograft recipients who often develop severe disseminated infections with HCMV in the post-transplant period. Virus is reactivated from an existing persistent infection, the transplant allograft, or rarely acquired by exposure to blood products. Virus replicates in susceptible cells free from immune control mediated by HCMV specific CD4+ helper and CD8+ cytotoxic T lymphocytes, antiviral antibodies and, possibly, natural killer cells (Quinnan *et al.*, 1982; Reusser *et al.*, 1991; Riddell *et al.*, 1992; Li *et al.*, 1994; Boppana and Britt, 1995; Boppana *et al.*, 1995; Walter *et al.*, 1995; Schoppel *et al.*, 1997, 1998; Boeckh *et al.*, 2003). Patients with AIDS or uncontrolled HIV infections not responsive to anti-retroviral therapy have very high levels of HCMV viral burden and exhibit invasive infections of the eye and gastrointestinal tract secondary to a loss of CD4+ lymphocytes. Similar mechanisms have been proposed to explain the disease seen in developmentally immunocompromised fetuses infected *in utero* following maternal infection during pregnancy.

In contrast to an apparent direct relationship between virus replication, virus burden and disease during acute HCMV infection, the role of virus replication in chronic diseases associated with HCMV such as transplant associated vascular sclerosis and atherosclerosis remains undefined. As noted previously, viral nucleic acids and viral antigens have been localised to specific regions of disease vasculature. However, only immediate viral gene expression has been shown to be sufficient for disease induction in some models of virus-induced vascular sclerosis, suggesting that replication and amplification of virus is unnecessary for the development of these diseases (Speir *et al.*, 1994; Zhou *et al.*, 1999; Suzuki *et al.*, 2002). Alternatively, treatment of CMV infected animals and transplant recipients with the antiviral drug ganciclovir can limit progression of the disease (Lemstrom *et al.*, 1997). Perhaps the most consistent interpretation of currently available data is that HCMV is a necessary cofactor in the development of vascular sclerosis in patients with underlying inflammatory vascular disease and is likely to contribute to the development of disease either by amplifying existing inflammation in transplant recipients or by dysregulation of a subclinical inflammatory response in normal individuals.

The intimate relationship between host derived immune responses and the biology of HCMV is well appreciated but is far from understood. Infection of susceptible cell types induces a wide variety of host responses, including expression of components of the host cell innate immune response (Child *et al.*, 2002). Responses such as those resulting from signalling through TLR-2 (toll-like receptor-2) receptors include the induction of the transcription factor NF-kB, a key element of the host immune response (Yurochko *et al.*, 1997; Browne *et al.*, 2001a; Compton *et al.*, 2003). The role of these early host responses in the control of HCMV replication and the ultimate outcome of HCMV infections are not well understood, but in murine models of HCMV disease, interferons appear to have a critical role in curtailing virus replication and organ involvement (Koszinowski, Del Val and Reddehase, 1990). However, it is somewhat paradoxical that this virus is frequently detected in areas of active inflammation. The explanation for the peculiar tropism of HCMV for cells in inflammatory lesions is unclear; however, it is well known that HCMV infection induces transcription factors such as NF-kB and the viral promoters of immediate early HCMV genes have multiple binding sites for NF-kB, raising the possibility that the inflammatory response may also positively regulate virus replication (Meier and Stinski, 1996). In addition, several studies have suggested that HCMV utilises cells infiltrating a site of inflammation as vehicles to disseminate both locally and to distant sites (Gerna *et al.*, 1998, 2000; Saederup *et al.*, 1999, 2001; Maidji *et al.*, 2002; Saederup and Mocarski, 2002). However, it is unclear how the virus persists in sites of inflammation. Over the last 10 years significant amounts of experimental evidence point to the importance of virus-encoded immune evasion mechanisms that can limit host derived effector functions that would otherwise eliminate virus. A discussion of these functions is beyond the scope of this chapter and the reader is referred to several recent reviews of this area of viral immunology (Miller, Cebulla and Sedmak, 2002; Mocarski, 2002; Saederup and Mocarski, 2002; Spencer *et al.*, 2002).

Although immune evasion functions of the virus appear to restrict effectively immune recognition and elimination of virus infected cells *in vitro*, in normal hosts these immune evasion functions can be overcome by the host immune response. The host immune response operates at several levels and includes cellular innate host responses such as the induction of double-stranded RNA-dependent protein kinase (PKR) and phosphorylation of key components of the protein translation machinery and cellular proteins that initiate programmed cell death (Samuel, 2001). Coupled to these responses are the release of inflammatory cytokines and chemokines from infected cells, which in some cases limit virus replication and can serve to recruit cellular components of the innate immune responses such as monocytes and NK cells (Salazar-Mather, Hamilton and Biron, 2000; Biron and Brossay, 2001). These immune effector cells recognise HCMV infected cells and mediate their elimination by either direct cytotoxicity or by the release of antiviral cytokines such as interferons. Severe HCMV infections have been reported in a small set of patients with a deficiency in NK cell function, indicating a key role of these early responses in the restriction of viral replication (Biron, Byron and Sullivan, 1989). Effector functions of the adaptive immune response have perhaps the most well-characterised role in the control of HCMV infections. Antiviral antibodies have been shown to react with a variety of virion and infected cell proteins (Zaia *et al.*, 1986; Alford, Hayes and Britt, 1988; Landini and LaPlaca, 1991). Although controversial, antibodies with virus neturalising activity are believed to be an important component of the protective immune response. These reports have included studies in HIV infected patients, in transplant recipients and in pregnant women with HCMV infections (Boppana and Britt, 1995; Boppana *et al.*, 1995; Schoppel *et al.*, 1997, 1998; Alberola *et al.*, 2000). The importance of virus specific CD8+ cytolytic T lymphocytes in resistance to severe HCMV infections has been well documented in allograft recipients (Quinnan *et al.*, 1982; Reusser *et al.*, 1991, 1997; Riddell *et al.*, 1993; Li *et al.*, 1994). Similarly, the loss of HCMV specific CD4+ T cell reactivity in patients with HIV infection has been correlated with susceptibility to invasive HCMV disease, and this susceptibility can be reversed by immune reconstitution of CD4+ T cell responsiveness in patients successfully treated with HAART (Autran *et al.*, 1997; Komanduri *et al.*, 2001a, 2001b). Interestingly, reconstitution of immune responsiveness in antiviral treated AIDS patients with high levels of viral burden can result in immune mediated disease such as immune recovery vitritis in patients with HCMV retinitis (Karavellas *et al.*, 1998; Holland, 1999; Mutimer *et al.*, 2002). Animal models of HCMV infections have provided findings consistent with the role of these various immune effector functions in the resistance to HCMV infections (Jonjic *et al.*, 1990, 1994; Koszinowski, Del Val and Reddehase, 1990; Koszinowski, Reddehase and Jonjic, 1991; Rapp *et al.*, 1993; Steffens *et al.*, 1998).

The equilibrium reached between host derived immune responses and viral evasion functions enables HCMV to persist for the life of the host. The high frequency of HCMV specific CD8+ T lymphocytes reactive with late gene products and the maintenance of stable titres of antilate protein antibodies suggest that the major function of the immune system is to restrict virus spread and dissemination but not to limit reactivation from latency. Thus, a range of immune responsiveness can control virus replication in most cell lineages, and only when this equilibrium is disrupted by pharmacological agents or immunosuppressive viruses can virus replication lead to viral dissemination and end-organ disease.

Congenital CMV infection and sensorineural hearing loss

It is estimated that one infant in 1000 is born with profound deafness and an additional 2 in 1000 will acquire hearing loss in early childhood (Davidson, Hyde and Alberti, 1989; Parving, 1993). In a study of significant hearing impairment in children in Metropolitan Atlanta, USA, the average, annual prevalence rate for moderate to profound hearing loss was 1.1 per 1000 (Naarden, Decouflé and Caldwell, 1999). The highest rate of hearing loss was seen in black male children (1.4 per 1000). Sensorineural hearing loss is the most frequent sequela following both symptomatic and asymptomatic congenital HCMV infection (Naarden, Decouflé and Caldwell, 1999). The importance of congenital HCMV infection as a cause of sensorineural hearing loss in children was recognised about 30 years ago (Reynolds *et al.*, 1974; Hanshaw *et al.*, 1976; Stagno *et al.*, 1977a). However, the exact contribution of this intrauterine infection to the hearing loss in children has been difficult to define because of the paucity of population based studies. Harris *et al.* (1984) conducted a population based study using virologic screening of 10 328 newborns for HCMV excretion and screening for hearing loss in Malmo, Sweden, over a period of 5 years and found 50 (0.5%) infected infants. Four of these children were found to have complete deafness. During the same 5 year period, a total of 10 children born in Malmo were found to have hearing loss severe enough to require amplification. Thus, in a population screened for intrauterine HCMV infection and hearing loss, 40% cases of severe hearing loss were due to congenital HCMV infection. The authors of that study suggested that many of the children labelled as probably hereditary or of unknown etiology were probably suffering from a congenital HCMV infection. The results of a longitudinal study of 860 children with congenital CMV infection who were seen as part of a natural history study over a 24 year period at the University of Alabama at Birmingham were recently summarised in a report by Dahle *et al.* (2000). Symptomatic congenital HCMV infection was observed in 209 (24%) of the children and the remaining 651 had asymptomatic infection. A summary of the results of the audiologic follow-up of the study children is shown in Table 4.5. Sensorineural hearing loss was observed in 85 symptomatic (40.7%) and 48 asymptomatic (7.4%) children (Table 4.5). The loss was bilateral in 48% of asymptomatic children with hearing loss and 67% of symptomatic children with hearing loss. The degree of sensorineural hearing loss varied from mild to profound loss, but the majority of both asymptomatic and symptomatic children had severe to profound loss (≤ 71 dB). Delayed onset hearing loss was observed in about a third of the children with hearing loss. The delay in onset of hearing loss occurred over a wide age range, from 6 months to 16.4 years, and the median age of onset of loss for children with symptomatic and asymptomatic congenital CMV infection was 33 and 44 months respectively.

The progressive nature of hearing loss in children with congenital CMV infection was first reported almost 30 years ago (Stagno *et al.*, 1977a; Dahle *et al.*, 1979). Subsequent studies have confirmed this observation and demonstrated that children with asymptomatic congenital HCMV infection are also at increased risk for progressive hearing loss (Williamson *et al.*, 1992; Fowler *et al.*, 1997). In a study of 59 children with asymptomatic congenital HCMV infection, Williamson *et al.* (1992) reported that nine children had hearing loss and, of those, five (55%) had continued deterioration of hearing function during early childhood. In a longitudinal study of 307 children with asymptomatic congenital HCMV infection by Fowler *et al.* (1997), the progression of

Table 4.5. Summary of audiologic findings for children with congenital CMV infection (Dahle *et al.*, 2000)[a]

Finding	Asymptomatic ($N = 651$)	Symptomatic ($N = 209$)
Number (%) with hearing loss	48 (7.4%)	85 (40.7%)
Characteristics of loss		
Unilateral loss	25 (52.1%)	28 (32.9%)
Bilateral loss	23 (47.9%)	57 (67.1%)
Delayed onset loss	18 (37.5%)	23 (27.1%)
Median age (range) delayed onset loss	44 months (24–182)	33 months (6–197)
Progressive loss	26 (54.2%)	46 (54.1%)
Median age (range) progressive loss	51 months (2–185)	26 months (2–209)
Degree of loss[b]		
Mild (21–45 dB)	8 (16.7%)	10 (11.8%)
Moderate (46–70 dB)	7 (14.6%)	11 (12.9%)
Severe (71–90 dB)	8 (16.7%)	26 (30.7%)
Profound (>90 dB)	25 (52%)	38 (44.6%)

[a] The results from a longitudinal study of congenital CMV infection.
[b] Degree of sensorineural hearing loss based on average pure-tone thresholds at the last audiologic evaluation (percentage of ears). If hearing loss was determined by the auditory brainstem response (ABR), hearing thresholds were calculated based on nHL as follows: mild (30–45 dB), moderate (50–70 dB), severe (>70 dB).

Table 4.6. Cumulative percentage of sensorineural hearing loss in children with congenital CMV infection according to age (Dahle *et al.*, 2000)[a]

Age	Asymptomatic ($N = 48$)	Symptomatic ($N = 85$)
Birth–1 month	25.5	43.5
3 months	31.4	55.3
6 months	43.1	67.2
2 years	47.1	82.4
3 years	58.8	88.2
4 years	72.5	89.4
6 years	86.6	95.3
7–15 years	100	100

[a] Results from a longitudinal study of congenital CMV infection. Hearing sensitivity was measured by either the auditory brainstem response (ABR) or pure-tone audiometry depending on the child's age and developmental level. The criteria for hearing loss for pure-tone audiometry was the presence of thresholds greater than 20 dB HL at one or more frequencies; for ABR, hearing loss consisted of thresholds greater than 25 dB nHL.

the hearing deficit was observed in 50% (11/22) of those with hearing loss during the study period (Table 4.6). The median age at first progression of the hearing impairment was 18 months (range, 2–70 months) (Fowler *et al.*, 1997). These studies have suggested that asymptomatic congenital HCMV infection is probably a leading cause of hearing loss in young children. The occurrence of delayed onset loss and progressive hearing loss also illustrate the need for continued monitoring of children with both symptomatic and asymptomatic congenital HCMV infection during early childhood.

The importance of screening of newborns for congenital HCMV infection to identify infants with hearing loss caused by congenital HCMV infection was demonstrated in a population based study by Harris *et al.* (1984). Screening newborns for hearing loss based on risk criteria fails to identify the majority of children with hearing loss caused by congenital HCMV infection, not only because most congenitally infected infants have subclinical or asymptomatic infection but also due to the fact that delayed onset and/or progressive hearing loss occurs frequently in congenitally infected children (Hicks *et al.*, 1993).

Following the endorsement of the universal newborn hearing screening (UNHS) to identify most or all children with hearing loss by the Joint Committee on Infant Hearing, UNHS programmes have been implemented across most of the United States (Statement, 1993; Joint Committee on Infant Hearing, 1995). In the United Kingdom, the newborn hearing screening programme (NHSP) was introduced in the year 2002 and by the end of 2004 the screening programme covered about 70% of the birth population (www.nhsp.info/). The deadline for full implementation of the programme in England is October 2005. To determine whether most children with hearing loss caused by congenital HCMV infection will be identified by UNHS, a cohort of 388 congenitally infected children born at the University of Alabama Hospitals between 1980 and 1996 were examined (Fowler *et al.*, 1999). Only 5.2% of congenitally infected infants were noted to have hearing loss at birth and hearing loss continued to occur throughout early childhood with 15.4% of the cohort developing hearing loss by the age of 72 months. Children with symptomatic congenital HCMV infection had 16.5% hearing loss in the first month of life compared with 2.9% in those with asymptomatic infection. By 72 months of age, 36.4% of children with symptomatic infection and 11.3% of those with asymptomatic infection had hearing loss. Hearing loss following a symptomatic infection occurs earlier, but delayed-onset loss continues to occur throughout the first few years of life in both symptomatic and asymptomatic children. These findings demonstrated that universal newborn hearing screening will only detect less than half of all hearing loss secondary to congenital HCMV infection. Thus, universal screening for the detection of congenital HCMV infection in addition to hearing screening will be a better approach for the identification of most infants at risk for hearing loss during childhood.

The occurrence of delayed-onset hearing loss and continued deterioration of the hearing deficit in the majority of children with congenital HCMV infection demonstrates the need for monitoring of infected children during early childhood. Since the vast majority of children with congenital HCMV infection develop normally without sequelae, an ability to identify children at risk for hearing loss early in life will permit better utilisation of resources by targeting these children for closer monitoring and intervention. The presence or absence of clinical abnormalities at birth has been recognised as an important determinant of outcome in children with congenital HCMV infection. The incidence of hearing loss in symptomatic children or those with clinically apparent disease at birth is between 40 and 60%, whereas only about 10% of children with asymptomatic infection develop hearing loss. Among the symptomatic children, the presence of neuroradiographic imaging abnormalities, especially the presence of intracerebral calcifications, has been associated with a significantly increased risk for hearing loss (Boppana *et al.*, 1997). Of children with an abnormal CT scan 72% (28/39) had hearing loss compared with 29% (5/17) of children with a normal imaging study. In a study of symptomatic congenital HCMV infection, the presence of intrauterine growth retardation, petechiae, hepatosplenomegaly, hepatitis, thrombocytopenia and intracerebral calcifications was associated with an increased likelihood of hearing loss (Rivera *et al.*, 2002). An evidence of CNS involvement at birth, including microcephaly or other neurological abnormalities, was not predictive of hearing loss. Logistic regression analysis revealed that only petechiae and intrauterine growth retardation independently predicted hearing loss. The children with hearing loss had higher urine HCMV titres than those with normal hearing. These findings suggested that in children with symptomatic congenital HCMV infection, evidence of disseminated infection with or without the neurologic involvement at birth was predictive of hearing loss.

The amount of systemic HCMV burden was shown to correlate with the risk of HCMV disease in immunocompromised hosts including AIDS patients and allograft recipients (Fox *et al.*, 1995; Gor *et al.*, 1998; Spector *et al.*, 1999). It has been reported that an increased amniotic fluid HCMV burden was predictive of intrauterine transmission (Lazzarotto *et al.*, 2000). In addition, studies have shown that infants with symptomatic infection excrete more HCMV in urine in the first few months of life and exhibit higher peripheral blood viral load than those with asymptomatic infection (Revello *et al.*, 1999; Guerra *et al.*, 2000). The amount of infectious HCMV in urine and the quantity of HCMV DNA in peripheral blood were determined in samples obtained during the first month of life from 83 congenitally infected infants (Boppana *et al.*, 2001). The group of 12 children with hearing loss had a significantly higher urinary HCMV excretion ($P = 0.003$) and peripheral blood virus burden ($P = < 0.0010$) during infancy than those with normal hearing. The results of that study also showed that none of 41 children with peripheral blood viral load $<1.0 \times 10^4$ copies/mL and only 1/33 children with urine HCMV titres $<5.0 \times 10^3$ pfu/mL had hearing loss, suggesting a dose–response relationship between virus burden and the risk of hearing loss. Among children with asymptomatic congenital CMV infection, the group of four infants with hearing loss had a significantly increased virus burden during infancy as compared to those with normal hearing, indicating that it may be possible to identify asymptomatic children who are at increased risk for hearing loss by measuring the virus burden in early infancy. These findings suggest that an increased virus burden and continued viral replication in the affected organ systems leading to the loss of nonregenerating inner ear hair cells and/or spiral ganglion cells play an important role in the pathogenesis of hearing loss in congenital HCMV infection. Furthermore, the demonstration of an association between the increasing amount of virus burden in infancy and the greater likelihood of hearing loss suggests a role for antiviral therapy in decreasing the incidence and severity of hearing loss in children with congenital HCMV infection.

PATHOLOGY OF CMV ASSOCIATED HEARING LOSS

Although the natural history of the sensorineural hearing loss associated with congenital CMV has been described in several large studies and the audiologic characteristics of the hearing loss is well documented, the pathogenesis of CMV associated hearing loss is poorly understood. Several reasons probably account for this lack of understanding, but perhaps the most obvious is the paucity of adequate histopathologic examinations of affected tissue from infected infants. A review of the literature revealed that less than 12 temporal bones from congenitally infected infants have been studied and reported in the medical literature. In addition, almost all of these were done with conventional histopathologic techniques and not with more sensitive techniques for the detection of viral nucleic acids and viral proteins. Furthermore, limited information about the nature of the maternal/fetal infection is available for most of these cases. Thus, it has been difficult to relate histopathologic findings from these few cases to the findings from larger natural history studies. However, even with these limitations, a framework of the pathogenesis of hearing loss in infants with congenital CMV infections can be proposed and aspects of this model have been studied with available animal models of congenital CMV infection. Finally, it should be noted that autopsy studies of AIDS patients with CMV central nervous system infections have provided little information in terms of the pathogenesis of sensorineural hearing loss in congenitally infected infants and will not be reviewed in this section.

The most comprehensive review of temporal bone pathology in infants with congenital CMV infections was published by 1990 (Strauss, 1990). This report reviewed temporal bone pathology from nine cases of congenital CMV infection in which labyrinthitis was present in most cases. These infants died between 3 weeks and 5 months in age. A more recent report described the findings in temporal bones obtained from a 14 year old female subject with severe neuromuscular sequelae resulting from congenital CMV. The original description has been modified and this additional case report has been included in a summary of published cases (Table 4.7) (Strauss, 1990; Rarey and Davis, 1993). Findings were reported for the inner ear, cochlea, vestibular system and auditory/vestibular neural structures. Five of the nine specimens

Table 4.7. Temporal bone histopathological findings associated with congenital HCMV infection. (Modified from the original by Strauss, 1990)

Age[a]	Diagnosis[b]	Vestibular/cochlear findings[c]		
		Cochlear	Vestibular	Neural
3 weeks	Symptomatic infection	Inclusion-bearing cells; hydrops	Inclusion-bearing cells; hydrops	Normal histology
6 weeks	Asymptomatic infection	Inclusion-bearing cells in Reissner's membrane	Inclusion-bearing epithelial cells	Normal histology
3 weeks[d]	Symptomatic infection	Inclusion-bearing epithelial cells	Inclusion-bearing epithelial cells	Normal histology
3–10 weeks (3 patients)[e]	Symptomatic infection	Rare inclusion-bearing cells; viral antigen detected (2 patients); inflammatory infiltrate	Inflammatory infiltrate	Viral antigen detected in spiral ganglion (2 patients)
4 weeks[f]	Symptomatic infection	Inclusion-bearing cells in epithelium; spiral ligament and Reissner's membrane with pathologic changes	Inclusion-bearing cells in epithelium; collapsed utricle and saccule; herpes virus particles by EM (electron microscopy)	Normal histology
1 week	Asymptomatic infection	No viral inclusions; normal histology	No viral inclusions; normal histology	No viral inclusions; normal histology
5 months	Symptomatic infection	No viral inclusions; normal histology	Exudates in endolymph	No viral inclusions; normal histology
14 years[g]	Symptomatic infection	Loss of cellularity in organ of Corti and spiral ligament; fibrous tissue in spiral sulcus; calcifications	Calcifications, cellular degeneration; fibrosis in perilymphatic spaces	Not described

[a] With the exception of studies of the temporal bones of a 14 year old patient, these results were originally compiled by Strauss (1990). The age listed indicates the age at death.

[b] The diagnosis of symptomatic congenital CMV infection was made based on typical clinical and pathologic findings of cytomegalic inclusion disease in the newborn period and in some cases virus isolation. No history was available on the nature of the maternal infection associated with these fetal infections.

[c] Routine histopathology was carried out on temporal bones except in the case of three patients in which immunological detection of viral antigen was also employed. The presence of viral inclusions and inflammatory infiltrates are listed along with notable pathologic findings.

[d] Autopsy findings in this premature infant indicated extensive involvement of endolabyrinth epithelium but sparing of the sensory neuroepithelium.

[e] Sections of temporal bones from these patients were examined by immunofluorescence for detection of viral antigens. The primary antibody was a high-titre antiserum from immune humans. Viral antigens were detected in two specimens in which viral inclusions could not be detected by routine methods.

[f] Virus was isolated from the perilymph from both ears in this patient and viral particles detected by electron microscopy.

[g] This study was carried out on temporal bones from a 14 year old patient with severe neuromuscular sequelae resulting from a symptomatic congenital CMV infection (Rarey and Davis, 1993).

had evidence of endolabyrinthitis and virus was isolated from the endolymph of three of the nine specimens (Strauss, 1990). Viral antigens were detected by immunofluorescence using a polyvalent anti-CMV antiserum in two of the cases in which routine histology failed to detect virus-induced cytopathology (Stagno *et al.*, 1977a). Virus was isolated from the perilymph in one case and viral particles were observed by electron microscopy (Sullivan *et al.*, 1993). Cochlear and vestibule findings were variable, ranging from an occasional inclusion bearing cell either in or adjacent to sensory epithelium of the cochlea or vestibular system to more extensive involvement of the nonsensory epithelium (Davis *et al.*, 1977; Strauss, 1990). Viral antigen was detected in the organ of Corti in the absence of cytopathology when viral antigens were assayed by immunologic methods (Stagno *et al.*, 1977a). Routine histology failed to demonstrate changes in the auditory/vestibular neural structures, but again using a more sensitive technique, virus could be detected in the spiral ganglion (Stagno *et al.*, 1977a). Perhaps the most interesting observation in these studies was that inflammatory infiltrates were minimal and only reported in three cases (Stagno *et al.*, 1977a). In contrast to findings in more acutely infected patients, extensive cellular degeneration, fibrosis and calcifications were seen in the cochlea and vestibular system in temporal bones obtained from a 14 year old patient with neurodevelopmental manifestations of congenital CMV (Sullivan *et al.*, 1993).

Although the limited number of temporal bone studies from infants with congenital CMV is insufficient to define the pathogenesis of hearing loss associated with CMV infection fully, they do point to a possible mechanism(s) of disease. Common to all but two of these reports was the presence of viral antigen or histopathologic findings (inclusions) in the cochlea and/or vestibular apparatus consistent with viral replication or viral gene expression (Table 4.7). These results suggest that CMV can readily infect the nonsensory epithelium (and perhaps the sensory epithelium) of these structures. Because viral-induced damage can occur as a result of bystander effects, hearing loss and damage to the vestibular function may develop in the absence of direct infection of the sensory neuroepithelium. Thus, the histopathological changes that were observed in all cases probably provide indirect evidence of virus infection of inner ear structures. A somewhat surprising observation in this series of patients was the lack of a significant inflammatory infiltrate in all but three of the reported specimens. This lack of an inflammatory infiltrate in most of these cases is unexpected, based on the role the host inflammatory response is thought to play in the end-organ disease associated with CMV infection. A possible explanation for these seemingly discordant results is that the host inflammatory response was delayed in these infants secondary to the immaturity of immune responses in young infants and that virus replicated in cells of the inner ear was unchecked by host immune responses. Furthermore, past studies have demonstrated a delay in the generation of specific cellular immune responses to CMV in congenitally infected infants, raising the possibility that infected infants may exhibit a delay in the development of an inflammatory response in the inner ear (Gehrz *et al.*, 1977; Starr *et al.*, 1979; Pass *et al.*, 1983). Thus, a delay in the inflammatory response to CMV infection of epithelium in the inner ear could slow the development of histologic changes associated with inflammation, such as infiltration of mononuclear cells, and ultimately the manifestations of cochlear and vestibular system damage.

An alternative explanation is that infection of the inner ear structures was a late, perhaps even postnatal, event in the natural history of congenital CMV infection. The relationship between the susceptibility of cells of the inner ear to infection and development is unknown and cells of the sensory neuroepithelium and supporting epithelium could be relatively resistant to infection until late in the fetal development. Thus, these cases may represent relatively recent infections of the inner ear structures without significant host derived inflammatory responses. Such an explanation is, however, inconsistent with the course of fetal CMV infection in other regions of the CNS.

The finding of extensive degenerative changes along with fibrosis and calcification in the temporal bones obtained from the oldest patient in this series (Table 4.7) probably reflects the natural history of CMV labyrinthitis and, depending on the rate of progression of these pathologic changes, could explain the progressive nature of the hearing loss associated with congenital CMV. The loss of the neuroepithelium, either secondary to direct virus-mediated cytotoxicity or indirectly as a result of loss of supporting structures, followed by fibrosis as a component of the inflammatory processes in the inner ear could lead to progressive hearing loss.

The finding of fibrosis is consistent with findings in experimental animal models of virus-induced hearing loss (see below). In addition, it has been suggested that deposition of extracellular matrix in the inner ear as part of the inflammatory response in this organ is exaggerated and possibly accounts for the ossification observed in the inner ear (Harris *et al.*, 1997; Chen, Harris and Keithley, 1998). The failure of the host immune response to clear virus infection in the inner ear rapidly is consistent with the persistence of CMV in a variety of epithelium, including the epithelium of the proximal renal tubule and the salivary gland. Virus-induced cytopathology and host-mediated destruction of virus-infected cells would have little consequence in organs with significant self-renewal, but in organs containing highly specialised sensory neuroepithelium, such as the inner ear, it could result in loss of function. The variability of hearing loss and differences in progression can probably be explained by the level and duration of virus replication and the intensity of the host inflammatory response.

EXPERIMENTAL MODELS OF CMV ASSOCIATED HEARING LOSS

The species restriction of human CMV replication has limited the development of animal models that closely recapitulate the natural history and pathogenesis of hearing loss associated with congenital CMV infection in humans. Several experimental animal model systems have been utilised with varying success. Small animal models include the mouse and the guinea pig, and a limited number of studies have been done on laboratory primates. A mouse model of congenital CMV infection has not been realised secondary to the difference in placental architecture that appears to effectively restrict the transmission of murine CMV to the developing fetus following maternal infection. Direct inoculation of murine CMV into the brain of newborn animals results in extensive virus replication in the CNS with widespread damage to most cell types in the CNS (Kosugi *et al.*, 1998; Tsutsui, 1998; van Den Pol, *et al.*, 1999; van den Pol, Reuter and Santarelli, 2002). Early attempts utilising direct inoculation of virus into the inner structures resulted in virus-induced histopathology, but it has been argued that it was not representative of human disease (Davis and Hawrisiak, 1977). Only limited effort has been directed towards developing the mouse as a model of hearing loss with congenital CMV infections.

In contrast to the limited results obtained with mouse models, the use of the guinea pig as a model of congenital CMV infection has been informative. Guinea pig CMV was initially recovered by Hsiung and colleagues (Hsiung *et al.*, 1978) and shown to replicate in normal, nonimmunosuppressed guinea pigs, and it could be transmitted to fetal guinea pigs *in utero* (Bia *et al.*, 1980, 1983; Griffith *et al.*, 1981, 1986). The transmission of guinea pig CMV to the fetus is more likely to be related to the anatomy of the guinea pig placenta rather than any specific tropism of this virus for placental tissue. Infection of fetal pigs can be modified by maternal immunity, both naturally acquired and vaccine induced (Bia *et al.*, 1984; Harrison *et al.*, 1995; Bourne *et al.*, 1996, 2001; Chatterjee *et al.*, 2001). Fetal infection with guinea pig CMV can result in widespread fetal infection in various organ systems, including the CNS, and a significant rate of fetal loss (Griffith *et al.*, 1982, 1986; Harrison *et al.*, 1995). Congenitally infected guinea pigs often exhibit end-organ infection and disease, including growth retardation (Bernstein and Bourne, 1999; Bourne *et al.*, 2001). Interestingly, congenitally infected animals have also been reported to have abnormalities in hearing (Woolf *et al.*, 1989; Woolf, 1991). In the most complete study of this model, Woolf and colleagues described the hearing abnormalities in offspring of infected pregnant guinea pigs (Woolf *et al.*, 1989). Inoculation of animals with guinea pig CMV in the first or second trimester of pregnancy resulted in a significant fetal loss (≈30%) and of the surviving offspring 64% were infected at birth (Woolf *et al.*, 1989). Guinea pig CMV antigens were localised in the inner ear in 45% of infected animals, with antigen being detected in spiral ganglion cells and cochlear modiolar vein endothelial cells. In addition, inflammatory infiltrates were present in the perilymphatic scalae in a small number of animals. About 30% of infected animals had guinea pig CMV in cells within the temporal bone marrow (Woolf *et al.*, 1989). Of the infected animals, 28% had abnormalities of auditory function as measured by auditory nerve action potentials (Woolf *et al.*, 1989). Subsequent studies by this same group of investigators demonstrated that not only was viral gene expression a prerequisite for damage to the inner ear and auditory abnormalities but that an intact host immune response was also required (Woolf *et al.*, 1985; Harris, Fan and Keithley, 1990). Immune suppression of animals inoculated with guinea pig CMV was associated with a decreased incidence of hearing abnormalities that correlated with a decrease in the inflammatory infiltrate in scala tympani (Harris, Fan and Keithley, 1990).

The pattern of auditory abnormalities suggested that guinea pig CMV damaged cells of the auditory spiral ganglion, a finding consistent with the auditory abnormalities associated with congenital CMV infection. The characteristics of hearing loss in congenitally infected guinea pigs suggests involvement of the auditory nerve and approximately 30% of infected animals had guinea pig CMV antigens detected in either the auditory or vestibular ganglion (Woolf, 1990). Virus-induced inclusions were not detected in these cells. This result is similar to results in the limited number of temporal bones, in that viral antigens were detected by immunohistochemistry in the spiral ganglion in two of three patients; however, viral inclusions were not detected by light microscopy in these two cases and nor in any of the reported cases listed in Table 4.3 (Stagno *et al.*, 1977a). Consistent with the findings in this limited number of cases, the hearing loss associated with congenital infection in humans is most frequently described by abnormalities in auditory brainstem responses, a pattern compatible with damage to the auditory neural tissue. From these studies in animal models and from studies of human temporal bones, it appears that virus (or viral antigen) can localise to both the epithelium and neural cells in the inner ear and that damage can occur as a result of direct virus-mediated damage to neural tissue or secondary to host derived inflammatory responses, depending on the balance achieved between virus replication and host clearance functions. Because virus replication was necessary for the development of hearing damage, it was not surprising that preexisting immunity in these animals as measured by serum antibody could modify the course of hearing loss in guinea pigs inoculated with virus (Harris *et al.*, 1984; Fukuda, Keithley and Harris, 1988; Woolf *et al.*, 1988). Although progressive hearing loss has not been reported in this small animal model, prolonged inflammation in the inner ear of virus-infected animals was associated with degenerative changes of cochlear structures including the organ of Corti and spiral ganglion as well as fibrosis, histopathological changes that have been associated with hearing loss (Keithley and Harris, 1996). Together, these studies support a model that includes virus infection and host derived inflammatory responses leading to both acute (viral-mediated) and chronic (virus and host derived) damage to the auditory apparatus of the inner ear. Effective therapy to limit this process will necessarily include both antiviral and anti-inflammatory components, depending on the duration of the infection in structures of the inner ear.

TREATMENT AND PREVENTION OF HEARING LOSS ASSOCIATED WITH CONGENITAL CMV INFECTIONS

Treatment

Although there are several antiviral agents that have been shown to be efficacious in the treatment of invasive CMV disease in the immunocompromised
host, only ganciclovir has been studied as a potential therapy for hearing loss
associated with congenital CMV infections. This agent is phosphorylated by
the virus encoded phosphotransferase, UL97, and when phosphorylated
inhibits virus replication by inhibiting the viral DNA polymerase and viral
DNA polymerisation. It has significant bone marrow toxicity and toxicity
requiring dose modifications is often observed. Fortunately, this toxicity is
reversible once the dosing has been modified.

Several case and series reports have been published that have detailed anecdotal experience with ganciclovir treatment of infants with congenital CMV
infection. In many of these reports, it was claimed that the drug modified the
disease; however, a sufficient number of controls were not available to provide
any meaningful comparisons. In some studies, efficacy was compared to historical controls or previous natural history studies that have been reported in
the medical literature (Michaels et al., 2003). The single trial that included a
control group was conducted as part of a National Institutes of Health supported study of ganciclovir treatment of congenital CMV infections. The
results of this trial were recently published and suggest a therapeutic benefit
in terms of stablilisation of hearing in infected infants (Kimberlin et al., 2003).
There have been numerous criticisms of the trial including the small number
of evaluable patients, limited follow-up of patients and the necessity of
analysing each ear in individual patients as an independent data point
(Kimberlin et al., 2003). Treatment was carried out for 6 weeks in the perinatal period and was associated with both adverse effects of treatment and dose-
limiting toxicity in nearly 50% of patients (Kimberlin et al., 2003). The results
of this trial suggested that postnatal treatment of congenitally infected babies
could modify the hearing loss associated with this infection; however, additional trials will be necessary prior to any firm recommendation of perinatal
therapy with ganciclovir for congenital CMV infection.

Prophylaxis

Vaccine prevention of congenital CMV infection has been considered since
the 1970s (Stern, 1984). To date, no trial of adequate size has been undertaken
that would allow a determination of the efficacy of a vaccine for the prevention of either fetal infection or fetal disease. Several vaccine candidates have
been studied including an attenuated, replication competent virus and an adju-
vanted glycoprotein subunit vaccine. Both appear to induce an immune
response and both produce at least some level of cellular immunity (Gonczol

and Plotkin, 1990; Plotkin *et al.*, 1991; Adler *et al.*, 1995, 1999; Pass *et al.*, 1999; Plotkin, 1999). Efficacy of the replicating virus vaccine was claimed in trials of renal allograft recipients in terms of modification of symptomatology but not infection (Plotkin *et al.*, 1991). Immunisation of normal women with this vaccine failed to prevent infection, raising the concern that live virus vaccines may not prevent maternal infection (Adler *et al.*, 1995). The study was not adequately powered to address the prevention of fetal infection or prevention of disease following intrauterine infection (Adler *et al.*, 1995). Recent studies in several species including man, rhesus macaques and mice have convincingly demonstrated that seroimmune hosts can be reinfected with CMVs, thus raising the question of whether protective immunity can be achieved with any vaccine (personal communication, Dr J. Nelson, Oregon Health and Sciences University, Portland, Oregon; Moro *et al.*, 1999; Boppana *et al.*, 2001). Perhaps more worrisome is that, in humans, reinfection in pregnant women appears to be common and can lead to fetal infection and disease, albeit at decreased frequency as compared to primary infection (Boppana *et al.*, 1999, 2001; Ahlfors, Ivarsson and Harris, 2001; Yamamoto *et al.*, 2001). Thus, it remains to be determined if a conventional vaccine strategy against CMV will alter the natural history of this infection in human populations.

5 RUBELLA

P. A. Tookey

Introduction

Maternal rubella infection transmitted to the fetus in early pregnancy can have devastating results, including miscarriage, stillbirth and serious and often multiple disabilities in the liveborn infant. However, the most common defect associated with congenital rubella following maternal infection in the first 16 weeks of pregnancy is sensorineural hearing loss (SNHL). It can occur as an isolated manifestation or, particularly if infection occurs in the first 10 weeks of pregnancy, in combination with other rubella damage. Rubella-associated SNHL can be present at birth, may be progressive and is sometimes of late onset.

Long-standing rubella vaccination programmes in North America, Australia, Scandinavia and much of Europe mean that congenital rubella is now a rare disease in these regions. Ambitious and comprehensive vaccination programmes, along with rigorous surveillance procedures, have been established more recently in many countries in South and Central America and the Caribbean (Castillo-Solorzano et al., 2003). The picture is variable in Africa and Asia, and at the beginning of the 21st century it is likely that at least 100 000 cases of congenital rubella syndrome (CRS) still occur each year in the developing world (Robertson et al., 2003).

According to an expert review late in 2004, rubella and congenital rubella have now been eliminated from the United States (MMWR, 2005). The European region of the World Health Organization (WHO) has developed a strategic plan for the prevention of congenital rubella infection by 2010, and enhanced surveillance is being established throughout the region in order to monitor progress towards this goal (WHO, 2005).

Infection and Hearing Impairment. Edited by V.E. Newton and P.J. Vallely
© 2006 John Wiley & Sons, Ltd

The National Congenital Rubella Surveillance Programme

The National Congenital Rubella Surveillance Programme (NCRSP) was set up in 1971 to establish a baseline for the annual incidence of congenital rubella births in England, Scotland and Wales, and to monitor the impact of the newly introduced rubella vaccination programme targeted at schoolgirls (Dudgeon *et al.*, 1973). Audiologists, microbiologists and doctors notified suspected and confirmed congenital rubella births to the NCRSP, providing clinical and laboratory details of maternal vaccination history, symptoms and investigations in pregnancy, and neonatal presentation. Follow-up information about the notified children was sought on an occasional basis, and for specific studies. By 1990 the annual number of births reported to the NCRSP had reduced substantially (Figure 5.1), and congenital rubella (CR) was then included on the British Paediatric Surveillance Unit's 'orange card'. This active surveillance scheme provides a means of monitoring selected rare conditions of childhood, involves most consultant paediatricians throughout the British Isles and has a consistently high response rate (Nicoll *et al.*, 2000).

Other sources of information about rubella in the UK and Ireland include the Office for National Statistics (ONS), from which the annual number of rubella-associated terminations of pregnancy in England and Wales is available, and the Health Protection Agency (HPA) and national equivalents in the other countries of the British Isles, which monitor laboratory notifications of rubella, rubella susceptibility in selected population groups and vaccination uptake.

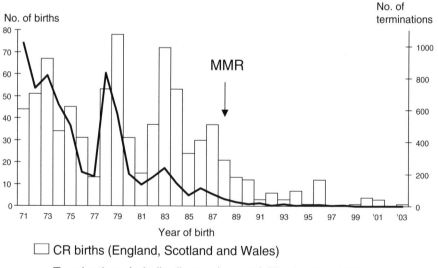

Figure 5.1. Congenital rubella births (NCRSP) and rubella-associated terminations (ONS) 1971–2003

Epidemiology of rubella

Rubella was only recognised as a disease in its own right, distinct from measles and scarlet fever, in the 19th century. Since it was generally a relatively mild disease it did not attract a great deal of attention until the 1940s, when the association between rubella infection in pregnancy and serious birth defects in newborn infants was first suggested. The virus itself – an RNA virus with an envelope, classified as a togavirus – was isolated in 1962, and vaccine development then proceeded quickly. The first vaccines were licensed in the United States in 1969 and in the UK in 1970, and were rapidly incorporated into many national vaccination programmes in the developed world.

Prior to the availability of vaccine, rubella was common virtually everywhere in the world, with infection rates peaking in the spring in temperate zones. Epidemics were superimposed on the endemic infection every 4 to 5 years in Europe, and there were major pandemics every 10 to 30 years. Infection was usually acquired in childhood, but about 10 to 20% of women in most countries would reach adult life still susceptible to rubella infection and at risk of acquiring the infection during pregnancy.

The incubation period ranges from 12 to 23 days. Virus can be isolated from nasopharyngeal samples and infection is spread by the respiratory route. Individuals are infectious from about a week before symptoms appear, to up to a week after, with the most infectious period being immediately before and on the first day of symptoms. Reinfection occurs occasionally, but in most cases infection seems to confer lifelong immunity.

Rubella is rarely an illness of much consequence, and if symptoms do occur they are usually mild and only last a few days. The infected individual might have enlarged lymph nodes, a mild fever, sore throat, coryza, cough and conjunctivitis. The rash, if it occurs at all, is nonvesicular, lasts for anything between a few hours and five days, and usually starts on the face, then spreads to the trunk and finally to the extremities. Some adults, especially women, have pain in their joints, but this is usually transient and long-lasting complications of rubella infection are very uncommon. About half of all rubella infections are nonspecific or without obvious symptoms, and as symptomatic infection is clinically indistinguishable from a number of other infections, including Erythrovirus B19 (parvovirus) and measles, a history of clinically diagnosed infection is unreliable.

The exception to this generally benign picture is congenital rubella infection where primary maternal infection in the early stages of pregnancy can seriously damage the developing fetus.

Rubella infection in pregnancy

Rubella infection in pregnancy was first associated with damage to the fetus in the early 1940s when Norman Gregg, an Australian ophthalmologist, published his classic paper linking women's reports of rubella infection in early pregnancy with cataracts in their infants (Gregg, 1941). He acknowledged at the time that: 'It is difficult to forecast the future for these unfortunate babies. We cannot at this stage be sure that there are not other defects present which are not evident now but which may show up as development proceeds.'

Quantifying the risks associated with rubella infection in pregnancy was difficult in the early years, before the virus was isolated. Researchers had to rely on clinical reports of symptoms in pregnant women and typical signs of rubella in their babies, and this could lead to both under- and overestimation of the risks of transmission and of defects: e.g. women who did not actually have rubella, only compatible symptoms, might be included and women with asymptomatic infection would be excluded; only infants with serious problems at birth were likely to be identified and progressive or late-onset health problems might easily be missed.

Not long after the rubella virus was first isolated a major rubella pandemic swept across the world, reaching the United States in 1964 where an estimated 20 per 1000 pregnant women were infected, thousands had their pregnancies terminated and at least 20000 babies were born with congenital rubella damage (Cooper, Preblud and Alford, 1995). The timely coincidence of the newly developed laboratory techniques and the dreadful effects of the pandemic provided a major impetus to vaccine development. The availability of reliable diagnostic tests also made it possible to carry out more rigorous studies to quantify the risks associated with rubella infection at different gestations.

TIMING OF INFECTION AND RISK OF TRANSMISSION

The likelihood of transmission of maternal infection to the fetus and of damage if transmission occurs are both related to the stage of pregnancy at which maternal rubella infection occurs. Maternal rubella infection before conception, and even just around the time of conception, is not associated with fetal infection (Enders *et al.*, 1988), but subsequently and up to about 10 weeks of pregnancy the risk of transmission is very high. It then declines during the second trimester before rising again during the third. If transmission does occur in the first 10 weeks, the likelihood of rubella defects is also very high, but the risk of damage drops substantially over the next 8 weeks as the fetus develops its own immune responses. Rubella-associated abnormalities have hardly ever been demonstrated following serologically confirmed maternal infection after 18 weeks gestation, and are very rare after 16 weeks.

A comprehensive, prospective study of the consequences of confirmed maternal rubella at different stages of pregnancy carried out between 1976 and 1978 involved over 1000 women in England and Wales with serologically confirmed rubella in pregnancy, 95% of whom were symptomatic (Miller, Cradock-Watson and Pollock, 1982). Just over half of the pregnancies ended in termination and about 40% in a live birth. These children were followed up for the first two years of life to establish whether they had congenital rubella infection and to allow time for any rubella-associated problems to be identified: 90% of infants whose mothers had rubella in the first 10 weeks of pregnancy were infected, and all of those had rubella damage. The transmission rate declined to 25% towards the end of the second trimester and then rose again during the third. The overall risk of infection and damage dropped to about 20% at 13–16 weeks. Although 40% of infants whose mothers had rubella between 17 weeks and term had congenital infection, none of them had rubella-associated manifestations.

REINFECTION IN PREGNANCY

Most prospective studies of the risk to the fetus have been carried out on women with symptomatic primary infection, but asymptomatic primary infection probably carries a similar risk. Reinfection in pregnancy is a different matter; while asymptomatic reinfection probably carries a very low risk, the risk of damage following symptomatic reinfection in early pregnancy is believed to be about 8% (Morgan-Capner et al., 1991). Although symptomatic reinfection is rare, viraemia is probably more likely than with asymptomatic reinfection, and this may explain the increased risk to the fetus (Miller, 1990).

INVESTIGATION AND MANAGEMENT OF SUSPECTED RUBELLA INFECTION IN PREGNANCY

The likelihood of a rash illness in pregnancy actually being rubella varies from country to country, depending on whether rubella is still an endemic disease and the local prevalence of other rash illnesses. In the present situation in the UK, with little rubella infection circulating, most clinically suspected rubella cases are not rubella at all. Although a rubella immunity test is part of the routine antenatal testing programme in the UK, the test employed is not designed to identify infection in pregnancy: its sole aim is to identify susceptible women who should be offered vaccination against rubella after delivery, in order to protect them in future pregnancies.

Guidelines have been established in the UK for investigating rash illness and exposure to rash illness in pregnancy, which lay out different algorithms for different situations in the context of the current low levels of circulating infection (Morgan-Capner and Crowcroft, 2002). These recommend that an asymptomatic pregnant woman with good past evidence of rubella immunity should not be investigated for rubella simply because she has been in contact with someone who has a rash illness. However, if a pregnant woman presents with a rash, specific diagnostic investigations, generally requiring at least two blood samples taken two weeks apart, should be carried out regardless of a history of immunity or vaccination, in case of past laboratory error or reinfection. Seroconversion between the first and second sample indicates primary infection, but if rubella-specific IgG is detected in the first sample it becomes more difficult to interpret the results. Although rubella-specific IgM antibody usually indicates recent rubella infection, this is not invariably the case; IgG avidity testing is also advisable, with low avidity being a sign of recent primary infection (Thomas *et al.*, 1992). Test results need careful interpretation in the context of full clinical details, including the date and type of contact, stage of pregnancy and history of previous immunisation (Best *et al.*, 2002). Simultaneous investigation for parvovirus infection, which is often difficult to distinguish from rubella and can also potentially affect the fetus, is also recommended (Morgan-Capner and Crowcroft, 2002). There is no evidence to support the use of immunoglobulin treatment for women with primary rubella infection in pregnancy, and there is currently no treatment to prevent or reduce mother-to-fetus transmission of infection. If maternal infection occurs during the first 12 weeks of pregnancy the risk of damage is high and the option of termination of the pregnancy should be discussed. However, it is difficult to predict the likely outcome when infection occurs between 12 and 18 weeks, even if fetal infection is confirmed by prenatal diagnosis. Infants known to have been exposed to maternal rubella in the first half of pregnancy should be monitored closely in the neonatal period, diagnostic tests should be performed and if infection is confirmed there should be early assessment of hearing and vision in particular.

CONGENITAL RUBELLA INFECTION

Since the rubella virus is transmitted through the placenta, the developing fetus may be malnourished: a proportion of affected pregnancies end in spontaneous abortion or stillbirth, and many infants with congenital rubella are of low birth weight. Other neonatal manifestations, which generally resolve, include enlarged liver or spleen, meningoencephalitis, thrombocytopenic purpura and pneumonitis; the presence of any of these symptoms following an otherwise asymptomatic pregnancy may provoke investigations that reveal congenital rubella infection.

If congenital rubella infection is suspected in early infancy and IgM antibody is detected, then the diagnosis is relatively straightforward as acquired infection is rare at this stage. Virus can also be isolated or detected by polymerase chain reaction (PCR) from many sites including the oropharynx, urine and conjunctival fluid during the first months of life. Congenitally infected infants shed a lot of virus and can be infectious for many months, although only about 10% are still shedding virus by the time they reach their first birthday. When abnormalities suggestive of congenital rubella are identified in an older infant or a young child, diagnosis is more difficult. IgG antibody in a baby is generally due to passively transferred maternal antibody, but persistence of IgG beyond 6 months of age probably indicates congenital infection.

Signs of congenital rubella

CLASSIC TRIAD
- Sensorineural hearing loss
- Heart abnormalities
- Eye abnormalities

OTHER SIGNS
- Growth retardation
- Microcephaly
- Neonatal signs
- Other signs in infancy

LATE APPEARING PROBLEMS
- Diabetes • Thyroid dysfunction • SNHL

Figure 5.2. Typical signs of congenital rubella infection

In a young child who has not yet been vaccinated, a presumptive diagnosis can therefore be made on the basis of a compatible clinical picture and the presence or persistence of rubella IgG antibodies.

Rubella infection in the first few weeks of pregnancy, while the lens and other structures of the eye are developing, can result in unilateral or bilateral cataracts, and microphthalmia; glaucoma is also reported, but more rarely. Pigmentary retinopathy (salt and pepper appearance of the retina) is associated with maternal infection at any time up to about 18 weeks, and although it is not usually sight threatening, its presence can be an aid to diagnosis. When maternal infection occurs during the second month of gestation, the developing structures of the heart are at risk, and patent ductus arteriosus, pulmonary stenosis and ventricular septal defect are the most likely heart defects. Development of the inner ear occurs over a longer period during the second to fourth month of gestation, and this is one reason why sensorineural hearing loss (SNHL) is the most common rubella-associated problem. Because the eye, heart and ear are all overlapping in their periods of development, multiple defects are common when infection occurs at this early stage and the term 'congenital rubella syndrome' (CRS) or 'classic triad' has conventionally been used to describe the devastating pattern of damage in the congenitally infected deaf–blind child with a heart defect (Figure 5.2).

Other less commonly reported rubella-associated features include dental defects, psychomotor delay and microcephaly. Some damage might only be recognised if specific investigations are undertaken; e.g. transient translucent areas in the long bones of the leg were detected by X-ray in 20% of congenitally infected infants in a study in the 1960s (Banatvala and Best, 1998). MRI scans carried out on some congenitally infected infants in recent years have revealed areas of intracranial calcification; since this technique was not available when the large prospective studies of congenital rubella were undertaken, it is not known how common this is or with what period of gestation it is associated (Chang, Huang and Liu, 1996).

Although children with congenital rubella do eventually stop excreting virus, it nevertheless persists in certain parts of the body and can continue to replicate in some organs and cause further damage, e.g. to the eye and ear. Some problems, particularly SNHL, may not develop or become apparent until later infancy or childhood, so it is vital that children and adults with congenital rubella have regular ophthalmological and audiological assessment. Families, including the congenitally infected individual if possible and those looking after their healthcare, should be aware of the diagnosis so that any late-onset problems are identified and managed appropriately. For example, people with congenital rubella are at increased risk of diabetes and thyroid disorders, although it is not yet clear whether these conditions are associated with infection at a particular stage of gestation (Forrest et al., 2002). More rarely autism and other learning, behavioural and psychiatric disorders are reported, and there are also case reports of progressive and ultimately fatal rubella panencephalitis (Townsend et al., 1975).

Rubella and the inner ear

Histopathological examination of the inner ear of individuals with hearing loss resulting from viral infection is rarely carried out, and so information on virus-induced pathology is sparse. However, the principal effect of congenital rubella is thought to be teratogenic, disrupting the development of normal organs. In the 1950s Lindsay and colleagues described abnormalities in the organ of Corti including a reduction in area of the stria vascularis. Additionally they noted a lack of development of hair cells and supporting cells, especially in the apical coil of the cochlea and cochleosaccular defects associated with congenital rubella infection (Lindsay et al., 1953; Lindsay and Harrison, 1954). Further reports exploring the pathology of congenital rubella deafness appeared in the 1960s (Friedman and Wright, 1966; Beal, Davey and Lindsay, 1967; Ward, Honrubia and Moore, 1968; Esterly and Oppenheimer, 1969). It is likely that rubella virus circulating during the first trimester acts on the epithelial cells of the developing labyrinth and causes cochleosaccular degeneration (Strauss and Davis, 1973).

The hearing loss can be unilateral or bilateral and range from mild to profound, and asymmetric loss is not uncommon (Jackson and Fisch, 1958). Rubella virus can persist in the fluid of the inner ear, and degenerative damage may then occur over the short and the long term. The hearing loss can be progressive, and a child with normal hearing at birth might experience late-onset loss. Diagnosis is frequently delayed, and the reported prevalence of hearing loss at birth following fetal infection at different stages varies from study to study. The picture might also be complicated by concurrent conductive hearing loss. Some children have more severe speech and language problems than their audiometric loss would suggest, probably because of central brain damage (Ames et al., 1970).

It is difficult to make an accurate estimate of the prevalence of SNHL in individuals with congenital rubella because of problems associated with comprehensive case ascertainment of both deafness and congenital rubella. Since hearing loss is often the only sign of congenital rubella, and maternal and congenital infection are both prone to underdiagnosis, in most populations a proportion of hearing loss of no known aetiology will be due to rubella infection in pregnancy. The size of its contribution will vary according to many different factors including the prevalence of other causes of congenital and acquired hearing loss, the level of susceptibility to rubella in pregnant women and the pattern of use of rubella vaccine, if available. A study of 568 deaf children aged under 4 years attending the Nuffield Hearing and Speech Centre in London in 1972–5 provided data suggesting that about 15% of SNHL in the UK was then due to congenital rubella, and probably considerably more in epidemic years (Peckham et al., 1979). A study of deafness in 1977 among 8 year olds living in the then nine countries of the European Community (Martin, 1982) provided a remarkably similar estimate of 16% for the region as a whole. Both these studies also showed clear evidence of an increased prevalence of hearing loss in children born in the winter, consistent with the increased circulation of rubella infection in the spring.

Among children born from 1978 to 1982 with confirmed congenital rubella who were reported to the NCRSP, 61% were classified as hearing impaired; their average age at confirmation of hearing loss was 11.6 months (Wild et al., 1989). Additional follow-up information was sought for the cohort in the 1990s, by which time at least 73% of children born from 1978 to 1982 had been diagnosed with SNHL. Overall, about half of the children reported to the NCRSP between 1971 and 1993 had SNHL when last followed up at a mean age of 10 years, and in a substantial proportion of cases hearing loss was only reported at a second or subsequent follow-up, not at initial registration.

Although about a quarter of all children ever reported to the NCRSP have SNHL as their only reported rubella-associated manifestation, virtually all infants reported in the last decade have either had multiple rubella defects or were born to women whose rubella infection was diagnosed in pregnancy. It seems likely that there is some underdiagnosis (and therefore under-reporting) of congenital rubella infection among children with isolated SNHL (Tookey and Peckham, 1999). In the 1970s and 1980s the presence of rubella antibodies in a young deaf child would, at the very least, have been suggestive of congenital infection. More recently, by the time hearing loss is identified and investigated many children will have had the MMR vaccine. There may also be a loss of professional awareness as congenital rubella has become rare, and other explanations for unexplained hearing loss appear more likely.

With the recent introduction of routine neonatal hearing screening in England and Wales it is possible that otherwise unsuspected cases of congenital rubella could be identified in the future.

Prevention of congenital rubella

VACCINE AND VACCINE STRATEGY

Three strains of live attenuated rubella vaccine were licensed in 1969, but only the RA27/3 strain is now in use, and this is the rubella component of the combined measles, mumps and rubella vaccine (MMR). Protective levels of antibody are produced in over 95% of recipients and long-term follow-up of vaccinees suggests protection is probably life-long in most individuals (O'Shea *et al.*, 1988; Christenson and Bottiger, 1994). Nonetheless, these studies were carried out at a time when vaccine-induced immunity could have been boosted by continuing exposure to wild virus circulating in the community. What would happen in a population with vaccine-induced immunity and no previous exposure to wild virus if the infection started to circulate freely again has not been tested.

In children, rubella vaccine causes few side-effects, although mild fever and rash are occasionally reported. Joint symptoms are common following vaccination of susceptible women, though they are less frequent and less severe than after rubella infection itself; symptoms are generally mild and do not persist, but there are a few case reports of apparently recurrent or persistent arthritis after rubella immunisation.

Once rubella vaccine was developed in the late 1960s different strategies were pursued in different countries. In the UK, concern about the duration of vaccine-induced immunity led initially to the adoption of a selective strategy of immunising schoolgirls after the age of peak incidence. Routine testing and immunisation of nurses and other health care staff who might be in contact with pregnant women was introduced, as well as antenatal screening for rubella susceptibility, with post-partum vaccination of susceptible women to protect subsequent pregnancies. This was also the strategy pursued in Australia and many European and Scandinavian countries: it allowed rubella infection to continue to circulate widely. This meant that most people acquired infection in childhood and therefore most women were protected by natural immunity. Girls who had escaped natural infection were 'mopped up' by the schoolgirl programme, as were susceptible women in the other targeted groups.

However, in the United States, mass immunisation of all young children with rubella vaccine was introduced straightaway in 1969 with the explicit aim of preventing the circulation of disease. This strategy not only protects those individuals who are vaccinated but also reduces the risk of infection in susceptible pregnant women.

Apart from considerations about the long-term persistence of vaccine-induced immunity, the main concern about mass vaccination in early childhood related to the uptake of vaccine over the long term. Mathematical models suggested that if vaccine uptake in early childhood were less than about 80%, the spread of wild virus would be reduced but not eliminated; this could lead to an increase in the average age at infection as it would take longer for those who escaped vaccination to acquire natural infection. In that case, the period between epidemics of rubella would lengthen, so that when an epidemic did occur, there could be many susceptible adults and the potential for a large number of congenital rubella cases (Knox, 1985).

An obvious solution to this problem is to combine the mass immunisation of young children either with a second dose for all children at a later age or with a selective programme of vaccination for schoolgirls. This type of strategy was implemented in Sweden in 1982, when MMR vaccine was introduced for all one year olds with a second dose at 12 years designed to reach those who did not receive vaccine previously or failed to respond. Similarly in the UK, reassuring data on the persistence of immunity after vaccination and high vaccine uptake levels led to the introduction in 1988 of MMR for all children in the second year of life, while still maintaining the schoolgirl vaccination programme. However, MMR uptake by the age of 24 months averaged about 92% between 1988 and 1992, and never reached the goal of 95% that was thought necessary to prevent outbreaks of measles, the most infectious of the three diseases.

By 1994 there was concern about the possibility of a measles epidemic and a mass campaign offering combined measles and rubella (MR) vaccine to all children was undertaken. Rubella was included in order to increase the proportion of the population immune to rubella. Since boys had not been offered rubella vaccine before 1988 and the circulation of rubella virus had substantially declined, a significant proportion of older and adolescent boys remained susceptible and could have provided a pool of susceptible individuals capable of sustaining rubella transmission among young adults. In 1996 a second dose of MMR was introduced for preschool children and the schoolgirl vaccination programme was abandoned.

VACCINATION IN PREGNANCY

There have been persistent concerns that the vaccine virus might be teratogenic if given during pregnancy. Although vaccinees cannot infect other susceptible individuals, the vaccine virus can cross the placenta, and in many countries women who were inadvertently vaccinated during pregnancy or close to the time of conception were advised to consider termination of the pregnancy. Data pooled from studies of children born to several hundred women inadvertently vaccinated around the time of conception, or in early pregnancy, show less than 3% with serological evidence of congenital infection, and no reported case of abnormalities attributable to congenital rubella. Over 80 of these infants were born to women vaccinated in the month of conception, probably the period of greatest vulnerability, and these data suggest that if a risk exists, it is likely to be well under 5% (Banatvala and Best, 1998). Although rubella vaccine should not be given to a woman who knows she is pregnant, and women are advised to avoid pregnancy for one month after vaccination, women are no longer advised to consider termination following inadvertent vaccination (Department of Health, 1996).

Continuing risk of congenital rubella

Since the mid 1990s when several papers were published suggesting a link between measles and/or MMR vaccine, bowel disease and autism (Thompson *et al.*, 1995; Wakefield *et al.*, 1998), public concern about the safety of the triple vaccine has led to a gradual decline in MMR uptake rates in the UK. Parental and professional anxieties persist despite subsequent studies that specifically set out to investigate the link between MMR vaccine, autism and bowel disease, and concluded that there was no such association (Peltola *et al.*, 1998; Taylor *et al.*, 2002; Smeeth *et al.*, 2004) and the consensus among most experts that the original studies were flawed (Elliman and Bedford, 2001; DeStefano and Thompson, 2004).

MMR uptake by the age of 24 months dropped from 92% in 1995–6 to 80% in 2003–4 in England (Government Statistical Service, 2004) and dipped well below 60% in parts of London (up-to-date vaccine uptake data are available at http://www.hpa.org.uk). If this decline in vaccine uptake is not reversed it is possible that outbreaks of rubella could occur once again, putting susceptible pregnant women at risk.

Antenatal screening for rubella susceptibility continues in the UK, but the delivery of post-partum vaccination is not routinely monitored. Through much of the 1980s and 1990s about 1% of women in a second or subsequent pregnancy were rubella susceptible, compared to 2–3% of women having their first baby (Figure 5.3) (Vyse *et al.*, 2002). This probably reflected not only the impact of the post-partum vaccination programme but also the higher prior exposure risk of women who already had young children compared to those who were pregnant for the first time.

There has been a well-documented disproportion in both rubella susceptibility rates and congenital rubella births between women of different ethnic origins in the UK over many years. In the 1960s rubella epidemic there was a higher prevalence of congenital rubella among Caribbean children, while in the 1980s a disproportionate number of children of Asian origin were being reported to the NCRSP (Miller *et al.*, 1991). A study of pregnant women in west London in the 1980s showed that Asian women were 2 to 3 times more likely than white women to be susceptible (Tookey *et al.*, 1988), and this was confirmed using national data in the mid 1990s (Miller *et al.*, 1997). A study of rubella susceptibility among pregnant women in London in the late 1990s revealed even greater variations in rubella susceptibility rates between women of different ethnic origins (Figure 5.4) (Tookey, Cortina-Borja and Peckham, 2002). Whereas only about 2% of British-born women were susceptible,

%

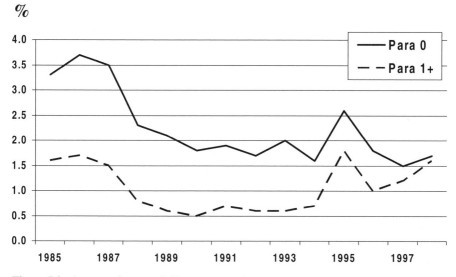

Figure 5.3. Antenatal susceptibility to rubella in England and Wales 1985–98, from routinely collected data. (Adapted from Figure 9 in Vyse *et al.*, 2002)

Ethnic group	Total number tested	Susceptible women (%)	Susceptible primip women
White British	94626	1.6	1.9
Other White	2480	3.4	3.8
Mediterranean	3715	3.7	4.4
Pakistani	4312	4.1	5.4
Indian	8469	4.4	6.7
Bangladeshi	2171	6.1	9.4
Sri Lankan	763	14.9	23.3
Other Asian	955	5.9	10.4
Oriental	1896	8.0	9.4
Black British	240	2.1	2.0
Black Caribbean	3242	3.1	3.2
Black African	4878	6.2	8.4
Other Black	651	4.3	6.5

Figure 5.4. Rubella susceptibility by ethnic group among women screened antenatally in North London 1996–99 (primip = first pregnancy). (Adapted from Tookey, Cortina-Borja and Peckham, 2002)

overall susceptibility for women born elsewhere was about 5%. African and Asian women had particularly high rates, and among women in their first pregnancy almost a quarter of those from Sri Lanka, 9% of Bangladeshi women and 8% of African women were susceptible. If rubella does start to circulate again in the UK, women who have arrived in the UK as young adults will once again be at particularly high risk of acquiring infection in pregnancy. Similar observations have been made in Spain with regard to Latin American women (Lemos *et al.*, 2004).

About 450 congenital rubella births were reported to the National Congenital Rubella Surveillance Programme between 1971 and 1980, and about 6000 rubella-associated terminations were recorded by the Office for National Statistics (2001). This compares with about 40 congenital rubella births reported between 1991 and 2004, and about 60 terminations (Figure 5.1). In this latter period about a third of the mothers of babies with congenital rubella had actually acquired their infection abroad, mostly in their countries of origin in Asia or Africa, but in a few cases elsewhere in Europe. Another third of the mothers were women who had migrated to the UK in adult life, from countries without established rubella vaccination programmes, and then acquired rubella infection in pregnancy in the UK (Tookey, 2004).

By 2004 MMR vaccine was being used in all but 7 of the 52 countries in the European region (WHO, 2005), usually given to young children with a second dose later in childhood. However, uptake varies both within countries and between them. Outbreaks of rubella, with consequent congenital rubella births, occurred in Greece in 1993 and 1999, due to inadequate uptake of MMR (Panagiotopoulos and Georgakopoulou, 2004). The 1999 Greek outbreak also led to a number of clusters of rubella infection in the UK, mostly in university settings, and a congenital rubella birth in Scotland in 1999 (the only one reported in the UK that year) was epidemiologically linked to the Greek outbreak (Tookey, Molyneaux and Helms, 2000). In Romania, where there was no national childhood rubella vaccination programme and only sporadic schoolgirl vaccination, a major outbreak in 2003 led to at least 17 congenital rubella births (WHO, 2005); consequently MMR for young children and selective vaccination of adolescent girls was adopted in 2004 (Rafila *et al.*, 2004).

Elsewhere in the world countries with successful measles immunisation programmes are increasingly likely to add rubella to measles vaccine, or move to MMR. The strategy to be adopted in any country seeking to control congenital rubella by vaccination must depend on the projected uptake of vaccination and the long-term prospects for continuing the programme. Rubella vaccination for young women will continue to be an important element of any control programme where a continuing high uptake of MMR among children cannot be guaranteed, as will the screening and immunisation of susceptible health personnel, particularly those in contact with pregnant women. Although well-implemented national vaccination programmes can lead to dramatic reductions in the number of rubella infections and congenital rubella births, the constant movement of people across national borders seeking work, recreation or refuge presents a major challenge to the control of all infectious diseases, including rubella.

Summary

Control of rubella by vaccination has substantially altered the national and international epidemiology of rubella and congenital rubella. Hundreds of thousands of congenital rubella births have been averted, but the infection continues to present an enormous challenge. The combination of its presentation as a mild and often asymptomatic infection, concerns about vaccine safety, economic and political impediments to high and prolonged vaccine uptake, and the potential for importing and exporting infection across national boundaries all mean that the eradication of this particularly devastating infection will be hard won, if at all. In the meantime, its contribution to childhood disability, and particularly to congenital hearing loss, must not be underestimated.

6 MUMPS

K. E. Wright

Introduction

Prior to the 1970s and the introduction of an effective vaccine, mumps was a common childhood illness. Infections with the mumps virus were a major cause of viral meningitis and encephalitis (Ritter, 1958; Gray, Moffat and Sangster, 1969; Strussberg *et al.*, 1969; Johnstone, Ross and Dunn, 1972; Jubelt, 1984), and caused a significant number of deaths each year, as many as 50 in the United States (Stokes, 1970). The virus was endemic in urban areas, but epidemics occurred every 2 to 7 years (Jubelt, 1984). In unvaccinated populations, the majority of cases occur in children under the age of 14 (Levitt, Kinde and Gates, 1970) and by adulthood 95% of individuals will be seropositive (Wolinsky, 1996; Batayneh and Bdour, 2002). Since 1967, when the first vaccine was available, the yearly incidence of mumps virus infections, and consequent disease, has declined in countries where routine vaccination takes place (Bakshi and Cooper, 1990; Nussinovitch, Volovitz and Varsano, 1995). However, the frequency of infections remains high in countries where vaccination is not available or is voluntary (Garty, Danon and Nitzan, 1985; Minja, 1998; Batayneh and Bdour, 2002; Gabutti *et al.*, 2002; Nardone *et al.*, 2003), and outbreaks also continue to occur in countries where routine vaccination has been in place for years. For example, since 1995, large outbreaks of mumps have been reported in Portugal (Dias *et al.*, 1996), Northern Ireland (Reaney *et al.*, 2001), Spain (Montes *et al.*, 2002) and England (Pugh *et al.*, 2002). In fact the figures released by the UK Health Protection Agency in February 2005 show a total of 4891 cases of mumps occurring in the first 4 weeks of 2005, compared with 358 for the same period in 2004. These cases are predominantly in older teenagers and young adults, particularly in higher education institu-

Infection and Hearing Impairment. Edited by V.E. Newton and P.J. Vallely
© 2006 John Wiley & Sons, Ltd

tions. These outbreaks have been attributed to reduced vaccine uptake in some countries, and vaccine failure, most evident when only one dose of MMR had been administered (as is likely to have been the vaccination situation for the UK teenagers) (Reaney *et al.*, 2001; Pugh *et al.*, 2002). Cases of mumps reinfections in the presence of neutralising antibodies have also been documented, and may account for some of these reported infections (Gut *et al.*, 1995; Crowley and Afzal, 2002).

Hearing loss and mumps virus

Sudden sensorineural deafness is defined as deafness that appears instantly or develops over a period of days (Snow and Telian, 1991). In the 1950s, the prevalence of sudden hearing loss was estimated to be one case per 5000 population per year (van Dishoek and Bierman, 1957). The majority of cases are unilateral, with 4 to 17% of patients showing involvement of both ears (van Dishoek and Bierman, 1957; Jaffe, 1967). Sudden hearing loss is known to be caused by vascular factors, acoustic neuromas, exposure to intense noise, autoimmunity, rupture of a labyrinthine membrane and some drug treatments. In the majority of cases an aetiology is not easily determined, and these cases are sometimes referred to as idiopathic sudden sensorineural hearing loss (ISSHL) (Yoon *et al.*, 1990; Yagi *et al.*, 1994).

A role for infections in causing sudden hearing loss has long been postulated. In early retrospective studies, a temporal association of hearing loss with a recent history of infection was reported in 30 to 40% of cases (van Dishoeck and Bierman, 1957; Everberg, 1960; Jaffe, 1970; Morrison and Booth, 1970; Rowson, Hinchcliffe and Gamble, 1975). The seasonal occurrence of ISSHL was suggestive of a role for viral infections (Rowson, Hinchcliffe and Gamble, 1975; Wilson *et al.*, 1983), and a drop in the prevalence of sudden deafness in children after the introduction of vaccination for the major childhood infections, from 2.2 per 1000 live births to 1.2 per 1000 live births, lends support to this hypothesis (Vartianinen and Karjalainen, 1998). Despite the availability of good vaccines, infections remain a significant cause of deafness throughout the world. Surveys of deaf children in China and Africa undertaken in the past 15 years demonstrated that 31 to 50% of cases had serological evidence of a recent infection (Viljoen *et al.*, 1988; Liu *et al.*, 1993; Minja, 1998). The proportion of these cases caused by virus infections will differ widely from study to study, depending on the vaccination status of the population examined and the method of establishing the infection. A review of the literature between 1970 and 1972 reported that 37 to 40% of total ISSHL cases were caused by viral infections (Bordley, Brookhouser and Worthington, 1972). Of cases attributable to viral infections, 60% showed seroconversion to a handful of viruses that included influenza, mumps, rubeola and rubella (Veltri *et al.*, 1981; Wilson *et al.*, 1983). Even in current times, in a population vaccinated for

measles, other postnatal viral infections cause about one-fifth of cases of childhood deafness in children (Minja, 1998).

In considering how significant mumps infections have been in causing deafness, it should be remembered that only a handful of cases have been
described where hearing loss was noticed during the acute phase of mumps
infections (van Dishoeck and Bierman, 1957; Bitnum, Rakover and Rosen,
1986), and in only one case has mumps virus been isolated from the inner ear
(Westmore, Pickard and Stern, 1979). There have also been unquestioned cases
of deafness attributed to the mumps vaccine, either alone or as a component
of the MMR vaccine (Nabe-Nielson and Walter, 1988; Stewart and Prabhu,
1993). Nonetheless, mumps is considered to have been the most common cause
of unilateral sudden hearing loss in children prior to the development of the
vaccine (Lindsay, 1973; Paparella and Schachern, 1991). Retrospective studies
attempting to determine the aetiology of deafness in large groups of ISSHL
patients have shown that infections with mumps account for a significant proportion of cases in children. Three early studies carried out prior to the introduction of routine childhood vaccinations reported that 4% (Everberg, 1957,
1960), 8% (Marschak, 1931, cited in Tarkkanen and Aho, 1966) and 11%
(Kinney, 1953) of cases of deafness in children and adolescents were attributable to mumps infections, as established largely by case history. Using serological evidence, van Dishoeck and Bierman (1957) reported that as many as
17% of patients of all ages with sudden deafness had evidence of a recent
mumps infection. It is generally accepted that these numbers are low. The
methodology was not always explained well in these studies, and serological
methods were less sensitive than current assays. In addition, unilateral hearing
loss in young children can go undetected until years after the mumps infection (Lindsay, 1973; Koga *et al.*, 1988), and it is now recognised that hearing
loss can occur even after asymptomatic mumps infections (Koga *et al.*, 1988).
This possibility was not considered in early studies. In Japan, surveys of ISSHL
cases for the presence of mumps-specific IgM antibody have shown that
asymptomatic mumps infections account for 5 to 7% of ISSHL cases (Nomura
et al., 1988; Okamoto *et al.*, 1994; Fukuda *et al.*, 2001), and in Italy, 17% of cases
with unilateral hearing loss had serological evidence of a recent mumps infection without any memory of illness (Tieri *et al.*, 1988).

Even after the development of a safe effective mumps vaccine, mumps infections continue to be a significant cause of deafness. The vaccine is still unavail-
able or immunisation is voluntary in many parts of the world. For example, in
Tanzania children are vaccinated for measles but not mumps, and 16.7% of
354 cases of childhood deafness in one study were attributed to mumps infections (Minja, 1998). Mumps infections were responsible for 7% of cases of
patients with sudden hearing loss over a 4 year period in Japan at a time when
mumps vaccination was voluntary (Kanzaki and Nomura, 1986). In other
countries vaccine coverage remains low for various reasons. Well after the
introduction of mumps vaccination to the UK, as many as one-third of the

cases of hearing loss in 33 children in Wales were associated with mumps infections, as determined by case history (Hall and Richard, 1987). In Italy, 15% of 280 cases of childhood deafness were ascribed to mumps infections, as determined by both serology and case history. This number rises to 32% if patients with serological evidence of asymptomatic mumps infections are included (Tieri *et al.*, 1988). The prevalence of mumps deafness is surprisingly high in these populations that are at least partially protected by vaccination, and may be due, at least in part, to improved methods for diagnosing recent infections, and also to the elimination of other causes of deafness, such as measles and rubella.

Mumps virus structure and replication cycle

Mumps virus is one of several viruses responsible for common childhood illnesses that are members of the virus family *Paramyxoviridae*. Within this family, mumps virus is in the subfamily *Paramyxovirinae* and the genus *Rubulavirus*.

Like other paramyxoviruses, mumps virus is a pleomorphic enveloped virus of 100 to 600 nm in diameter (Carbone and Wolinsky, 2001). Virions contain a single stranded negative sense RNA genome of 15 300 nucleotides in length (Wolinsky, 1996). The genome contains seven open reading frames (ORF) separated by short intergenic regions: NP, P, M, F, SH, HN and L. Nine proteins are encoded by the genome (Table 6.1). The genome is encapsidated along its entire length with the nucleoprotein, NP, and with a few copies of the polymerase complex containing the viral polymerase, L, and the phosphoprotein,

Table 6.1. Mumps virus proteins

Gene	Protein	Molecular weight (kilodaltons)	Function
NP	NP – nucleoprotein	68–73	Protection of genome from cellular RNases
P	V	28	Associated with NC
	P – phosphoprotein	45–47	Co-factor for polymerase
	I	19	Non-structural protein
M	Matrix	38.5–42	Alignment of nucleocapsids with cytoplasmic domains of HN and F
F	Fusion protein	65–72	Fusion of viral and cellular membranes
SH	Small hydrophobic	6	Membrane association; unknown function
HN	Hemagglutinin-neuraminidase	74–80	Attachment and release of virions from the host cell
L	Polymerase	180–200	RNA-dependent RNA polymerase

P, to create a helical nucleocapsid. The lipid envelope contains the viral gly-coproteins hemagglutinin-neuraminidase, HN, the fusion protein, F, and the SH protein, complexed to the matrix protein, M, on the luminal side.

Mumps virus is considered to exist as a single serotype, but several geno-types of mumps have been defined based on the sequence of the SH gene, which varies most between strains of virus (Johansson, Tecle and Örvell, 2002). Recently, evidence for lack of cross-protecting neutralising antibodies between genotypes suggests the evolution of additional serotypes of mumps virus (Nojd et al., 2001; Örvell, Tecle and Johansson, 2002).

Mumps virus binds to sialic acid-containing cell surface molecules via the HN protein. Upon binding, a change in conformation of HN is thought to trigger a conformational change in the F protein, resulting in the release of a hydrophobic peptide that inserts into the cellular membrane to mediate fusion (Lamb and Kolakofsky, 2001). The nucleocapsids are then released directly into the cytoplasm of the cell, where all subsequent stages of replication take place. Primary transcription of message by the viral polymerase begins at the 3' end of the genome. At the end of each gene the polymerase is released and reinitiates at the start site for the next gene. The further the gene is from the 3' end, the less abundant the mRNA (messenger RNA). At the P ORF, three mRNAs are produced. The V mRNA is directly transcribed from the gene, while mRNAs for P and I are generated by the addition of extra nucleotides at an internal site that shifts the reading frames. After translation, the HN and F undergo modification in the ER and Golgi, which includes cleavage of F into two segments, F1 and F2, which are disulfide linked. The mature forms of the glycoproteins are transported to the cell membrane, where they mediate cell-to-cell fusion allowing spread of the virus to neighbouring cells. M and NP accumulate in the cytoplasm. The function of the SH glycoprotein is unknown, but it does not appear to be necessary for replication, at least in tissue culture cells (Takeuchi et al., 1996). At a certain point during the infection, presum-ably triggered by the accumulation of structural proteins, the polymerase shifts from transcription of mRNA to replication of genomes. Full-length antigenomes are produced that serve as templates for the synthesis of new negative-sense genomes. NP and the polymerase/P proteins associate with the genomes to produce new nucleocapsids. The M protein is central in the assem-bly of virions, directing nucleocapsids to sites where viral glycoproteins are inserted in the cell membrane. New virions then bud out of the membrane and are released from the cell through neuraminidase activity of HN.

Mumps virus infection usually, but not always, results in cell lysis (McCarthy et al., 1980). There is no correlation between effects in tissue culture and the severity of the disease caused. One of the most striking effects is the forma-tion of large syncytia. Other effects include vacuolisation, pyknosis and cell lysis (Carbone and Wolinsky, 2001). Mumps virus can establish persistent, noncytolytic infections in some cell types or under certain growth conditions (reviewed in Carbone and Wolinksy, 2001). Persistence in vitro has been linked to a decrease in the cellular response to interferon via reduced amounts of STAT1α (Yokosawa, Kubota and Fujji, 1998).

Pathogenesis of mumps infections

Mumps virus displays a restricted host range. Natural infection occurs only in humans, although experimentally monkeys, hamsters, suckling mice, neonatal and suckling rats and chick embryos can all be infected. The virus is transmitted via droplets and directly from saliva. The incubation period from first exposure to earliest clinical signs is generally around 18 days, but ranges from 14 to 24 days. The virus replicates locally in mucosal epithelial cells of the respiratory tract and in draining lymph nodes, and can be shed from about 6 to 7 days prior to the onset of symptoms and for as long as 9 days afterwards (Jubelt, 1984). Early symptoms include fever, headache, malaise and upper and/or lower respiratory tract symptoms. The disease is most often characterized by swelling of the parotid glands, although as many as half the patients do not have parotitis (Azimi, Cramblett and Haynes, 1969; Gray, Moffat and Sangster, 1969; Levitt, Kinde and Gates, 1970; Jubelt, 1984), and 7 to 30% of infections may be totally asymptomatic but still infectious (Gray, Moffat and Sangster, 1969; Jubelt, 1984). Mild or asymptomatic infections occur more often in females than males, although the reason for this is unknown (Johnstone, Ross and Dunn, 1972).

After the primary round of replication, there is spread to secondary sites of infection via the blood, evident about one week after the first symptoms but often at the same time as parotid involvement. The kidney is infected, and virus is excreted in urine for up to 2 weeks after the appearance of symptoms and after the development of neutralising antibodies (Utz et al., 1957; Wolinsky, 1996). Spread of mumps to testes occurs in 10 to 35% of cases, most often in postpubertal males (Jubelt, 1984; Wolinsky, 1996; Carbone and Wolinsky, 2001). Although testicular atrophy occurs in about half the cases, sterility is rare (Jubelt, 1984). Infection of ovaries has been less often documented and may be underreported (Carbone and Wolinsky, 2001), but it has been estimated to occur in 5% of females (Jubelt, 1984). Pancreatic involvement occurs in approximately 5% of cases (Azimi, Cramblett and Haynes, 1969; Feldstein et al., 1974; Jubelt, 1984), resulting in transient functional abnormalities (Dacou-Voutetakis et al., 1974) and rarely in hemorrhagic pancreatitis (Feldstein et al., 1974). Mumps infections have been implicated, along with other infections, in the development of type I diabetes, but there is little support for a direct causative role (reviewed in Carbone and Wolinsky, 2001). Other tissues, including thyroid, mammary and prostate glands, and the eye and heart, can be affected (Jubelt, 1984). Abnormal electrocardiograms have been reported in patients hospitalised with mumps infections (Arita, Ueno and Masuyama, 1981), and cases of fatal myocarditis have been reported in children (Ozkutlu et al., 1989; Kabakus et al., 1999). Infectious virus has been isolated from the heart of one fatal case (Brown and Richmond, 1980) and detected by PCR in more than 70% of myocardial samples from cases of fatal endocardial fibroelastosis (Ni *et al.*, 1997). Arthritis and thrombocytopenia are other rare complications of mumps infection (Graham *et al.*, 1974; Lacour *et al.*, 1993; Nussinovitch, Volovitz and Varsano, 1995).

There are few reports of the effects of mumps infection during pregnancy. Infections within the first trimester appear to cause fetal wasting (reviewed in Carbone and Wolinksy, 2001). Mumps virus has been isolated from fetal tissues following spontaneous abortion on the fourth day of a maternal mumps infection (Kurtz *et al.*, 1982). There has been one report of an infant with severe pulmonary symptoms whose mother had developed mumps 4 weeks prior to delivery (Yakahashi *et al.*, 1998).

SPREAD TO THE CNS

Mumps virus spreads readily to the CNS, and is thought to do so even in patients who display no symptoms of meningitis or encephalitis. CSF pleocytosis has been demonstrated in 40 to 65% of patients with parotitis but no CNS symptoms (Bang and Bang, 1943; Azimi, Cramblett and Haynes, 1969). The percentage of total mumps infections that show clinical signs of CNS involvement has been reported to be anywhere from 0.5 to 30% (Levitt, Kinde and Gates, 1970; Smith and Gusson, 1976). Interestingly, meningitis and encephalitis often occur in patients showing no signs of parotitis (Meyer *et al.*, 1960; Azimi, Cramblett and Haynes, 1969; Gray, Moffat and Sangster, 1969; Levitt, Kinde and Gates, 1970), and indeed in many cases the only symptoms of infection are the CNS symptoms (Gray, Moffat and Sangster, 1969; Koskiniemi, Donner and Pettay, 1983).

The majority of cases of CNS disease are classified as meningitis (Strussberg *et al.*, 1969; Johnstone, Ross and Dunn, 1972), which is estimated to occur in 23% of total mumps cases (Russell and Donald, 1958) and which has a benign course with complete recovery. Symptoms include high fever, lasting for 4 to 7 days, a stiff neck and headache (Gray, Moffat and Sangster, 1969; Jubelt, 1984). The electroencephalogram (EEG) is usually normal (Wolinsky, 1996). High cell counts in CSF (pleocytosis) are characteristic of mumps meningitis (Gray, Moffat and Sangster, 1969), and inclusions consistent with mumps virus have been visualised in ependymal cells collected from the CSF of patients with mumps meningitis (Herndon *et al.*, 1974). Pleocytosis can persist for several weeks after the disappearance of symptoms (Tashima, 1969). Infectious virus has been isolated from the CSF in at least 50% of cases with clinical CNS disease (Utz *et al.*, 1957; McLean *et al.*, 1967; Bistrian, Phillips and Kaye, 1972) and by a reverse transcriptase polymerase chain reaction (RT-PCR), mumps virus has been detected in the CSF of 96% of patients with a clinical diagnosis of mumps CNS disease (Poggio *et al.*, 2000).

The incidence of true encephalitis, with penetration of the virus into the brain and/or spinal cord and infection of neurones, is more difficult to determine because patients have been classified as having meningoencephalitis when there have not been clear signs of parenchymal involvement (Jubelt, 1984). Estimates of the incidence of encephalitis range from 0.01 to 0.2% of total mumps infections (Levitt, Kinde and Gates, 1970; Smith and Gusson, 1976; Koskiniemi, Donner and Pettay, 1983; Ito *et al.*, 1991). The ratio of males to females showing signs of encephalitis can be as high as 4:1 (Koskiniemi, Donner and Pettay, 1983). Of hospitalized patients, a much higher percentage have signs of encephalitis, but again the numbers range widely, from 4% (Johnstone, Ross and Dunn, 1972) to 13% (Gray, Moffat and Sangster, 1969; Levitt, Kinde and Gates, 1970) to as high as 35% (Azimi, Cramblett and Haynes, 1969). Primary encephalitis resulting from infection of neurones occurs about 1 week after the first symptoms of infection. In addition to fever and headache, symptoms are confusion, drowsiness, slurred speech, hallucinations and seizures. There are few pathological studies from patients with primary encephalitis, as this condition is rarely fatal (Taylor and Toreson, 1963; Azimi, Cramblett and Haynes, 1969; Jubelt, 1984). However, where examinations were possible, edema, perivascular cuffing and neuronal cytolysis were observed, indicative of infection and destruction of neurones (Taylor and Toreson, 1963; Bistrian, Phillips and Kaye, 1972). Mumps virus has been isolated from the brain of at least one fatal case (de Godoy *et al.*, 1969, cited in Bistrian, Phillips and Kaye, 1972).

Postinfection encephalitis can also develop, usually appearing one to three weeks after the first symptoms of infection (Strussberg *et al.*, 1969; Levitt, Kinde and Gates, 1970; Johnstone, Ross and Dunn, 1972). Clinically, postinfectious encephalitis is difficult to differentiate from primary disease, except that there may be a sudden onset of additional signs such as ataxia, dizziness, double vision and paralysis (Tan, Manickam and Cardosa, 1992), stupor and coma (Jubelt, 1984). The mortality rate of this disease is estimated at 20 to 22% (Johnstone, Ross and Dunn, 1972; Tan, Manickam and Cardosa, 1992). Pathological analysis reveals demyelination, thought to result from an immune response directed to breakdown products of destroyed neurones (Bistrian, Phillips and Kaye, 1972; Tan, Manickam and Cardosa, 1992).

Patients surviving acute mumps CNS disease, especially those with encephalitis, often continue to experience neurological symptoms for several years (Oldfelt, 1949; Meyer *et al.*, 1960; Koskiniemi, Donner and Pettay, 1983; Julkunen *et al.*, 1985). Sequelae are more frequent and severe in patients who were adult at the time of primary mumps infections (Azimi, Cramblett and Haynes, 1969; Julkunen *et al.*, 1985). In one study, almost half of 47 patients experienced symptoms as long as 15 years after the primary episode (Julkunen *et al.*, 1985). Problems range from headache and irritability to severe problems such as loss of vision, difficulties with learning and memory, focal motor and sensory signs, and paralysis (Meyer *et al.*, 1960; Koskiniemi, Donner and Pettay,

1983; Julkunen *et al.*, 1985). Some of these problems may result from chronic infection with mumps, which has been marked by the continued production of mumps specific antibody in the CSF (Vaheri, Julkunen and Koskiniemi, 1982; Julkunen *et al.*, 1985; Ito *et al.*, 1991). These patients often suffer from progressive mental deterioration. Hydrocephalus, resulting from aqueductal stenosis after shedding of infected ependymal cells, is a rare complication that can occur during primary infection (Ogata, Oka and Mitsudome, 1992; Viola *et al.*, 1998) or several years later (Timmons and Johnson, 1970; Johnson, 1975; Koskiniemi, Donner and Pettay, 1983; Julkunen *et al.*, 1985). Worsening headaches, changes in mental status and gait abnormalities may arise from hydrocephalus (Carbone and Wolinsky, 2001).

There are no animal models of mumps infection that represent natural infection and disease in humans, but some aspects of mumps virus replication and spread to the CNS *in vivo* have been examined in neonatal hamsters. Intraperitoneal inoculation of suckling animals with a wild-type mumps virus resulted in virus replication in the liver and spleen, and then spread to the pancreas, thymus, heart, lungs and kidney, but virus did not enter the brain (Wolinsky and Stroop, 1978). Primary viraemia declined by 7 days postinfection (p.i.), and virus was cleared from all organs except the kidney by day 9 to 11. Results were similar with the Jeryl Lynn vaccine virus, a virus highly attenuated for humans, except that this virus did establish a transient infection of the brain. Kilham virus is a strain of mumps selected for enhanced neurovirulence for hamsters by passage through neonatal hamster brain (Kilham and Overman, 1953). When inoculated intraperitoneally, this virus spread throughout the visceral organs, and readily penetrated the CNS. Ependyma and parenchyma of the brain were infected and 90% of the animals died. In the surviving animals, virus persisted in the ependymal cells of the brain and in the kidney until 50 days p.i. (Wolinsky *et al.*, 1974; Wolinsky and Stroop, 1978).

Intracranial inoculation of suckling hamsters with several mumps virus strains also resulted in infection of the ependyma and cells of the choroid plexus (Johnson, 1968; Wolinsky and Stroop, 1978; Takano, Takikita and Shimada, 1999). In these cases, ependyma was damaged with a loss of cilia (Johnson, 1968; Wolinsky *et al.*, 1974). There was very little inflammation, but perivascular infiltration of lymphocytes and small haemorrhages were observed (Johnson, 1968). Most virus strains did not infect neurones, and depending on the dose of inoculum, 50 to 100% of animals survived (Johnson, 1968; Wolinsky and Stroop, 1978). With Jeryl Lynn virus and Kilham virus, viral antigen was present in the neurones of the hippocampus in addition to the ependymal cells, and, ultrastructurally, Kilham virus was visualised budding from the free surfaces of ependymal and choroidal cells and neurones (Wolinsky *et al.*, 1974; Margolis, Kilham and Baringer, 1974; Wolinksy and Stroop, 1978; Takikita *et al.*, 2001). Viral antigen was distributed throughout the dendritic branches of infected neurones, indicating that virus could spread easily along neuronal pathways (Schwendemann *et al.*, 1982). Interleukin 1β production in areas of the cortex positive for mumps virus antigen has been hypothesised to cause neuronal apoptosis (Takikita *et al.*, 2001). In animals surviving inoculation with all strains of virus, healing of ependymitis resulted in hydrocephalus with or without aqueductal stenosis (Johnson and Johnson, 1968; Margolis, Kilham and Baringer, 1974; Wolinsky and Stroop, 1978; Sarnat, 1995). Destruction of ependymal cells has also been observed in monkeys after intracutaneous inoculation with various isolates of mumps virus (Rozina and Hilgenfeldt, 1985), and invasion of neurones has also been demonstrated in monkeys (Levenbuk *et al.*, 1979; Rozina *et al.*, 1984). Based on these studies, the virus is assumed to enter the CNS through infection of the choroid plexus during viraemia. It is not known whether the virus crosses the endothelium of the choroid plexus directly from the plasma or whether activated lymphocytes harbouring virus cross the endothelium to initiate infection of the epithelium (Carbone and Wolinsky, 2001). Virus is then shed into the CSF, and from there can infect ependymal cells and possibly neurones (Wolinsky *et al.*, 1974; Wolinsky, Klassen and Baringer, 1976; Takano, Takikita and Shimada, 1999).

In the hamster model, the ability to penetrate the brain and infect neurones varies from virus to virus, and the changes in the Kilham virus responsible for increased neurovirulence have not been documented. The F protein may play a role in the pathogenesis of necrosis in the brain, as preincubating Kilham virus with antibody to F-moderated CNS disease after intracranial inoculation (Löve *et al.*, 1986a, 1986b). HN has also been implicated in the neurovirulence of Kilham virus. A neutralising antibody escape mutant of this virus, with a single amino acid change at position 360 of HN, lost the ability to penetrate and infect neurones (Kövamees *et al.*, 1990).

The relevance of these observations for humans is questionable. It is presumed that different isolates of mumps will differ in their ability to enter the CNS and cause meningitis and to infect neurones, but almost nothing is known about these aspects of mumps biology in humans. It is clear that virulence in the hamster model does not correlate with virulence in humans, as Jeryl Lynn virus, the most attenuated mumps vaccine strain, is more neuroinvasive in neonatal hamsters than wild type isolates of mumps (Wolinsky *et al.*, 1974; Wolinksy and Stroop, 1978). A model in neonatal rats that measures the extent of hydrocephalus after intracranial inoculation appears to be a better indicator of attenuation or virulence for humans, but whether virulent viruses can be further differentiated into those causing more or less severe disease has not yet been tested (Rubin, Pletnikov and Carbone, 1998; Rubin *et al.*, 2000).

In support of a role for HN in the virulence of mumps virus for humans, an isolate of the Urabe vaccine virus that is highly attenuated (Wright, unpublished results) has a unique amino acid change at position 335, while viruses causing postvaccination meningitis have a unique change at position 464 (Afzal, Yates and Minor, 1988; Brown, Dimock and Wright, 1996; Wright, Dimock and Brown, 2000) and 498 (Afzal, Yates and Minor, 1988). However, these amino acid substitutions in HN are not the only differences between the virulent and attenuated Urabe viruses, and they are not universal markers of attenuation or virulence applicable to other mumps strains (Brown and Wright, 1998; Örvell, Tecle and Johansson, 2002). The SH protein has been hypothesised to affect neurovirulence for humans, as some genotypes, defined by SH sequences, are associated with higher incidences of meningitis (Örvell, Tecle and Johansson, 2002). On the other hand, there is considerable variation in virulence of viruses within a genotype. In a recent outbreak of mumps in Europe, viruses associated with parotitis had two unique amino acid changes in the SH protein that were not found in viruses of the same genotype isolated from cases of meningitis, suggesting that mutations in SH can be attenuating (Örvell, Tecle and Johansson, 2002; Tecle, *et al.*, 2002). A virus that fails to produce SH has been isolated from a patient with mumps meningitis (Takeuchi *et al.*, 1996), and the Urabe isolate associated with meningitis has one amino acid change in SH compared to the published sequence for this protein (Wright, unpublished results). Virulence has also been associated with changes in the P protein; in an outbreak in Japan, isolates from patients with meningitis lacked a *BamHI* restriction site in this gene compared to virus from patients without CNS symptoms (Saito *et al.*, 1996). Although these findings are suggestive that SH and HN, and possibly F, all affect the ability of mumps virus to enter the CNS, no conclusions can be made about the significance of these proteins without comparison of the complete genomes of closely related attenuated and virulent viruses.

IMMUNE RESPONSES

Infection with mumps elicits a full spectrum of immune responses: interferon (IFN), CD4+ and CD8+ T cells and mucosal and serum antibody directed to all viral proteins except M (Carbone and Wolinsky, 2001). Type I interferon is measurable in sera and CSF of patients with mumps meningitis and encephalitis (Morishima *et al.*, 1980; Dussaix *et al.*, 1985). During the normal course of infection, IFN titres decline within one week (Morishima *et al.*, 1980). Specific cytotoxic T cell (CTL) responses are detectable in purified peripheral blood lymphocytes (PBL) and CSF after natural infection and immunisation with mumps (Chiba *et al.*, 1976; Tsutsumi *et al.*, 1980; Kreth *et al.*, 1982). Unlike the situation with other paramyxoviruses, clearance of primary infection is dependent on the development of neutralising antibody rather than on cell-mediated responses (Carbone and Wolinsky, 2001). However, the persistence of CTL activity in the CSF for as long as 3 weeks after the onset of meningitis has led some to speculate that mumps-specific CTL play an immunopathologic role (Kreth *et al.*, 1982). Shedding of virus from the upper respiratory tract is limited by the development of virus-specific IgA, while disappearance of viraemia coincides with the appearance of serum neutralising IgG (McLean *et al.*, 1967). *In vitro* neutralising responses are directed to both HN and F (Örvell, 1984), but neutralising antibody to HN alone is protective in an animal model of mumps meningoencephalitis (Wolinsky, Waxham and Server, 1985). Serum neutralising antibody persists indefinitely (Carbone and Wolinsky, 2001), and natural infection with mumps generally provides life-long protection against disease but not necessarily against infection, as both asymptomatic and symptomatic reinfections have been reported (Gut et al., 1995).

Cell-mediated responses to nonmumps antigens are transiently suppressed after immunisation against mumps (Kupers et al., 1970) and presumably during natural infection (Carbone and Wolinsky, 2001). Mumps virus infects both T and B lymphocyte cell lines and peripheral blood mononuclear cells (PBMC) and displays a preference for T lymphocytes (Fleischer and Kreth, 1982). However, infection of T lymphocytes during natural infection has never been demonstrated, and the mechanism of suppression of cellular responses has not been elucidated.

Mumps virus and the ear

Deafness after mumps infection manifests itself during or shortly after acute infection, but occasionally appears months later (Kayan and Bellman, 1990; Fuse et al., 1996). Deafness is usually unilateral (Everberg, 1960; Westmore, Pickard and Stern, 1979; Koga et al., 1988) but can be bilateral in about one-fifth to one-third of cases (Everberg, 1960; Lindsay, 1973; Bitnum, Rakover and Rosen, 1986). It has been estimated that hearing loss will occur in 0.005 to 0.3% of total mumps patients (Everberg, 1957; Vuori et al., 1962; Morrison and Booth, 1970). It has been recommended that routine audiology tests be conducted on all patients after mumps infections (Kanra et al., 2002). In the subset of patients with mumps meningitis or encephalitis, the incidence of deafness has been reported to be very similar (Azimi, Cramblett and Haynes, 1969; Levitt, Kinde and Gates, 1970; Julkunen et al., 1985), or slightly higher, at 3 to 4% (Vuori, Lahikainen and Peltonen, 1962; Garty, Danon and Nitzan, 1985). As the majority of patients suffering from infections with the virus are young, about half the cases of deafness caused by mumps occur in children less than 9 years of age (Mizushima and Murakami, 1986; Yanagita and Murahashi, 1986; Koga et al., 1988). One study found that children under 3 years of age were more susceptible to hearing loss than older children (Jensema, 1975). In this same study, slightly more males were affected than females (1.3 to 1.0), but others do not report this gender difference (Mizushima and Murakami, 1986).

Hearing loss caused by mumps infections is generally severe and permanent (Lindsay, 1973; Bitnum, Rakover and Rosen, 1986; Kanzaki and Nomura, 1986; Tieri et al., 1988), but can also be mild, with partial or total recovery (Vuori, Lahikainen and Peltonen, 1962; Nomura et al., 1988; Yamamoto, Watanabe and Mizukoshi, 1993; Hydén, 1996). Total mumps deafness does not respond to treatment (Morrison and Booth, 1970; Bitnum, Rakover and Rosen, 1986; Unal et al., 1998). Vestibular symptoms and tinnitus may or may not be present

(Tarkkanen, and Gho, 1966; Bordley, Brookhouser and Worthington, 1972; Lindsay, 1973; Tieri et al., 1988) and occur more often in patients over 10 years of age (Mizushima and Murakami, 1986; Yanagita and Murahashi, 1986). Dizziness in particular is reported in about half the cases (Hydén, Ödkvist and Kylén, 1979; Yanagita and Murahashi, 1986; Yamamoto, Watanabe and Mizukoshi, 1993). Delayed development of endolymphatic hydrops, or Ménière's syndrome, with symptoms of episodic vertigo, has been associated with previous mumps infections in a handful of patients (Schuknecht, Suzuka and Zimmermann, 1990; Hydén, 1996). It has been proposed that this may result from inner ear damage sustained during the primary infection (Schuknecht, Suzuka and Zimmermann, 1990).

Neurotologic testing of patients during the acute phase of deafness shortly after mumps infection reveals inner ear disturbances (Mizushima and Murakami, 1986; Yamamoto, Watanabe and Mizukoshi, 1993). Those with partial deafness experience loss in the high frequencies, consistent with basal cochlear damage (Morrison and Booth, 1970). The functioning of the inner ear and auditory nerve has been assessed in 15 patients with mumps deafness (Sawada, 1979). None of the cases responded to pure-tone audiometry, but they could be divided into three types of cochlear impairment based on electrocochleographic responses. One group had deficiencies at the neural level but continued functioning of the organ of Corti, one group showed severe impairment of the neural regions and partial functioning of organ of Corti, while in the last group both neural regions and the organ of Corti were impaired.

As the fatality rate for mumps infections is low, there have been few opportunities to examine directly the pathology of the temporal bone in cases of mumps-induced deafness. Temporal bones from two such individuals with bilateral hearing loss have been examined, in both instances several years after the mumps infections. The first case was that of a 6 year old child who died 4 years after becoming deaf (Figure 6.1). In both ears the perilymphatic system, the vestibular sense organs and the meninges in the internal meatus appeared normal, and the damage was limited to the cochlear ducts and the peripheral cochlear neurones in the basal coil (Lindsay, Davey and Ward, 1960). In the less affected ear, there was degeneration of the organ of Corti and of the stria vascularis, with the most atrophy in the basal coil and lesser amounts of damage in the upper and middle coils. The tectorial membrane was detached in the basal coil and part of the middle coil, and there was some decrease in the number of nerve fibres in the lower half of the basal coil. In the other more severely affected ear, atrophy of the stria vascularis was more extensive, the organ of Corti was absent in the basal and lower middle coils, and Reissner's membrane had collapsed (Lindsay, Davey and Ward, 1960). The nerve fibre loss was moderate. The damage to the tectorial membrane and the organ of Corti was considered to be secondary to the destruction of the stria vascularis (Lindsay, 1973). The second case was an adult who died 13 years after the

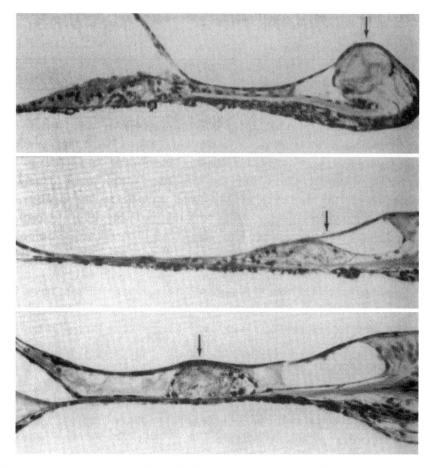

Figure 6.1. Apical (top), middle (middle) and basal (bottom) coils showing the degenerated tectorial membrane (arrows). In the apical coil, the cells of the organ of Corti can be identified. The organ of Corti is missing in the middle and basal coils. (Photo from Lindsay, Davey and Ward, 1960, printed with permission of Annals Publishing Company)

mumps infection (Figure 6.2). In neither ear was there damage to the stria vascularis or the tectorial membrane, but there was degeneration in the organ of Corti, mainly in the basal turn, with nerve fibre loss in the affected areas (Smith and Gussen, 1976). There was also marked degeneration of the outer sulcus area, evident in the basal turn. There was some disturbance in the utricle and saccule, but these changes were not thought to result from the mumps infection (Smith and Gussen, 1976). These observations are consistent with other studies examining temporal bones from adults who had suffered sudden deafness presumed to be due to viral infections but where no specific virus was

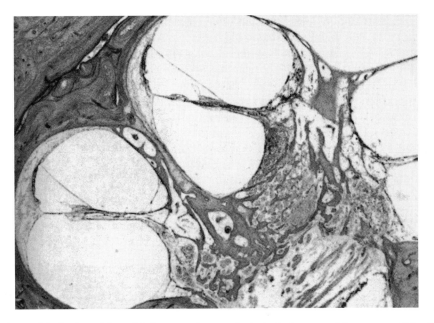

Figure 6.2. Left cochlea with intact stria vascularis, but absence of the organ of Corti in the basal turn (bottom left). (Photo from Smith and Gusson, 1976. Copyright American Medical Association © 1976)

implicated. Varying degrees of atrophy of the organ of Corti, stria vascularis and tectorial membrane were observed in the majority of these cases (Sando *et al.*, 1977; Schuknecht and Donovan, 1986). Temporal bones from patients with deafness associated with another paramyxovirus, measles, showed similar pathology in the cochlea, but measles infection also affected vestibular structures (Lindsay, 1973; Yoon *et al.*, 1990).

Early presumptions were that deafness after infection was due to the encroachment of the meningitis lesions on the acoustic nerve (Everberg, 1957; Lindsay, 1973). It is now generally accepted that the damage is more direct, and that virus reaches and infects the inner ear. There has been one instance of mumps virus isolation from the perilymph of a patient with sudden deafness during mumps infection (Westmore, Pickard and Stern, 1979). The possible routes of infection are: (a) via the blood during viraemia (haematogenous), (b) via the CSF that reaches the perilymphatic space through the internal auditory meatus or the cochlear aqueduct, (c) via the eighth cranial nerve or (d) directly from the middle ear (Smith and Gussen, 1976; Sawada, 1979; McKenna, 1997). There has never been any evidence supporting the latter route, from the middle ear after viral otitis media (Mizushima and Murakami, 1986). The recognition that only one-third of patients with hearing loss display CNS symptoms and that asymptomatic infections can result in deafness

(Vuori, Lahikainen and Peltonen, 1962; Mizushima and Murakami, 1986; Yamamoto, Watanabe and Mizukoshi, 1993) has led many to conclude that the major route of spread is haematogenous (Lindsay, 1973; Mizushima and Murakami, 1986). The fact that the major lesions in the ears are within the cochlear duct supports this. The stria vascularis may be particularly susceptible to infection because of the slow circulation and the location of the capillary network in these cells (reviewed by Lindsay, 1973).

Direct neural spread of virus, or spread via the CSF after infection of the meninges, cannot be ruled out. Given that mumps virus enters the CNS readily without causing overt CNS symptoms, meningeal spread remains a possibility, even in mild infections (Bang and Bang, 1943; Azimi, Cramblett and Haynes, 1969; Schuknecht, Suzuka and Zimmermann, 1990; Yamamoto, Watanabe and Mizukoshi, 1993). The isolation of mumps virus from the perilymph of a patient with sudden deafness lends support to this route (Westmore, Pickard and Stern, 1979). Sawada (1979) proposes that the virus spreads via the CSF, or along the eighth cranial nerve, after the development of viral neuritis and ganglionitis, even in cases with no clinical signs of meningitis. Unlike the majority of early studies, a recent survey found a group of 50 children with mumps meningoencephalitis, who had higher hearing level thresholds at most frequencies than the children with uncomplicated mumps, providing evidence for a higher risk of hearing loss after meningoencephalitis (Kanra et al., 2002). Pathological changes consistent with meningogenic invasion of mumps into the ear have yet to be described, although such changes have been noted in ears after meningoencephalitis caused by another paramyxovirus, measles (Lindsay, 1973). Infection of the cranial nerve is even less likely. Encephalitis caused by mumps is quite rare, and occurs at a male–female ratio of 4:1. Deafness after mumps does not follow the same pattern, occurring equally in both sexes. There has been some evidence of eighth nerve involvement in patients with ISSHL using magnetic resonance imaging (MRI). In one case of deafness linked to mumps infection, imaging indicated a pathological labyrinth and signs of inflammation of the eighth cranial nerve (Comacchio, D'Eredità and Marchiori, 1996). However, damage to the nerve could be secondary to infection in the labyrinth. In a second case associated with mumps infection, there were no signs of labyrinthine changes, but the cochlear nerve was reduced in size relative to the unaffected ear, also suggesting that the primary insult is at the level of the nerve (Furuta et al., 2000). Because of the limited ability to study the pathology of mumps infection in the ear in humans, mumps virus infection of the inner ear in various animals has been studied. When neonatal hamsters were inoculated with the Kilham mumps virus intracranially, viral antigen was detected by immunofluorescence in the endolymphatic cells, specifically both layers of Reissner's membrane, the stria vascularis and the organ of Corti (Davis, Shurin and Johnson, 1975; Davis and Johnsson, 1983). Similar results were obtained when the virus was introduced directly into the labyrinth (Davis, Shurin and Johnson, 1975). Antigen was also observed in the macula of the saccule, the endolymphatic membrane and in cochlear and vestibular ganglia (Davis, Shurin and Johnson, 1975). When nonneurotropic strains of mumps virus were inoculated, a similar distribution of viral antigen was noted, except that ganglia were not infected (Davis and Johnson, 1976; Davis, 1990). No viral antigen was detected in cells of the perilymphatic structures or within sensory cells of the labyrinth (Davis and Johnson, 1976; Davis, 1990). Histologically, very little inflammation developed in ears and no specific lesions were observed in the inner ear (Davis, Shurin and Johnson, 1975; Davis and Johnson, 1976). Experiments in neonatal guinea pigs resulted in similar results. After intravascular or intralabyrinthine inoculation of virus, a proportion of animals were positive for virus antigen in the cochlea, most often in the stria vascularis, and in some animals in the organ of Corti and Reissner's membrane (Tanaka *et al.*, 1988a). By electron microscopy (EM), evidence of virus replication and budding was observed in the marginal and intermediate cells of the stria vascularis. If the infection was productive, degeneration of the organ of Corti in the lower turns of the cochlea could be detected by EM (Tanaka *et al.*, 1988a).

Infection of the ear has also been examined in monkeys. Karmody (1975) did not observe any histological signs of labyrinthitis in the ears of Rhesus monkeys inoculated directly into the labyrinth, even though infection had occurred in eight of the nine monkeys, as detected by seroconversion. In a smaller study of three Macaque monkeys, virus was inoculated directly into the cochlea, and temporal bones were examined by EM 14 days later (Tanaka *et al.*, 1988b). As in the other animal studies, viral antigen was located in the stria vascularis of the basal turn of the cochlea, while ultrastructurally, virus shedding into the endolymph was evident in the marginal cells of the lower basal turn. Pathological changes were most severe in the organ of Corti and stria vascularis. Specifically, marginal and intermediate cells of the stria vascularis were swollen, and fibrosis and infiltration of macrophages and lymphocytes were observed. The outer hair cells were degenerated or lost, consistent with the observations made in human mumps deafness, while the inner hair cells were less affected. Nerve endings and nonmyelinated nerve fibres had also disappeared.

The animal studies confirm the tropism of mumps virus for epithelial cells of the membranous labyrinth, the stria vascularis, Reissner's membrane and cells of the organ of Corti. In studies where virus was inoculated intracranially, a similar distribution of virus antigen was observed, but neurones were not infected. These results demonstrate that virus in the CSF can reach the stria vascularis via the cochlear aqueduct. The fact that the neurotropic Kilham virus did infect neurones of the spiral and vestibular ganglia in neonatal hamsters does leave open the possibility of neural spread of some strains of mumps that may be particularly neurovirulent.

Summary

During infection with mumps, the virus initially replicates in the respiratory tract, then spreads via the blood to many other sites in the body. Spread to the ear occurs via this route, although virus in the CSF can gain access to the inner ear via the perilymph. Spread via the eighth cranial nerve is also possible but is probably a rare occurrence. Within the ear, the membranous structures of the cochlea are susceptible to infection. Deafness results, either from direct damage to these structures by the infection or by indirect damage from inflammatory responses that would impair the endolymphatic system (Mizushima and Murakami, 1986). In the rodent models of mumps infection in the ear, very few inflammatory changes were observed, even when the organ of Corti was degenerated (Tanaka et al., 1988a). In nonhuman primates, on the other hand, pathological changes in the inner ear after infection were accompanied by infiltration of macrophages and lymphocytes (Tanaka et al., 1988b). However, in cases where deafness was discovered very shortly after mumps infection, steroid treatment did not prevent further deterioration of hearing (Okamato et al., 1994).

Prior to the introduction of the mumps vaccine over 30 years ago, infections with mumps virus were a major cause of deafness in children and adolescents. Although a safe effective vaccine for mumps exists, immunisation is not available in many parts of the world. Even in countries where the vaccine has been in use for decades, epidemics and outbreaks of mumps continue to occur due to poor vaccine uptake. Consequently, mumps infections continue to cause avoidable cases of deafness. The International Task Force for Disease Eradication has identified mumps as a candidate for global eradication (cdc.confex.com/cdc/nic2002/techprogram/paper_307.htm).

7 MEASLES

B. Rima

Introduction

Measles virus is the cause of a major childhood disease, which, until vaccination reduced the incidence, was a major cause of morbidity and mortality in children. The number of cases worldwide is still estimated to be approximately 30 million per annum with a death toll of over 700000 children per annum. The mortality primarily occurs in the developing world, where vaccination coverage is low and where secondary infections are often the direct cause of the lethal complications of the infection. Vaccination has controlled the infection in many countries and several countries including the United Kingdom have been able to break transmission of the virus by mass vaccination campaigns. However, such efforts only bear fruit temporarily as imported cases rapidly bring the virus back. Measles virus infection has been associated with hearing loss in a minority of infected children and vaccination has reduced the incidence of this. However, the scale of the reduction in acquired deafness due to measles virus infection has not been assessed. The mechanism(s) involved in the induction of hearing loss by measles virus is unclear. Several potential ones will be discussed in this chapter, which will begin with a molecular description of the virus, its clinical symptoms and sequelae, epidemiology and pathogenesis. These are of importance in consideration of the postulated involvement of the virus in otosclerosis (OS). No clear understanding of the way in which the virus can cause that disease, sensorineural hearing loss (SNHL) or otitis media (OM), emerges from these considerations, though in the latter case the association with infection is beyond question. In essence one can say that the major strategy for the reduction of measles-induced hearing loss should be to prevent measles infection in the first place. Effective vaccination strategies

Infection and Hearing Impairment. Edited by V.E. Newton and P.J. Vallely
© 2006 John Wiley & Sons, Ltd

exist that could lead to the eradication of the virus, provided there is the political will to implement them fully. In this chapter, recent reviews are sourced to describe the virus and its clinical effects and complications (Rima, 1999; Griffin, 2001). The role of measles in OM, SNHL and OS, however, is reviewed here using primary research references.

The virus

Measles virus is classified in the family *Paramyxoviridae* and in the genus *Morbillivirus*. Measles virus is a large RNA virus with a pleomorphic appearance in the electron microscope (EM) (Figure 7.1(a)). It is an enveloped virus with a diameter of between 100 and 300 nm. The lipid bilayer envelope is derived from the host cell and is surrounded by a fringe of spikes formed by the two viral glycoproteins. All spikes are about 5 nm in diameter and up to 15 nm in length and of a uniform appearance. The spikes probably consist of complexes of both viral glycoproteins. Inside the envelope there is a ribonucleoprotein structure (RNP), which is the basic replicating structure delivered into the cells after fusion of the viral membrane with that of the host. It consists of a helical nucleocapsid of about 1 μm in length and 18–21 nm in diameter, with a central core of 5 nm in diameter. In the EM after negative staining the RNP displays the herringbone structure characteristic of all paramyxovirus nucleocapsids. The distribution of the viral protein in the virion is indicated diagrammatically in Figure 7.1(b). The virus contains six structural proteins, the nucleocapsid (N), phospho- (P), matrix (M), fusion (F), hemagglutinin (H) and large (L) proteins. The functions of each are detailed in Figure 7.2. The genome organisation of the virus is also depicted in this figure. The genome of measles virus is an RNA molecule of negative polarity, i.e. opposite polarity to the viral

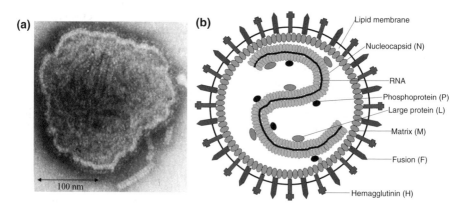

Figure 7.1. (a) Electron micrograph of a disrupted measles virion. (b) A schematic representation of the virion and the structural proteins contained in it

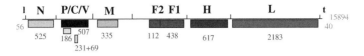

N protein: nucleocapsid protein; structural phosphoprotein of the ribonucleoprotein core
P protein: phosphoprotein; element of RNA transcriptase and / or replicase complex
L protein: large protein; RNA polymerase and other functions in replication
              and transcription (capping, methylation; polyadenylation; helicase?)

M protein: matrix protein involved in budding (and transcriptional control?)

F protein: type I glycoprotein; fusion activated by proteolytic cleavage; acylated
H protein: hemagglutinin protein type II glycoprotein; receptor binding

C protein: nonstructural protein; control of IFN response? other?
V protein: Zn binding protein of unknown function; mRNA generated by editing
              (host transcription?), IFN response

Figure 7.2. Measles virus gene order; size and functions of proteins. A diagrammatic scale representation of the measles genome indicating the size of the genes and the open reading frames. The small numbers under each gene indicate the number of amino acid residues in each of the viral proteins; the length of the leader (56) and trailer (40) regions and the complete genome (15894) are also indicated but as numbers of nucleotides

messenger RNAs. It is a single nonsegmented RNA molecule with a length of 15 894 nucleotides. It consists of six transcribed regions (genes), each of which encodes a major structural protein of the virus, and which are separated from each other by three nucleotide long intergenic sequences. The six transcription units are preceded by a region coding for the so-called leader RNA of 56 nucleotides and are followed by a trailer region of 40 nucleotides (Figure 7.2). The entire nucleotide sequence has been determined for the measles prototype strain Edmonston, which was isolated in 1954 and passaged in tissue culture by John Enders. Complete genome sequences have also been determined for several vaccine viruses derived from the Edmonston strain as well as for a number of wild-type strains.

The MV genome encodes, besides the six structural proteins, two nonstructural proteins, C and V. The C protein is translated from the P mRNA from an overlapping reading frame. The V protein is generated from an 'edited' transcript of the P gene. During transcription of the P gene about 30–50% of the transcripts are edited by insertion of a single G residue, which allows access to an overlapping reading frame after the editing site. Thus V is aminocoterminal with the P protein for the first 231 amino acids and then has a 69 residue cysteine-rich tail that contains a zinc-binding domain and represents one of the most conserved products encoded by the 'P' genes of paramyxoviruses. It is likely that at least V or C plays a role in the viral inhibition of the innate immune responses of infected cells. Virus mutants lacking V or C protein can be propagated successfully in tissue culture, but they are less able to replicate in human tissues.

The replication cycle of measles virus is outlined in Figure 7.3. MV attaches to the host cell by interaction of the viral glycoprotein spikes with cellular receptors. The H protein is the most important attachment protein but the full spike complement including interactions between the H and F with cellular receptors and possibly coreceptors are required for fusion of the viral envelope with the host cell membrane. CD46, one of the complement decay accelerating factors that protects cells from lysis, is a cellular receptor for some measles virus strains including the vaccines and other laboratory-adapted strains. It is, however, clear that many wild-type viruses use a different receptor, which has been identified as SLAM or CD150. Fusion occurs at the cell membrane and apparently not in endocytotic vesicles, and in a pH-independent manner. In analogy to other viral systems, it probably involves complex rearrangements of residues in the F proteins.

After fusion of the virion with the cell membrane, the nucleocapsid RNP is introduced in the cytoplasm where it acts as a template for the transcription

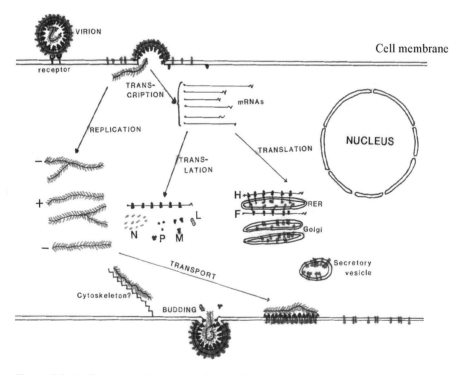

Figure 7.3. A diagrammatic representation of the replication cycle. The cycle involves entry of the virus, transcription and replication and viral egress by budding (see the text for details) (RER, rough endoplastic reticulum)

of mRNAs as well as a template for replication of the negative stranded genome RNA into positive antigenome RNA (Figure 7.3). Transcription involves the binding of the RNA polymerase complex of the virus to the 3′ end of the RNP and the sequential copying of the genome sequence into positive stranded mRNA. The intergenic sequences are not transcribed and transcription begins at the start of a consensus sequence present at the 3′ end of each gene. At each gene junction there is a finite chance for the polymerase complex to leave the template and this gives rise to a gradient of gene expression in which the promoter proximal (e.g. N and P/V/C) genes are transcribed much more frequently into mRNA than the promoter distal H and especially the L gene.

The RNP introduced into the cell contains a negative strand RNA molecule encapsidated by N protein. In the replication process, the RNA polymerase complex binds again at the 3′ end of the genome, as in transcription, but during replication the nascent RNA molecule is immediately encapsidated by N protein and the intergenic signals for polyadenylation; stop and start and editing are entirely ignored in this process. This gives rise to positive stranded RNA molecules in Y formed nucleocapsid complexes as intermediates (Figure 7.3). The positive antigenome containing nucleocapsids have strong promoter sequences at their 3′ end, which in the same manner allow the generation of more nucleocapsids containing the negative (genomic) RNA. These are transported via cytoskeletal elements to the cell membrane where the viral M protein and the glycoproteins form patches through which the nucleocapsids bud out to form new virus particles.

Transmission and molecular epidemiology

Previously measles virus gave rise to epidemic patterns, presumably due to the need to accumulate sufficient numbers of susceptible individuals in the population whose maternal antibody levels had waned enough to allow infection and systemic virus replication to cause disease. The spatial and temporal distribution of measles in the UK has been described in exquisite detail by Grenfell, Bjornstad and Kappey (2001). Their analysis of the extensive UK database demonstrated the two-yearly cycle of measles in the large population centres and the more sporadic epidemic patterns in the small towns, as well as the disease radiating out in waves from large centres such as London and Liverpool into the English countryside. In order to remain endemic, measles virus requires human populations in excess of 300000 individuals so as to be supplied with adequate numbers of susceptible individuals to maintain the chain of transmission. The virus is transmitted by aerosol. Measles is an extremely infectious virus. One measure of transmissibility of a virus is the so-called R_0 value, which indicates the number of secondary cases that can occur from a single index case. In the case of measles this is estimated to be about 40, one of the highest values reported for any virus. It has been estimated that one tissue culture infectious dose is sufficient to infect a rhesus monkey.

Measles virus is a monotypic virus. This means that there is only a single serotype and infection with one strain of measles appears to provide life-long protection from measles disease. Nevertheless, with the development of DNA sequencing techniques and reverse transcription polymerase chain reaction, it has become clear that strains vary in their nucleotide sequences, especially where it concerns the area of the genome encoding the last 150 amino acids of the N protein and the entire sequence of the H protein gene. Sequences for these variable regions of the genomes of over 250 strains and isolates have been determined during the last decade and these show that more than 22 different genotypes exist which belong to eight different clades. These virus clades may have been geographically restricted in their distribution at earlier times, e.g. before worldwide vaccination campaigns. Especially, the increase in travel by children who are the prime reservoir for virus replication has now allowed worldwide distribution of some of the genotypes. The study of the actual present-day distribution of genotypes over the globe is hampered by the fact that surveillance is poor precisely in those countries in which the virus is endemic and in which specific genotypes might be sustained.

In the USA and the UK mass measles vaccination campaigns have allowed transmission of the virus to be broken for short periods. However, afterwards the virus is quickly reimported by infected children from other parts of the world. In the USA and UK it has been possible to link the origin of the imported strain with travel by specific index cases. Thus knowledge of the different genotypes has made it possible to establish transmission chains for a number of outbreaks. It will also be important for future eradication campaigns.

Vaccines

Measles virus vaccines are live-attenuated virus strains derived from the Edmonston virus isolated in 1954. These have been derived by passage of the virus in nonhuman primate host cells or in embryonated chicken eggs. All currently used vaccines appear to be related to the Edmonston strain. Formalin or tween-ether inactivated virus preparations were introduced as a killed vaccine in 1964, but these were withdrawn in 1967 as cases of exacerbated measles disease became apparent in recipients of this vaccine when they contracted wild-type measles. Since that time, live-attenuated strains derived from the Edmonston strain have been used exclusively. Nowadays, measles virus vaccine has been incorporated into the trivalent measles–mumps–rubella vaccine, which is a mixture of three live viruses. This vaccine is safe and efficacious and has been used to control measles in developed countries successfully by a two-dose schedule in which the first dose is given at 15 months of age and the second to children aged 4 or 5.

The prospects for eradication of measles are good. The World Health Organization hopes to achieve control of the infection by the year 2007. Since there is no animal reservoir and transmission does not involve arthropod vectors, successful immunisation of the human population should theoretically allow the chain of transmission to be broken. For this to be achieved, over 95% of the susceptible population has to be effectively vaccinated, i.e. show seroconversion. Whether the programmatic ability to deliver such campaigns exists in those developing countries where they are most needed and whether the political will exists to spend the money required for such campaigns are open questions. The lack of exposure of the population, especially in the developed world, leads people very wrongly to consider the disease not to be a very serious one. However, in Africa and other developing regions the virus is still recognised as a major killer.

Clinical syndromes

Measles virus causes a severe disease in childhood characterised by a maculopapular rash, dry cough, coryza, conjunctivitis and photophobia. This may be preceded by the appearance of Koplik's spots in the mouth of the patient. Its incubation period is 10–14 days. It was not distinguished from infections caused by small poxvirus until the 7th century AD. In the developed world the infection is usually mild and, apart from rare but severe sequelae, usually has no lasting after-effects. In developing countries, however, the situation is very different. There the infection can have high mortality rates (5–10%) and severe morbidity is associated with the virus. The causes of these differences in clinical outcome of the infection are not well understood although several hypotheses have been put forward to explain them, such as the dose rate of infection, immunological challenge by other infections, vitamin status and strain differences. However, at present none of these offer a satisfactory explanation for the striking differences in the clinical symptoms manifested in the infected child.

SEQUELAE OF MEASLES VIRUS INFECTION

One of the main complications of measles is interstitial pneumonitis and mucosal inflammation in the respiratory tract. Giant cell pneumonia is much more clinically significant and is primarily a feature in immunocompromised people (see below). Another common occurrence in measles is diarrhoea. However, it is not clear whether this is caused by infection of the virus in epithelia in the gastrointestinal tract or results from the virus-induced immunosuppression, which allows secondary infections to become manifest. It is most common in the developing world where intercurrent bacterial and parasitic infections are frequent. OM (see below) and laryngotracheobronchitis are possibly other manifestations of secondary infection.

IMMUNE SUPPRESSION

Measles virus infection causes a pronounced immunosuppression in patients, which may be the cause of secondary bacterial and viral infections that are more life-threatening than the virus infection itself. The mechanisms by which this immunosuppression occurs are not clear, but long-lived cytokine imbalances as well as direct effects on the proliferation of lymphocytes have been postulated. The latter are the probable cause of the marked lymphopenia associated with the disease. Delayed-type hypersensitivity responses to pre-existing antigens such as the tuberculin reaction may transiently disappear during acute measles infection and convalescence. However, the immunosuppression does not appear to affect the development of an immune response to the virus itself. Antibody responses are detectable at the time of onset of the rash. The earliest are IgM responses, which switch to IgG1, IgG4 and IgA, the latter especially noted in mucous secretions and saliva. The earliest antigens that are recognised are the N and P proteins of the virus, and during the acute phase these can be the only antigens to which antibody is demonstrable. Antibodies to the H and F protein develop later. Thus hemolysis inhibiting and neutralising responses are delayed. Antibody responses to the M protein are difficult to demonstrate in many human infections and no immune response to the L protein has been observed. Antibody can protect against disease, as witnessed by the protective effect of maternal antibody in infants, but its role in control of the virus is not clear as patients with dysgamma-globulinaemia usually overcome measles infection without problems. The cellular immune response is probably more important as patients who are defective in this are more prone to severe sequelae and widespread virus infection in many tissues. During the acute phase of the infection CD8+ T cells are apparent. Measles-induced interferon beta induction upregulates HLA class I expression *in vitro* so that infected cells are more easily recognised. The target antigens are probably the F protein and the N proteins of measles virus (MV). In the later stages of infection CD4+ T cells predominate. The proliferation-stimulating antigens appear to be H, N, P, F and M proteins of the virus. A typical change from a Th1 to a Th2 response seems to occur in MV infection, leading to early activation of cytolytic T cells followed by the later stimulation of Th2 cells which, via cytokine IL4, stimulate antibody production. The immune responses are very long-lived. Early island studies carried out by Panum in 1846 indicated that life-long protection from disease follows after infection with 'wild-type' virus. After contact with wild-type virus the immune response to measles is boosted. It is unlikely to induce a sterilising immune response.

NEUROLOGICAL SEQUELAE

Acute measles infection is associated with severe neurological symptoms in a very small minority of the cases. About 1 per 1000 cases will suffer postinfection encephalitis, which is often fatal. It appears to be autoimmune in nature as no virus can be demonstrated in the brain of such patients. A rare, but invariably fatal, late complication of measles is subacute sclerosing panencephalitis (SSPE) which occurs in 1 per 10–300000 cases. It occurs 2 to 30 years postinfection, with an average time of appearance of symptoms of eight years after the acute infection. Acute infection below the age of two years is a risk factor in this disease. It predominates in males (2.5 males to 1 female) and practically disappears where the disease is effectively controlled by measles vaccination campaigns. It is caused by a persistent infection with an aberrant measles virus, which finally manifests itself in demyelination and severe neuronal infection leading to neuronal death. Depending on the neural systems affected, severe neurological deficits and death of the patient occurs between 3 months and 3 decades after the onset of symptoms. The virus found in the brain is characterised by mutations, which render it defective. The mutations are concentrated in the cytoplasmic tail of the F protein and in the M protein. Some mutations are caused by biased hypermutation, possibly involving a double-stranded RNA-dependent adenosine deaminase (DRADA). A further feature of the transcription process of measles virus in SSPE is that the slope of the transcription gradient appears especially steep (little L expression) in human CNS cells infected with the virus. In SSPE, the slope of the gradient of gene expression is so steep that little F and H protein is produced. This may aid the virus in escaping detection by the immune system.

In immunosuppressed patients measles can give rise to another CNS infection called measles inclusion body encephalitis (MIBE). In contrast to SSPE, MIBE is not associated with a hyperimmune antibody response to measles proteins, but mutations in the M proteins, similar to those in SSPE, are found.

Other suggested sequelae of measles virus infection are multiple sclerosis, Paget's disease, OS (see below) and, more recently, Crohn's disease and autism. However, no confirmed evidence has been presented to substantiate these associations, let alone prove a causal relationship.

Hearing loss and measles infection

Lindsay and Hemenway (1954) reviewed the importance of measles as a cause of hearing loss and cited studies that estimated the proportion of cases of deafness that might be attributed to measles. This ranged from 4 to 9.3%. There is uncertainty about the criteria that were used to attribute cases to measles infection. Nevertheless, the figures demonstrate the importance of measles virus infection in hearing loss.

Otitis media (OM) occurs as a complication in acute measles in a substantial minority of patients. In hospitalised cases the rate of occurrence was found to be 9.8% in an unselected group of cases in Israel (Leibovici *et al.*, 1988) and 8.5 and 10% in two studies of hospitalised cases in the USA (Gremillion and Crawford, 1981; Markowitz *et al.*, 1987). However, in another US study of 3220 measles cases in military recruits, 106 cases were complicated by pneumonia, of which 30% also had OM. Thus OM appears to be enhanced in measles cases that have severe respiratory involvement. It has been estimated that 35 years of measles vaccination in France has prevented one million cases of OM and 600 cases of deafness (Reinert, Soubeyrand and Gauchoux, 2003). There have been many studies that suggest that vitamin A treatment reduces the severity of measles infection. A recent Cochrane review concludes that vitamin A affects the morbidity but not the mortality of measles, with the exception of pneumonia associated mortality, which is reduced (D'Souza and D'Souza, 2002). There is a single study (which has not been replicated) that suggests that the incidence of OM may be reduced by 74% by treatment of measles patients with vitamin A (Ogaro et al., 1993).

Sensorineural hearing loss (SNHL) has been primarily associated with post measles infection encephalitis, but reliable estimates of its incidence are lacking. The virus has also been implicated in otosclerosis (OS), but the evidence for this remains weak and unconfirmed.

PATHOLOGY OF HEARING LOSS

Target tissues for virus replication

In order to evaluate the potential role of measles virus in hearing loss it is important to review the properties of the virus that may influence its pathogenesis, such as receptor usage, cytopathic effect, recognition by the immune system and ability to establish persistent infections, etc. The virus is carried in aerosol and infects cells in the upper and lower respiratory tract. It has been suggested that it may replicate transiently in epithelial cells in this area. However, direct evidence to support this is not very strong and it cannot be ruled out that the major site of primary replication is in cells of the reticulo-endothelial system, such as macrophages and dendritic cells present in the lung. The virus reaches the draining lymph nodes and from there establishes a transient viraemia through infection of monocytes primarily and some lymphocytes. Receptors for measles virus are of importance for the spread of the infection and in the mid 1990s, CD46 was identified as a receptor molecule for the virus that is uniformly expressed on most nucleated cells in the body. However, it became clear in the late 1990s that the many wild-type strains of the virus, in contrast to laboratory adapted strains, cannot use this receptor. Instead they use CD150 or SLAM. This molecule is expressed only on dendritic cells and mature lymphocytes and its expression can be induced in cells of the monocyte/macrophage lineage. This raises the question 'Are wild-type measles virus strains restricted to these cells or can they infect other cells using other receptors?' The answer is currently not clear since it is possible that there are low-affinity interactions with CD46 and possibly other as yet unidentified receptors. The 'classical' description of the pathogenesis of measles states that the viraemia allows spread of the virus infection to all epithelial cell types and surfaces, including the endothelium of small blood vessels. Infection in dermal endothelium spreads to the overlaying layers of the epithelium, which results in the formation of the characteristic rash, due to local inflammation. Whether infection of these cell layers involves direct cell-to-cell interactions with immune cells or whether free virus can infect these cells is not clear. All lymphoid organs including the thymus, spleen and lymph nodes as well as the appendix and the tonsils show severe virus infection. Other target organs include the lungs, where a severe infection of the mucosa may lead to bronchopneumonia, the liver (although not giving rise to clinical hepatitis), the gut, where gastroenteritis is a common manifestation, and the kidney, which gives rise to shedding of virus-infected cells into the urine. The genital mucosa can also be infected. Thus the virus causes a very widespread systemic infection. In most tissues multinucleated Warthin–Finkledey cells appear and signs of local inflammation are prevalent. Whether it is epithelial infection in the lung or whether alveolar macrophages and lymphocytes are the source of the virus that is transmitted is not clear.

The role of measles virus in otitis media

The mechanisms by which measles causes OM are not understood and most of what follows is therefore speculative. Indirect and direct mechanisms can be put forward. Indirectly, the immunosuppressive effect of measles virus infection may play a role in allowing secondary bacterial infections to cause the disease. In the course of acute measles a temporary immune suppression occurs affecting T and B lymphocyte reactions. This makes the patient susceptible to secondary viral, bacterial and parasitic infection. Whether protection against middle ear bacterial infection is B or T cell mediated is not clear (reviewed by Bernstein, 2002). The main protective mechanism appears to involve IgG and IgM as bacteriocidal agents in combination with nonspecific mechanisms. The role of T lymphocytes is not clear, but T cells appear to be few in number in the middle ear fluid (MEF). The origin of the B lymphocytes that produce the immunoglobulins may be from the mucosal associated lymphoid tissue or the cells may enter the middle ear mucosa from the vasculature.

If antibody secreted into the MEF is derived from serum antibody then it is unlikely that measles infection will be able to suppress this significantly unless the virus infects the B cells directly involved in local production of the antibodies. Sloyer et al. (1977) suggested that the mucosa lining the middle ear cavity is an active epithelium that locally produces antibodies. They described evidence for local production of IgA against measles virus in 16 out of 41 cases of OM. However, in an equal number of cases the IgA detected was against poliovirus and in four and five cases, respectively, against mumps and rubella virus. Some papers have suggested that the ratio of IgA antibodies in serum and MEF is so skewed on occasion that this may be taken as evidence for local production.

The normal immune mechanisms that maintain the sterility of MEF could well be compromised if local inflammation caused by viral infection can alter the cytokine milieu in the middle ear. However, no evidence to support this mechanism is available in the case of measles virus.

The possibility that direct pathology associated with the viral infection in the middle ear may also be involved cannot be excluded. Bordley and Kapur (1977) described histopathological changes in the middle ear of children who died as a result of bronchopneumonia secondary to measles virus. The children all suffered from severe necrotising OM and in one out of four cases Warthin–Finkeldey multinucleate giant cells were observed in the middle ear. These cells are characteristic of measles infections elsewhere in the body. However, the presence of viral antigen or RNA was not demonstrated, and these studies do not appear to have been replicated.

In conclusion, it appears that too little is known about the immune control of OM to explain how measles virus could cause it and speculation about a direct or indirect role for measles virus is premature.

The role of measles virus in sensorineural hearing loss

That the loss of sensorineurons and other damage to the inner ear would lead to hearing loss is self-evident. Only 5–10% of all cases of SNHL have been estimated to be measles induced (McKenna, 1997). Friedmann (1974) in his classical treatment of the pathology of the ear states that endolymphatic labyrinthitis is well recognised in measles, and destruction of the neuroepithelium may give rise to deafness. The disease is primarily associated with the neurological sequelae of measles postinfection encephalitis. His overall conclusion that the knowledge of the pathology of measles infection and its role in deafness is scant still holds today. Other authors who have reviewed this area of research give the same message. Davis and Johnsson (1983) conclude that although it is known that viruses can cause several forms of deafness, 'the pathogenesis of the hearing loss is poorly understood'. McKenna (1997), in a review of the role of measles and mumps virus in SNHL concluded that:

> Despite the well established *association* between certain specific viruses and corresponding characteristic cochlear and vestibular pathology, the mechanisms by which some of these viruses results in end organ pathology has not been determined. Specifically, it is not known whether the damage that occurs within the cochlea and vestibular labyrinth is the result of viral infection of specific target cells or the sequela of a reactive inflammatory response to viral infection or the presence of viral antigens or some combination of both.

There are only a few cases in which the time elapsed between the hearing loss and the availability of tissue for histopathological assessment is small enough to approach such questions. Furthermore, none of these studies have used direct methodology such as immunocytochemistry with measles-specific monoclonal antibodies or *in situ* hybridisation to determine the presence of viral antigen or RNA; rather most have concentrated on explaining the hearing loss by looking at the pathological changes in the inner ear (Lindsay and Hemenway, 1954; Lindsay, 1973; Davis and Johnsson, 1983; Yoon *et al.*, 1990). Thus although several of the investigators have described pathology, some of which is commensurate with possible measles infection, its specificity is unknown. Richard Johnson and his collaborators (Davis, Shurin and Johnson, 1975; Davis and Johnson, 1976) have described similar pathology in labyrinthitis induced by measles virus in hamsters. In this model, infection of cochlear and vestibular neurones is observed. Measles-induced syncytia were seen in the organ of Corti and spiral ganglion cells (Davis and Johnsson, 1983) independent of the route of infection. Hence, it is clear that the pathology observed in SNHL could be measles induced; the association of measles infection with SNHL is undisputed, but evidence for direct viral infection is lacking. While at one stage there was a consideration that the inner ear was an immuno-privileged site (Harris and Ryan, 1995) it is now clear that this tissue is under immune surveillance and that humoral and cell-mediated immunity is operating. Hence, the inflammation that was observed in the histopathological studies of SNHL could have occurred as a result of immune responses to specific antigens. However, at present inflammatory mechanisms in response to the past or persistent presence of viral antigen cannot be distinguished from bystander effects and virally-induced autoimmunity (Harris and Ryan, 1995) as potential causative mechanisms.

In conclusion, as far as the role of MV in SNHL is concerned, apart from studies in animal models, we have not progressed significantly beyond the description of gross pathology and speculation about mechanisms.

The role of measles virus in otosclerosis

Otosclerosis (OS) is a disease that involves aberrant bone metabolism, which causes acquired deafness. It primarily affects the stapes bone in the middle ear. Excessive osteoclast function and/or reduced osteoblast activity leads to an imbalance in bone turnover. When the stapes is affected it may lead to conductive hearing loss. The disease is similar to Paget's disease (PD), which also appears to be caused by an imbalance between bone resorption and bone formation. The similarity with PD is important since there is a controversy about a role for measles virus in this disease as well as in OS. It is clear that both diseases have a strong genetic component and for OS a number of chromosomal locations have been identified (reviewed by Menger and Tange, 2003). These include, among others, sites on chromosome 15 (15q25–26) and on chromosome 7 (7q34–36). These are different from the seven sites with significant

LOD (logarithm of the odds of gene linkage) scores in PD. The nature of the genes involved has not been elucidated.

A number of groups have postulated a viral aetiology for OS and, as is the case with many viral diseases, there have been suggested associations between particular HLA (histocompatibility leucocyte antigen) haplotypes and development of OS. These might be explained by specific susceptibilities or resistances to virus infection (Menger and Tange, 2003). However, these studies are not conclusive and some studies have found no linkage to particular HLA haplotypes. A number of groups have published evidence for and against the involvement of measles virus in OS. The evidence is primarily based on histopathology and humoral immune responses in the serum and the perilymph as well as electron microscopy. Attempts to demonstrate the presence of a specific virus have used techniques to identify viral antigens by immunocytochemistry and viral RNA by various reverse-transcription polymerase chain reaction (RT-PCR) technologies. Instructive parallels exist with the postulated role and persistence of measles virus in PD. These parallels extend to the weakness of the evidence for measles virus involvement.

The pathology of the bone found in OS indicates that an inflammatory process of long duration has taken place, which may have given rise to the formation of spongeolytic bone (Arnold and Friedmann, 1988; Harris and Keithley, 1993). The latter is most probably the cause of the hearing loss in OS patients. However, whether this is caused by the aforementioned imbalance in bone turnover or by inflammatory reactions, i.e. which is cause and which effect, is not clear. Long-term viral persistence has been advanced as a potential explanation for the inflammatory process (Niedermeyer et al., 2001a). Hence, several studies have searched for the presence of enhanced viral antibody levels that may be associated with inflammation and local antibody production. The results have been inconclusive. One study demonstrated enhanced levels of measles IgG in the perilymph and suggested local antibody production (Arnold et al., 1996). Other studies have not been able to confirm this (Lolov et al., 2001) and in the most recent study no difference was seen between levels of measles antibodies in the perilymph and serum in OS patients and controls (Niedermeyer et al., 2001a). More direct evidence for viral involvement is provided by the detection of paracrystalline arrays in the electron microscope, which were interpreted as virus-like structures in the osteoblast of OS patients and seemed to look like typical paramyxoviral nucleocapsids in osteoblasts (McKenna and Mills, 1990). It must be stressed, however, that such arrays are also found in osteosarcoma and other diseases with a clear genetic origin, such as familial extensive osteolysis (Dickson et al., 1991). Since measles and mumps viruses are the two main paramyxoviruses that give rise to systemic human infection, and since measles is able to persist at least in SSPE (see above), a role for measles virus has been postulated in both PD and OS. Similar observations of paracrystalline arrays of nucleocapsids of paramyxoviruses have been made for PD (Mills and Singer, 1976).

However, in contrast to OS, in PD these are more prevalent in osteoclasts than in osteoblasts. Immunohistochemical techniques were then applied to identify the virus involved and several groups obtained conflicting results implicating the presence of measles virus, mumps virus or respiratory syncytial virus, again similar to observations in PD (Mills *et al.*, 1984). McKenna and Mills (1990) provide immunocytochemical evidence for the presence of measles virus but that was not confirmed by Roald *et al.* (1992). The next technology that was employed was RT-PCR. This involves reverse transcription of the measles RNA with specific or nonspecific primers resulting in the formation of cDNA, which is then amplified by PCR. This method can be applied to RNA samples extracted from bone or *in situ* (IS-RT-PCR). The IS-RT-PCR study technique is open to artefacts and many control experiments need to be carried out before one can draw valid conclusions from it. Only one IS-RT-PCR (Grayeli *et al.*, 2000) has been reported for OS and this did not provide evidence for the presence of measles virus. However, in the absence of any data on the sensitivity of the technique and its specificity, it is difficult to evaluate the meaning of such negative data. Absence of evidence is not evidence of absence. Conflicting data have also been obtained for both PD and OS using RT-PCR on extracted bone RNA samples. Early users of this technology were often not aware of the power of the technique to detect single DNA molecules and insufficient precautions were exercised in the early studies to avoid cross-contamination from DNA present in the laboratory, especially when nested RT-PCR is performed. This is a serious problem that has beset many studies. Niedermeyer and Arnold's group (Niedermeier *et al.*, 1994, 2000, 2001a) provided evidence for the presence of measles RNA in active lesions in bone derived from stapedectomies. Similar observations have been reported by McKenna, Kristiansen and Haines (1996). However, other groups have not been able to confirm the presence of measles virus sequences in RNA extracted from OS bone samples.

How can we progress in this area and firm the data up? Firstly, because of the potential for contamination, it is important that the presence of measles RNA in RT-PCR products is confirmed with nucleotide sequence data; in the absence of this, nested RT-PCR data must be questioned. Furthermore, depending on the area of the genome that has been amplified, it will be possible to subject the sequences of the measles virus to phylogenetic analyses and to determine the genotypes of the viral strains that are present in the sample. If all sequences from all patients in a given study are the same, contamination from DNA must be considered as an explanation of the data. If the sequences are not the same and they represent RNA from wild-type viruses that have circulated in the countries in which the patients have resided, then that would indicate that acute measles virus infection is a potential factor in the disease. It is noteworthy that in SSPE the virus genotypes that are found in the CNS are those of the acute early-in-life infection and not those of viruses circulating at the time of appearance of first symptoms. Hence, superinfection is unlikely to be involved. If the sequences of measles virus found in OS turn out to be those of the vaccine Edmonston strain, then there is a difficulty in explaining the reported suggestion that the vaccination programmes in Germany have been responsible for a delay in the first presentation of OS (Niedermeier *et al.*, 2001b). In PD so far only vaccine-like sequences have been reported (Rima *et al.*, 2002). The results that have implicated a role for measles virus in OS so far are at best inconclusive and similar to the situation in PD.

Summary

It is clear that otitis media is a significant complication of acute measles infection. However, how the virus does this is not clear. A plausible mechanism may be the generalised long-lasting immunosuppression associated with measles. There is also an association between measles and sensorineural hearing loss. The mechanisms by which this occurs can only be speculated about. In a hamster model of infection, tissues involved in the human pathology are directly infected by measles virus whether it is introduced in the labyrinth or intracerebrally. The role of the virus in otosclerosis is controversial. Analogies to Paget's disease have to be applied with care as the cell type in which the virus-like inclusions have been observed is not the same in both diseases and in any case the inclusions may not be due to viruses. Furthermore, the persistent infection in osteoclasts or osteoblasts would have to explain a disease that in this case only affects the middle ear bones, whereas Paget's disease can be a multifocal disease, affecting a variety of bones. Altogether, it is clear that measles infection can cause hearing loss and deafness. However, precisely how this occurs is unclear.

8 TOXOPLASMA INFECTION AND THE EAR

B. Stray-Pedersen

Introduction

It is well known that sensorineural hearing loss may be caused by infections that damage the inner ear, the auditory nerve or the nerve pathways in the brain. Deafness due to congenital and perinatal infections is often missed and the frequency underestimated since the diagnosis is difficult to make in infancy and early childhood and the connection to a maternal infection is not clear. In addition, all infections causing meningitis in the newborn baby may lead to damage of the auditory nerve.

The critical period of the embryonic development of the internal ear is during the seventh to eighth gestational week. Viral infections such as rubella and cytomegalovirus acquired by the mother during the developmental period may have a devastating effect on the hearing ability of the offspring. For rubella the ear might be affected even if the infection occurs up to 18–20 weeks of gestation. In an American study 17% of 59 children where the mother acquired CMV during pregnancy suffered from sensorineural hearing loss (Stagno *et al.*, 1977a).

Deafness has also been connected to parasitic infections. An association between malaria and hearing loss are being discussed today, but the status is not clarified. It has been proposed that the high fever occurring during malaria episodes may lead to convulsions and cerebral involvement, which may again cause hearing impairment (Chukuezi, 1995). However, the actual mechanism of causation is not clearly understood and the complications may equally well result from the adverse affect of antimalarial drug treatment.

The role of the parasite *Toxoplasma gondii* in causing hearing loss has been discussed for almost 40 years. The presence of the parasite in the mastoid and

Infection and Hearing Impairment. Edited by V.E. Newton and P.J. Vallely
© 2006 John Wiley & Sons, Ltd

inner ear and the accompanying inflammatory and pathologic changes have been considered to be the cause of deafness in *Toxoplasma gondii* infection.

This chapter focuses upon toxoplasmosis and its association with hearing impairment.

Toxoplasmosis

Human infections with *T. gondii* occur worldwide. The frequency varies greatly depending on geographical location, social–economic status and food habits (Stray-Pedersen, 2003). The seroprevalence rises with age and in central and southern Europe, and in many countries in Africa and South America more than half of the adults are infected. In some tropical countries up to 95% are infected, while in northern Europe, the UK and the USA 10–30% of the pregnant population has antibodies (Figure 8.1). However, the prevalence of *T. gondii* infection has been steadily falling in some countries over the past few decades (Stray-Pedersen, 2003).

Infection with *T. gondii* is usually benign and asymptomatic in children and adults, but can lead to severe complications if it occurs in an immunocompromised patient or in a developing fetus.

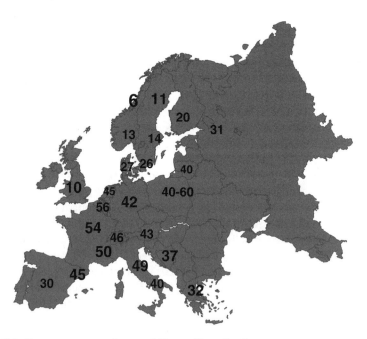

Figure 8.1. Percentage prevalence of *T. gondii* antibodies among pregnant women in Europe

TRANSMISSION OF THE ORGANISM

Toxoplasma gondii is a parasite that exists in three forms: the oocyst, the tachyzoite and the cyst (for a review see Montoya and Liesenfeld, 2004). The cat represents the main host and reservoir (Figure 8.2). Replication of the parasite happens in the intestine of the cat, resulting in production of several million oocysts. The oocyst in the cat faeces becomes infectious after one to five days and remains so for years. Once the parasite has been orally ingested in humans, parasitemia occurs and the tachyzoite may invade different organs throughout the body.

The immune response, with development of antibodies, leads to formation of tissue cysts that contains thousands of parasites. These cysts may persist in

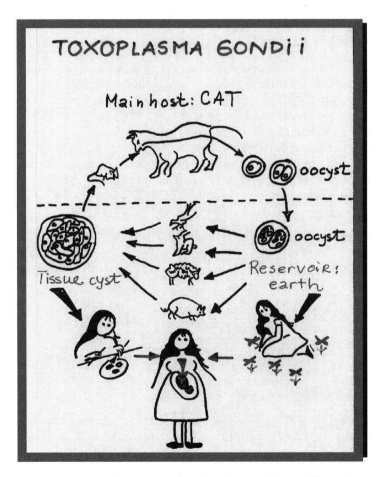

Figure 8.2. The life cycle and mode of transmission of *T. gondii*

a dormant state for years in skeletal or heart muscles, brain or eye, or they may reactivate. When reactivation occurs in an immunocompromised individual the cysts may rupture and release viable organisms that induce necrosis and inflammation resulting in the appearance of disease.

T. gondii tissue cysts are frequently found in pork and lamb, and rarely in beef and chicken. Freezing below −12 °C or cooking until the meat changes colour (66 °C) renders the parasites nonviable. The oocysts are destroyed by freezing or exposure to dry heat and boiling water, but are resistant to the usual detergents (Stray-Pedersen, 1993).

Human infection results from digestion of raw meat containing tissue cysts or from contact with cat faeces directly or by eating contaminated fruit or vegetables (Figure 8.2). Direct human-to-human transmission other than from mother to fetus has not been recorded.

CLINICAL MANIFESTATIONS OF ACQUIRED TOXOPLASMA INFECTION

Primary infection with *T. gondii* is usually asymptomatic or produces only mild symptoms, which are often ignored. The incubation period varies between 4 and 21 days. Vague flu-like symptoms such as fatigue, headache and fever may appear together with nucheal lymphadenopathy. The condition may resemble the common cold, influenza or infectious mononucleosis.

Ocular toxoplasmosis usually manifests itself as chorioretinitis or optic neuritis, often as a result of reactivation of congenital *T. gondii* infection. The debut age is around 15–25 years. The patient complains of blurred vision and pain. Relapses often occur.

IMMUNOCOMPROMISED PATIENTS

Toxoplasmosis also affects people who are immunosuppressed (AIDS, cancer or patients on immunosuppressive therapies). The disease may involve the brain, lung, heart, eyes or liver. Toxoplasma encephalitis develops in up to one-third of the seropositive AIDS patients (Montoya and Liesenfeld, 2004). Headache is a prominent symptom, as well as alterations in mental status, seizure and hemiparesis. Overt disease with fatal outcome may occur. The condition is usually caused by reactivation of a previous toxoplasma infection.

Congenital toxoplasmosis

Primary infection with *T. gondii* acquired during pregnancy may cause congenital disease in nearly half of the cases. During the maternal parasitemia, the parasites infect the placenta and then the fetus. The rate of transmission from mother to fetus increases from 10 to 80% with increasing gestational age (Dunn *et al.*, 1999). Frequency of transmission and severity of congenital disease are inversely related. Early maternal infection (first and second trimester) may result in severe congenital toxoplasmosis, while late infection (third trimester) usually results in newborns who appear normal. The clinical consequences include intrauterine death, brain damage with mental retardation and chorioretinitis with impaired vision (Stray-Pedersen, 1993). Many subclinically infected infants, if not treated, will develop symptoms later in life (Remington *et al.*, 2001). None of the signs described in children with congenital disease is pathognomonic for toxoplasmosis and the disease can mimic other congenital infections including rubella and CMV. Maternal infection acquired before pregnancy poses no risk to the fetus. Thus the frequency of congenital infection depends on the incidence of susceptible (seronegative) pregnant women, the infection risk in the geographical area and the gestational stage at the time of maternal infection.

Diagnosis of toxoplasmosis

The diagnosis of toxoplasmosis depends either on identification of parasites in body fluids and tissues (usually by PCR of *T. gondii* DNA) or on detection of specific antibodies. In pregnancy, the diagnostic challenge lies in differentiating between the primary maternal infection, which may cause fetal infection, and past latent infection, which is without importance (Gross and Pelloux, 2000). In the neonate, the challenge is to identify infected cases at an early stage, while in patients presenting with chorioretinitis it is important to decide if *T. gondii* is involved. In all situations reliable laboratory techniques are fundamental.

Various serologic tests can be used for detection of IgG antibodies that arise within 1–2 weeks after acquisition of the infection and persist for life (Figure 8.3). The test for IgG avidity has become standard to discriminate between newly acquired infection and 'old infection'. A test to identify IgM is usually added. The IgM antibodies typically indicate recent infection, but the interpretation has to be carefully considered since these antibodies may persist for more than 18 months after acquisition and many commercial kits give a high false positive rate (Remington *et al.*, 2001; Montoya and Liesenfeld, 2004).

Therapy

Acquired toxoplasmosis infections are not treated unless significant organ dysfunction occurs or there are systemic symptoms. The drug of choice is still a combination of pyrimethamine (25 mg daily) and sulfonamides with folinic acid for a period of 3–4 weeks. Where the eye is affected (acute chorioretinitis) long-term clindamycin (2 g/day) is also used, but the effect is dubious since none of these drugs kills the tissue cysts.

In pregnancy antiparasitic treatment is offered to every woman with a primary infection (Stray-Pedersen and Foulon, 2000). It is acknowledged that

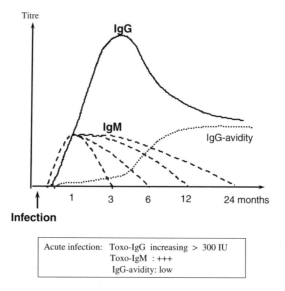

Figure 8.3. Serological response to acquired toxoplasmosis

prenatal treatment has *no impact* on the maternal–fetal transmission rate, but a beneficial effect of such treatment is seen on severe sequelae in infected infants at 1 year of age (Foulon *et al.*, 1999). Early implementation of treatment in pregnancy is important. If the fetus is infected, pyrimethamine-sulfadiazine-folinic acid is offered as a 3 week course, alternating with spiramycin. In France, two tablets weekly of pyrimethamine-sulphadoxine (Fansidar) are given. Infected infants should receive therapy during the first year of life.

Toxoplasma infection and the ear

ANIMAL MODEL STUDIES

In a series of investigations guinea pigs have been infected with *T. gondii*. The parasite was inoculated into the cochlea directly or via the hematogenous or intracisternal route (Falser, 1981). In three out of ten guinea pigs that were directly inoculated, and in one out of five hematogenously infected pigs, severe labyrinthitis was observed by electron and light microscopy. It was thus concluded that *T. gondii* was a potent pathogenetic factor in acute inner ear disturbances in laboratory animals.

ACQUIRED INFECTION

In the world literature there are only a few reports about acquired toxoplasmosis as a cause of inner ear damage. In 1991 an 18 year old Danish woman, while suffering from acute toxoplasmosis, experienced sudden deafness and a total loss of vestibular functions, first in the right ear and, three months later, also in the left ear (Katholm *et al.*, 1991). Following antitoxoplasma treatment the hearing was retrieved to such a degree that the patient was able to communicate by means of a body-worn hearing aid and lip-reading.

The authors discussed the different diagnostic possibilities and concluded that toxoplasmosis was the most probable cause of the severe hearing loss. They recommend that in patients with acute bilateral sensorineural hearing loss of unknown origin, the patients should be examined for acute *T. gondii* infection with the aim of instituting chemotherapy.

Some years later, in 1996, there was a report from Germany where a 9 year old boy was reported to be suffering from unilateral hearing loss and tinnitus (Schlottmann *et al.*, 1996). The boy had a very high *Toxoplasma* antibody titre of 1:120400; he was treated with pyrimethamine and sulfadiazine. The antibody titre decreased and he lost the tinnitus, but the sensorineural hearing loss remained. In both cases the *T. gondii* infection may have been accidental: the infection was serologically diagnosed and the parasite was not detected in any body samples.

CONGENITAL INFECTION

In the historical studies by Eichenwald (1960) the clinical spectrum of congenital toxoplasmosis was described and profound hearing loss was a prominent finding in infants with severe clinical toxoplasmosis. Of 105 children with neurological or generalised disease followed for more than 4 years, 15 (14%) were found to have 'deafness' as a major sequela. Unfortunately the term 'deafness' was not defined further.

Some years later, audiometric evaluation of 7 out of 12 American children with congenital infection revealed no hearing impairment in those infected with *T. gondii*, only in children with congenital CMV infection (Stagno *et al.*, 1977a). The toxoplasma-infected children, however, suffered from visual impairment and ocular defects.

In the US, studies to investigate the involvement of the ear in congenital toxoplasmosis continued. Wilson and colleagues (1980) evaluated 24 infants with serologic evidence of congenital toxoplasmosis. They were all asymptomatic at birth, but out of 19 children tested by audiometry up to 8 years after the diagnosis, 5 (26%) had unilateral or bilateral hearing loss. Of these, between 10 and 15% had educationally significant hearing loss.

In the US (Chicago) during the National Collaborative Treatment Trial (1984 to 1990), 30 infants and children with congenital toxoplasmosis were evaluated for hearing loss (McGee *et al.*, 1992). A total of 28 of the children were treated for congenital toxoplasmosis during their first year of life. The children were tested by high frequency ABR (auditory brainstem response) beginning within 2 months after birth. Six (20%) of the 30 infants had mild or moderate conductive-type hearing loss associated with otitis media. No infant or child had sensorineural hearing loss. This was the case for all tests including those for eight children who were retested with an additional lower frequency stimulus: a 500 Hz tone burst with subsequent ABR and MLR (middle latency responses) recording. When this better outcome with no deafness is compared with the incidence of 15–26% sensorineural hearing loss and 10–15% incidence of educational bilateral hearing impairment in the historical controls, the differences are statistically significant ($p = 0.02$).

It is, however, possible that an intensive one year treatment may diminish the development of hearing defects during the first year of life. The children studied by Wilson and colleagues (1980) received antimicrobial therapy only for a short time (i.e. one month) and Eichenwald's patients (1960) were also treated for only one month or not treated at all. The children in the National Collaborative Treatment Trial were treated extensively for the first year after birth. Continued follow-up to date in a larger number of children has not revealed progressive hearing impairment in any child (McLeod et al., 2000) and thus appears to verify the findings of the 1992 study (McGee et al., 1992).

From Israel, a retrospective study of 95 children aged 1–15 years who suffered from either epilepsy, cerebral palsy or nerve deafness were compared with 109 age-matched controls (Potasman et al., 1995). The prevalence of Toxoplasma gondii IgG seropositivity was 22% in the test groups versus 9% in the controls. A significant relationship was found between nerve deafness and T. gondii serology status ($p = 0.01$). They concluded that a deaf child was 7.1 times more likely to test positive than a hearing child. The deaf children had no other signs of congenital toxoplasmosis. Their mothers were not tested. No relationship between epilepsy or cerebral palsy and T. gondii specific serology was found. However, it is not stated how many children suffered from deafness alone, in the absence of any of the other conditions.

Another study from Saudi Arabia (Muhaimeed, 1996) found that 49 out of 70 T. gondii IgM positive children suffered from hearing impairment. However, in this study the quality of the serological method has to be questioned since 7% of 1054 tested children were T. gondii IgG positive and 6.8% were IgM positive, and only some of those who were IgM positive were also IgG positive. It would be expected that all IgM positive children should also be IgG positive as there is only one week after initiation of the infection when IgM appears alone before IgG is demonstrated (Figure 8.3), and in cases of congenital infection, IgM always appears together with IgG.

Several further studies suggesting that toxoplasmosis may not be a significant cause of hearing loss have recently emerged from Europe. For example, among 327 congenitally infected but treated children from the Lyon area in France, monitored for up to 14 years, no hearing loss was mentioned, although 24% had at least one retinochoroidal lesion in the eye (Wallon et al., 2004).

Conclusion

There is today not enough evidence to state that congenital toxoplasmosis is connected to hearing loss. Previously, 30–40 year old historical data reported a significant connection. However, more recent studies, even given that in these the pregnant mother and the congenitally infected child would now typically have received antitoxoplasmosis therapy, do not suggest that hearing loss is a complication of congenital toxoplasmosis. In acquired infection, impairment of the ear is very uncommon and may be coincidental.

9 SEXUALLY TRANSMITTED INFECTIONS

P. Turner

Introduction

Sexually transmitted infections have been ubiquitous across the World throughout history. Up until the 20th century there were no safe effective treatments available. Mercury had been used to treat syphilis since the late 15th century but it was not until 1909 when Ehrlich introduced arsphenamine (Salvarsan) that a truly effective treatment was available. However, it was the discovery of penicillin that led to the key advance in the treatment of sexually transmitted bacterial infections. Thus, by the 1960s, most of the common sexually transmitted infections could be relatively easily treated. However, in the late 1970s it was clear that a hitherto unrecognised sexually transmitted infection was in the ascendancy. This was named Acquired Immune Deficiency Syndrome (AIDS). Its cause, the human immunodeficiency virus (HIV), was discovered in 1984 (Montagnier, 2002).

Most sexually transmitted infections are not associated with hearing loss. HIV and syphilis, however, are notable exceptions. Both have many clinical manifestations. Indeed syphilis has long been recognised as the 'great imitator' of disease and HIV, by destruction of the immune system, makes those it infects susceptible to myriad opportunistic infections. Both these diseases can be asymptomatic at the time hearing loss presents. For this reason, syphilis and HIV must be considered in the differential diagnosis when a patient presents with sudden onset of sensorineural hearing loss.

Infection and Hearing Impairment. Edited by V.E. Newton and P.J. Vallely
© 2006 John Wiley & Sons, Ltd

General features of sexually transmitted infections

KEY CHARACTERISTICS

Most sexually transmitted infections share three common features. Firstly, the organisms are fairly labile and do not survive long outside the host and, therefore, are not easily transmissible other than by sexual means. Secondly, they do cause symptoms but are often associated with long periods where there are either no symptoms or nonspecific manifestations that do not always lead to the suspicion of a sexually transmitted infection. Thirdly, they are either non-fatal in their interaction with the host or kill at a late stage of the infection. These latter two features ensure that sexually transmitted infections are present in the host long enough to be transmitted to another person and, frequently, to many people.

EPIDEMIOLOGY

Since adolescents and young adults are the most sexually active in society, the incidence of sexually transmitted infection is highest in these groups. The main risk factors for acquiring a sexually transmitted infection are early age of first intercourse, multiple sexual partners and unprotected intercourse with a partner whose sexual history is unknown. These risk factors tend to concentrate in areas of deprivation and, therefore, the prevalence of sexually transmitted infection is higher in deprived areas. Internationally, this is reflected by the greater incidence and prevalence of sexually transmitted infections in sub-Saharan Africa, South Asia and South America. The World Health Organization (WHO) estimates that in 1999 there were 340 million new cases of curable sexually transmitted infection across the world (WHO, 2001e). Of these, 258 million (76%) were estimated to occur in the above three regions alone. Part of the problem, in this instance, is that timely, effective treatment is less accessible than in more affluent parts of the world. Therefore, the risk of transmission is greater. The highest prevalence of curable sexually transmitted infection is in sub-Saharan Africa. The World Health Organization has estimated this to be 119 per thousand population in 1999, i.e. about 12% of the population. This compares to an estimate of around 20 per thousand population in Western Europe and North America.

PREVENTION

The prevention of sexually transmitted diseases is proving a challenge in both the developed as well as the developing world. The best way to avoid sexually transmitted infection is to be in a monogamous relationship with someone whose prior sexual history you know and, therefore, the risk can be assessed. However, if either through lifestyle choice or circumstance this is not possible, then the next best means of protection is the judicious use of a barrier method such as a condom.

Syphilis and hearing loss

CAUSATIVE ORGANISM

Syphilis is caused by the spirochaete bacterium *Treponema pallidum*. These organisms are narrow (<0.15 μm diameter), making them impossible to see by light microscopy, but on dark-field microscopy the bacterium can be seen to have a corkscrew appearance with between 6 and 14 windings and a characteristic pattern of motion. Electron microscopy shows them to have tapered ends and regular spirals (Figure 9.1).

Treponema pallidum is a microaerophilic organism, tolerating only low levels of oxygen. It has limited biosynthetic capabilities and is therefore highly dependent on its host for provision of nutrients. Unsurprisingly, then, the genome of the organism, which has been fully sequenced (Fraser *et al.*, 1998), has been shown to use 5% of its genome to code for 18 distinct transporter proteins. These allow it to obtain and utilise the host amino acids, carbohydrates and cations that it requires for survival.

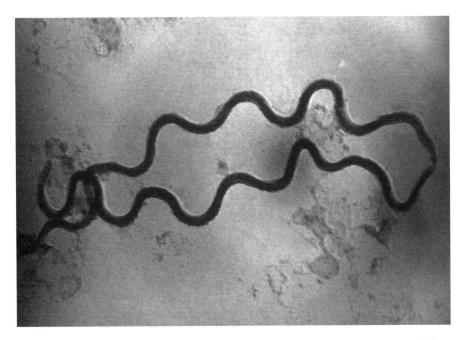

Figure 9.1. Scanning electron micrograph of two spiral-shaped *Treponema pallidum* bacteria (×368 000). (Provided courtesy of CDC/Joyce Ayers)

The importance of motility is reflected by the highly conserved nature of the genes coding for this activity, and the flagellar structure is produced from proteins encoded by 36 genes. There are a number of lipoproteins integrated into the bacterial membrane and it is thought that these may play a role in evasion of host immunity (Cox *et al.*, 1992). Analysis of the genome shows a considerable number of duplicated genes encoding putative membrane proteins (*tpr* genes), and this may represent the mechanism used by the organism to bring about antigenic variation; indeed, these are likely targets for vaccine development (Singh and Romanowski, 1999).

EPIDEMIOLOGY

Prior to the early 20th century syphilis was common. With the introduction of antimicrobial treatment the incidence of syphilis and the prevalence of the chronic stages of the disease fell in the Western World. However, hopes of eradication were unrealistic and, in the 1990s, the incidence of syphilis increased again, particularly in Eastern Europe and Russia, but also in many areas of the developed world such as the large cities in Western Europe and Northern America (Borisenko, Tichonova and Renton, 1999; Brown, Yen-Moore and Tyring, 1999; Weir and Fishman, 2002). Although the increase has been seen in both men and women, there has been a particularly explosive increase in homosexual men. Indeed, the incidence of syphilis in homosexual men in England has risen over 3000% from 1996 to 2002 (Figure 9.2). This rise

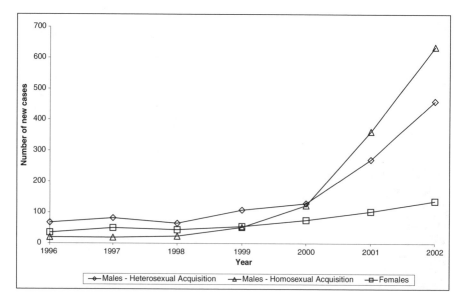

Figure 9.2. Trend in frequency of new cases of syphilis presenting to GUM clinics in England. (Source: Health Protection Agency, UK)

seems to indicate an increase in risky sexual behaviour and the decreased use of condoms that can reduce, though not eliminate, the likelihood of transmission.

However, despite this, syphilis remains a substantially more common disease in South America (3 million new cases in 1999), sub-Saharan Africa (4 million new cases in 1999) and South Asia (4 million new cases in 1999). This compares with 100000 new cases in North America and 140000 new cases in Western Europe in 1999 (WHO, 2001e). However, with the continuing increase in foreign travel by people in the developed world it is likely that there will be increased numbers of syphilis acquired abroad in the future.

TRANSMISSION AND INCUBATION

Humans are the natural host for *Treponema pallidum* and also act as the vector for transmission. The principal route of transmission between adults is via sexual contact as other forms of direct contact rarely result in infection, although transfusion of blood from donors in the incubation phase of the disease can also result in transmission. During sexual transmission, the organism from an infected individual penetrates through mucosal membranes or small breaks in the skin of the uninfected contact. At the point of entry an ulcer usually develops together with epidermal hyperplasia and an inflammatory infiltrate of lymphocytes and plasma cells in the dermis (Singh and Romanowski, 1999). The result is the classic chancre of primary syphilis.

Syphilis is also vertically transmitted from an infected mother to her fetus, presumably by transplacental transfer. Alternatively, infection may occur during passage of the baby through the birth canal as a result of direct contact with an infectious lesion. The incubation period is highly variable. In an adult, the primary chancre may develop within three days of sexual contact with an infected individual. However, it can take as long as 90 days after exposure to appear (Singh and Romanowski, 1999). The congenitally infected infant, however, typically shows no clinical signs of syphilis at birth, but if untreated symptoms will develop weeks, months or even years later.

CLINICAL MANIFESTATIONS

There are four stages in the natural history of untreated syphilis, although they are not always distinct. These are primary, secondary, latent and tertiary syphilis.

Primary syphilis

Primary syphilis typically presents with the chancre on the genitals (glans penis of the male and cervix or external genitalia of the female). This is a single rounded, firm ulcer with well-defined margins and is usually painless. Occasionally, multiple lesions are present. Hearing loss is rarely a feature of primary syphilis unless there is concomitant secondary syphilis or neurosyphilis. However, classical primary syphilis does not always manifest and the primary infection may go unnoticed by the patient, so that hearing loss, often sudden, with or without vestibular symptoms, can sometimes be the first presenting feature of the disease (Hungerbuhler and Regli, 1978). As such hearing loss is potentially reversible with early treatment, it is very important syphilis is considered as a possible cause in sexually active patients presenting with sudden hearing loss (Balkany and Dans, 1978).

Secondary syphilis

Typically, the chancre of primary syphilis has been healed for about two months prior to the development of secondary syphilis. However, in up to a third of cases of secondary syphilis the chancre is still present. Conversely, as mentioned above, in many cases of secondary syphilis patients do not recall having had a primary lesion. The key feature of secondary syphilis is a skin rash, occurring as the presenting complaint in more than 70% of patients and present on examination in 90% (Zeltser and Kurban, 2004). The rash can vary in appearance and may be macular, maculopapular, follicular and sometimes pustular, thus mimicking a number of dermatological conditions. For this reason the diagnosis of syphilis may often be obtained via referral from a dermatologist.

Secondary syphilis is a multisystemic disease, affecting many organ systems in the body including the kidneys, liver and gastrointestinal tract and central nervous system. That the disease may also affect the inner ear has been long recognised and otosyphilis is most often a feature of secondary syphilis. Hearing loss caused by otosyphilis is usually sensorineural in nature. The symptoms can be varied: acute or fluctuating hearing loss, hearing difficulty, bilateral tinnitus, vertigo, giddiness/unsteadiness and sometimes spontaneous or provoked nystagmus (Kobayashi *et al.*, 1991). Some of these symptoms are similar to those of Ménière's disease and it is estimated that up to 7% of patients diagnosed as having Ménière's disease may have undiagnosed syphilis (Ammerman *et al.*, 2000). Similarly, occasional case reports suggest that a diagnosis of syphilis can be missed initially because neurosyphilis can mimic other neurological diseases (Ahmad and Lee, 1999).

It is thus important to recognise syphilis as a cause of hearing loss particularly because it causes one of the few forms of sensorineural hearing loss that can be reversed if diagnosed early enough and treated appropriately (Darmstadt and Harris, 1989). With the increased incidence of syphilis in Europe, North America and elsewhere, the medical profession is again having to familiarise itself with the many facets of this disease, including hearing loss. This is illustrated by a recent study in Germany by Klemm and Wollina (2004). A retrospective analysis of patients seen by a cooperating team of ear, nose and throat (ENT) and dermatology specialists over the period 1986–2000 was carried out. The team identified six cases of otosyphilis; none of these were HIV positive and although one had known congenital syphilis, none of the other patients had been aware of a sexually transmitted disease. Five of the six patients were being seen by a GP, or ENT or dermatology specialist because of skin rash and/or hearing impairment of varying degrees. The remaining patient who was initially diagnosed with familial hearing difficulty was identified as having syphilis during blood donor screening. Most of the patients were in the secondary stage of syphilis although one patient was in the early stage of the disease, suggesting that primary syphilis may also interfere with hearing. The authors concluded that clinical cooperation between dermatologists, sexually transmitted disease specialists and audiologists will be essential to ensure cases of otosyphilis are recognised and treated at the earliest opportunity to ensure the best outcome for the patient.

Tertiary syphilis

Secondary syphilis may resolve spontaneously, but approximately one-third of untreated patients develop late sequelae, typically 3–15 years, but possibly considerably longer, after the initial infection (Zeltser and Kurban, 2004). There are three common presentations of tertiary syphilis, late benign, cardiovascular or neurological, all of which are caused by a delayed-type hypersensitivity (DTH) response to treponemes present in tissue.

Late benign syphilis is the most common form (approximately 50% of cases). In this form of the disease almost any organ can be affected although skin lesions are the most obvious feature. The lesions may be varied and include granulomatous nodules, plaques, papules and gummas. The latter are painless red nodules that often ulcerate and, depending on the site, can cause severe tissue damage; e.g. upper respiratory gummas can cause perforation of the nasal septum or palate. It is known as late benign syphilis because the lesions themselves are rarely fatal or even very incapacitating, but clearly when they occur in organs such as bone or brain the term benign is a misnomer and serious sequelae will result.

Cardiovascular syphilis usually presents 10 to 30 years after the initial infection. The most common manifestation is syphilitic aortitis; although in the early stages it is usually asymptomatic, it may present as dull substernal ache in some patients or as heart failure in others. If untreated, clinical presentation with angina or aneurysm will occur after 10 or 20 years.

Neurosyphilis results from invasion of the cerebrospinal fluid by the spirochetes, although not all cases where the organism enters the CSF lead to neurosyphilis and the infection may resolve spontaneously or an asymptomatic meningitis may result. If an acute syphilitic meningitis does develop it can progress to meningovascular syphilis, or parenchymatous neurosyphilis, which usually manifests as tabes dorsalis or paresis (Singh and Romanowski, 1999).

Hearing loss in tertiary syphilis can be as a result of osteitis of the temporal bone that involves the membranous labyrinth (Ammerman *et al.*, 2000) or the presence of an intraauditory canal gumma (Little *et al.*, 1995). These primarily cause a conductive hearing loss. If neurosyphilis is present, then the eighth cranial nerve (cochlear-vestibular nerve) may be affected, which can result in a sensorineural hearing loss associated with tinnitus and vertigo.

Congenital syphilis

Congenital syphilis results from maternal syphilis and infection occurs when spirochetes present in the mother's blood cross the placenta and enter the blood and tissues of the developing fetus (Donley, 1993). It used to be thought that infection could not occur until after the fourth month of gestation (Darmstadt and Harris, 1989) as pathologic changes in the fetal tissue could not be demonstrated before this time and Langhaus cell layer of the cytotrophoblast was thought to form a barrier preventing the organism crossing the placenta. However, the Langhaus cell layer is known to persist throughout pregnancy (Benirschke, 1974), making this mechanism unlikely, and spirochetes have been detected in fetal tissue from spontaneous abortions occurring at 9 and 10 weeks gestation (Harter and Benirschke, 1976). Thus, it appears that infection can occur at any stage during gestation and the highest rate of fetal mortality and morbidity are reported when infection occurs and is untreated during the first and second trimesters. Third trimester infection is more likely to result in asymptomatic disease (Wendel, 1988). Congenital syphilis is rare in developed countries. This is consistent with the relatively low incidence of untreated syphilis in women in these countries and widespread screening for the disease during antenatal care.

The pathogenesis of congenital syphilis and in particular the role of the mother's immune system in relation to infection of the fetus is not fully understood. Transmission can occur at any stage of pregnancy but the risk of transmission is highly dependent on the mother's stage of disease. During primary syphilis the rate of vertical transmission in untreated women is 70 to 100%, which drops to 40% in early latent syphilis and 10% in late latent syphilis (Singh and Romanowski, 1999). Similarly, the outcome of infection in the infant is dependent on the mother's disease stage. The most affected infants are those conceived in (rather than born to) a mother with primary or secondary syphilis, whereas those conceived in a mother in the late stages of disease are less affected. Thus the poorest prognosis is for an infant infected during the first or second trimester by a mother in the primary or secondary stages of disease (Wicher and Wicher, 2001). This relationship is described by Kassowitz's law, which states that the longer the interval between infection and pregnancy, the more benign is the outcome in the infant. This phenomenon has been explained by some as related to treponeme load. Thus, in the early stages of disease a higher number of organisms is present in the mother, and a poor immune response in the early embryo/fetus permits increased bacterial replication in the first and second trimesters. However, this disregards the fact that the organism is actually quite rare in aborted fetuses or amniotic fluid from early pregnancy (Harter and Bernischke, 1976; Nathan *et al.*, 1997). As stated above, sequencing of the genome of *Treponema pallidum* revealed the high dependency of the organism on its host because of its limited biosynthetic capabilities (Fraser *et al.*, 1998). This suggests that survival of the pathogen in the embryo/fetal environment would be limited and explains the low numbers of organisms found; it does not, however, explain why infection early in gestation often results in fetal death whereas infection later in pregnancy, although just as likely to occur, often produces an asymptomatic infant. An interesting theory has recently been put forward to explain these findings (Wicher and Wicher, 2001). It is known that cytokine production is an active part of the process of implantation, growth and survival of the fetus (Robertson *et al.*, 1994). Production of these cytokines occurs locally and is a delicate balance; on the one hand, the cytokines produced must act to help to protect the developing fetus from infection and, on the other, must help to prevent rejection of the fetus as an allogeneic implant. Normally, in early pregnancy this balance is tilted towards protecting the fetus from the harmful effects of systemic or local inflammation, so that the antiinflammatory cytokines IL-10, IL-4 and TGF-β (a Th2-type immune response) are predominantly produced. Such a response is designed, not to be protective against infection but to limit damage to the fetus caused by inflammation (Lin *et al.*, 1993). In contrast, in the situation where a recently infected mother becomes pregnant, the inflammatory cytokines IL-2, IFN-γ and TNF-α (a Th1-type immune response) will be produced in response to her infection. Such a response at the maternal/fetal interface in early pregnancy is associated with fetal death, growth retardation and pre-term delivery (Hill, Polgar and Anderson, 1995). Thus the cytokine environment induced in the early gestation fetal–placental unit of a mother with a recent infection is likely to lead to fetal death. However, later in pregnancy when the fetal cytokine response may be stronger and tilted towards preservation of the pregnancy the maternal infection may not produce such a pronounced alteration in the local cytokine environment. This would help to preserve the fetus, but not protect it against infection. It might be further speculated that this scenario would favour an asymptomatic infection in the newborn infant and that only as its own postpartum immune response developed would symptoms of the infection appear. Similar mechanisms have been postulated for some other intrauterine infection; e.g. depressed cellular immune responses have been demonstrated in the second and third trimesters for both CMV (cytomegalovirus) and HSV (herpes simplex virus) (Gehrz *et al.*, 1981). However, as yet the hypothesis must be proven for syphilis.

Although the pathogenic mechanisms underlying the process remain to be elucidated it is known that transmission of syphilis from mother to fetus can result in fetal death, premature delivery or congenital syphilis. The manifestations of congenital syphilis at birth are varied, and again the factors underlying this are incompletely understood. Often the neonate is asymptomatic, or there may be clear multiorgan involvement. The manifestations of congenital syphilis are arbitrarily divided into early (those occurring in the first two years of life) and late (symptoms of disease occurring after the first two years). Early manifestations typically develop within the first few months of life. One of the earliest of these is persistent rhinitis with profuse nasal discharge (Figure 9.3). The discharge may be blood-tinged and is highly infectious. Other features include hepatomegaly, erythematous maculopapular rash and lymphadenopathy; indeed, the appearance of a newborn with congenital syphilis has been described as 'a little wrinkled potbellied old man with a cold in his head' (Nabarro, 1954). Hydrops fetalis may also be a manifestation of congenital

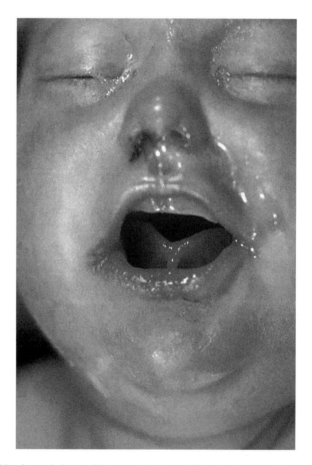

Figure 9.3. Newborn infant with congenital syphilis showing persistent rhinitis with profuse nasal discharge. (Courtesy of CDC/Dr Norman Cole)

syphilis in newborns. Late manifestations of congenital syphilis are malformations or stigmata, which represent scars induced by initial lesions of early congenital syphilis or result from ongoing inflammation. These include 'Hutchinson's triad' (Fiumara and Lessell, 1970), which consists of interstitial keratitis, peg-shaped upper incisors (Hutchinson's teeth) and eighth cranial nerve deafness. Hearing loss is the least common component of Hutchinson's triad and is typically present in around 3% of children with late congenital syphilis. It typically appears when the child is 8–10 years of age, although occasionally it may be delayed until adulthood. Onset is sudden and damage to the cranial nerve is thought to result from a persistent and ongoing inflammatory response to the infection. Mononuclear leukocytic infiltration and obliterative endarteritis are seen around the temporal bone and osteochondritis affects the otic capsule, which may lead to cochlear degeneration and fibrous adhesions. This results in eighth nerve deafness and vertigo (Ingall, Sanchez and Musher, 1995). Loss of hearing may be unilateral or bilateral and initially involves higher frequencies, with normal conversational tones affected later.

MANAGEMENT OF INFECTION

Laboratory diagnosis of syphilis is dealt with elsewhere (Chapter 14). Bone involvement by syphilis has a radiological picture that is consistent with the underlying pathology of an inflammatory resorptive osteitis. This results in patchy areas of bone resorption first replaced by fibrous tissues and then with fatty marrow, and gives rise to the 'motheaten' radiological appearance that is considered characteristic of syphilis osteitis (Sonne, Zeifer and Linstrom, 2002). Involvement of temporal bone and the ossicular chain is thought to be caused by such an osteitis and this can be seen as patchy lucencies by means of computed tomography. However, one must keep in mind that the differential diagnosis of otic capsule lucencies includes Paget's disease, otosclerosis and osteogenesis imperfecta. In addition, normal radiology does not exclude otic syphilis involvement.

The mainstay of treatment for syphilis is penicillin. The earlier penicillin is given, the greater the likelihood that the gross manifestations of syphilis will be prevented. However, even at a relatively late stage penicillin treatment can be beneficial. In order to ensure high levels of penicillin in the blood, it is given via the intramuscular route. For neurosyphilis and congenital syphilis the intravenous route is used (Singh and Romanowski, 1999). For individuals allergic to penicillin, there are alternatives such as doxycycline, erythromycin and ceftriaxone. For a full account of the management of syphilis the reader is referred to the *Sexually Transmitted Diseases Treatment Guidelines 2002* (Centers of Disease Control and Prevention, 2002). Because of the inflammatory element in otosyphilis systemic steroids are often used, in addition, when there is evidence of otologic disease. However, this has not been proven to be beneficial (Centers of Disease Control and Prevention, 2002).

HIV/AIDS and hearing loss

THE AIDS EPIDEMIC

A mysterious illness made its appearance in the late 1970s and early 1980s. It appeared to affect mainly homosexual men and caused severe immunodeficiency, leaving individuals highly susceptible to opportunistic infection which, in the absence of an effective immune response, often had a fatal course. The term Acquired Immunodeficiency Syndrome (AIDS) was coined to describe the disease. The aetiological agent of AIDS was identified in 1984 as a retrovirus, later named human immunodeficiency virus (HIV) (Montagnier, 2002). At that time the disease appeared largely confined to North America and Western Europe. However, it rapidly became apparent that the major focus of the disease was sub-Saharan Africa and that its principal route of transmission was via heterosexual contact.

By December 2004, the WHO estimated that 39.4 million people are living with HIV/AIDS, including 2.2 million children. In the same year 4.9 million new HIV infections occurred and 3.1 million, including 510 000 children, died from the disease (WHO, 2004c). The disproportional spread of the disease can be seen from the fact that sub-Saharan Africa is home to just over 10% of the World's population, but around 60% (25.4 million) of the total people infected with HIV come from this region. In 2004, 3.1 million people there became newly infected and 2.3 million died.

Although HIV/AIDS in North America and Western Europe continues to be most prevalent in gay men and injecting drug users, cases resulting from heterosexual transmission are increasing in number; e.g. in the UK, surveillance figures show that from 1999 onwards more new infections have been acquired via heterosexual than homosexual contact (Health Protection Agency, 2004b). Foreign travel and contact with an infected individual from a high prevalence area are key risk factors.

HEARING LOSS IN AIDS PATIENTS

HIV has a tropism for T helper lymphocytes. These cells are key orchestraters of the cell-mediated and humoral immune response. The virus infects and destroys these cells, effectively disabling the immune system and leaving the host susceptible to infection (Bankaitis and Schountz, 1998). In this situation, infection with normally nonpathogenic or mildly pathogenic organisms can result in severe opportunistic disease (Table 9.1). It is the effects of such opportunistic infection and sometimes malignant disease on the central nervous system and ear that most often causes hearing loss in people with HIV.

It is still unclear whether HIV can directly cause hearing loss. However, there have been a number of case reports of sensorineural hearing loss in

Table 9.1. The most common opportunistic infections
contracted by HIV-infected individuals

1. Candidiasis
2. *Pneumocystis carinii* infection
3. Cytomegalovirus
5. *Cryptococcus* infection
6. Toxoplasmosis
7. *Mycobacterium* infections
8. Syphilis
9. *Staphylococcus aureus*
10. Herpes zoster

Adapted from Bankaitis and Schountz, 1998.

patients found to be HIV positive, but with no other clear cause for their hearing loss (Timon and Walsh, 1989; Grimaldi *et al.*, 1993). HIV is neurotropic as well as lymphotrophic and a high proportion of AIDS patients demonstrate central nervous system involvement. It is certainly plausible that HIV could have a direct effect on the eighth cranial nerve that results in sensorineural hearing loss. A correlation of pure-tone hearing loss and clinical stage of HIV disease has been demonstrated, but only in advanced cases (Birchall *et al.*, 1992). This study had strict inclusion and exclusion criteria, excluding individuals where hearing loss was likely to have a cause not directly related to HIV infection. The correlation found may indicate hearing loss that is due to the direct neurological effects of HIV.

It is clear, though, that most cases of hearing loss associated with AIDS arise not from the effects of the virus itself but from infection with one of the numerous opportunistic pathogens to which these immunocompromised patients are susceptible. A summary of the various reports of involvement of some of these agents with hearing loss in AIDS patients is given below.

Aspergillosis

Aspergillosis is caused by a fungus (*Aspergillus*), which is commonly found growing on dead leaves, stored grain, compost piles or in other decaying vegetation. In individuals with AIDS it typically causes an invasive infection characterised by pneumonia. However, a case where the organism was thought to cause hearing loss has been reported in a 28 year old man (Linstrom *et al.*, 1993). In this instance there was fungal involvement of the middle ear, mastoid and petrous apex cells. Following radical mastoidectomy and petrous apicectomy, pathologic examination of removed tissue revealed chronic osteomyelitis. *Aspergillus* grew on culture. It is likely that this is a rare manifestation of *Aspergillus* infection.

Cryptococcosis

Cryptococcosis is infection caused by the fungus *Cryptococcus neoformans*. *Cryptococcus* infection is largely confined to immunocompromised patients and was relatively rare until the AIDS epidemic began. Cryptococcosis is the most frequent fungal infection of the central nervous system and mainly occurs in the tissues covering the brain and spinal cord (meninges), resulting in meningitis (Prada *et al.*, 1996), although it is also sometimes found in the lungs and on the skin. Other organs are occasionally involved. Cryptococcal meningitis can cause blindness, possibly through a direct effect on the optic nerve. It can also affect other cranial nerves including the eighth cranial nerve, which can result in hearing loss. This nerve damage may be due to direct infection of the nerve or compression from infection around it, or simply the indirect effect of raised intracranial pressure from the meningitic infection.

Cytomegalovirus (CMV)

CMV is a common cause of meningoencephalitis and peripheral nerve infection in people with AIDS, which often presents as central and peripheral neurological manifestations. Cranial nerves can be involved, though involvement of the eighth cranial nerve is unusual. However, two cases of CMV in patients with HIV that involved the eighth cranial nerve have been described (Meynard *et al.*, 1997). Both cases presented with hearing loss, tinnitus and dizzy spells.

Kaposi's sarcoma

Kaposi's sarcoma is an opportunistic mesenchymal malignancy associated with HIV-infected persons. It is characterised by brown/purple lesions appearing on the skin and affects capillaries, lymph nodes and connective tissue. It can also cause otological manifestations, either by growth of the lesions on the external ear or growth within the nasopharynx, which can affect the inner ear (Morris and Prasad, 1990). This latter involvement may result in conductive hearing loss (Rarey, 1990).

Herpes zoster oticus

Infection with the varicella zoster virus (VZV) occurs frequently in immuno-compromised patients, including those with AIDS. As with all herpes virus infections, VZV establishes latency in its host after the primary infection. In the case of VZV the site of latency is the trigeminal and dorsal root ganglia. The primary infection with this virus is varicella or chickenpox and reactivation causes herpes zoster or shingles.

Patients with HIV are more prone to reactivation and when this occurs in the geniculate ganglion of the seventh cranial nerve it causes a condition known as Ramsay Hunt syndrome or herpes zoster oticus (Mishell and Applebaum, 1990). An acute facial paralysis occurs in association with herpetic blisters of the skin of the ear canal and/or the auricle. As well as deep otalgia on the affected side, other symptoms include vertigo, ipsilateral hearing loss, tinnitus, and facial paresis. These symptoms are due to involvement of the geniculate ganglion, which is located near the petrous pyramid portion of the temporal bone where the ear apparatus is located, and to that of the ganglia of Corti and Scarpa, which are located in the inner ear and involved with hearing and balance (Byl and Adour, 1976). The facial paresis is caused by inflammation of the facial nerve, which runs through the inner and middle ear.

Extrapulmonary pneumocystosis

Pneumocystis carinii infection was a very rare cause of human disease prior to the present HIV epidemic. However, prior to the widespread introduction in the developed world of combination antiretroviral therapy it was estimated that between 66 and 85% of all HIV-1 infected individuals would have at least one episode of *Pneumocystis carinii* pneumonia (PCP) in their lifetime (Ng, Yajko and Hadley, 1997). This incidence has dropped considerably because of effective treatment regimes, but PCP remains a major problem in AIDS patients. In contrast, extrapulmonary *Pneumocystis* infection is comparatively rare. In HIV-infected individuals, *Pneumocystis* can infect a variety of extrapulmonary sites including the ear, eye, thyroid, spleen and liver. Infection of the ear can manifest as hearing loss and aural pain and therefore should be considered when an HIV patient presents with hearing loss. In most reported cases it is the middle ear that is involved, sometimes associated with an aural polyp protruding through the tympanic membrane (Wasserman and Haghighi, 1992; Ng, Yajko and Hadley, 1997). The presentation, therefore, is a conductive hearing loss.

Syphilis

Syphilis and HIV are both sexually transmitted diseases so it is unsurprising that syphilis is more common in HIV-infected individuals compared to the general population. Syphilis can cause hearing loss (see the section above on 'Syphilis and hearing loss'), but there is evidence that the progression of hearing loss due to syphilis is accelerated in HIV patients (Smith and Canalis, 1989). Otosyphilis needs to be considered in any HIV patient with fluctuating, asymmetric or sudden hearing loss.

CHILDREN WITH HIV/AIDS

Hearing loss can be the presenting feature in a child infected with HIV as well as being a later feature in established HIV disease. Recurrent otitis media and chronic sinusitis are common presenting symptoms of paediatric AIDS (Matkin, Diefendorf and Erenberg, 1998), particularly in young children. Eustachian tube maturation appears to reduce the prevalence of otitis media in older children with HIV infection as it does in uninfected children. Sensorineural hearing loss in HIV-infected children is mainly due to opportunistic infections and the ototoxicity of drugs used to treat HIV and its sequelae. This is much the same as in adults.

DRUG-RELATED HEARING LOSS

In the 25 years since the AIDS epidemic began, many drugs have been developed to treat people with an HIV infection. None of these drugs yet provide a cure for HIV infection and development of viral resistance against individual drugs is a considerable problem. However, enormous advances have been made, most notably the implementation of the drug combination regimen known as highly active antiretroviral therapy (HAART). Such regimens have resulted in HIV-infected individuals remaining AIDS free for much longer periods and increasing their life expectancy, in some cases, to normal terms. However, all anti-HIV drugs have side-effects and one relatively common side-effect is hearing loss, usually sensorineural in nature. For example, didanosine is an antiviral agent used to treat patients with HIV, often in combination with Zidovudine. This combination has been found to be effective in treating children, improving growth and weight gain as well as improving declining cognitive function and motor skills (Christensen *et al.*, 1998). However, both these drugs have been associated with hearing loss in HIV patients and are, therefore, potentially ototoxic. Zalcitabine is used as an anti-HIV treatment both as a single agent and in combination with Zidovudine. The main side-effect associated with this agent is a peripheral neuropathy. However, there have been case reports of an associated sensorineural hearing loss (Monte, Fenwick and Monteiro, 1997).

It is not just anti-HIV drugs that have to be considered when faced with drug-related hearing loss in HIV patients. Drug treatment for opportunistic infection may also be related to hearing loss. For example, most of the mycobacterial infections in HIV patients are due to *Mycobacterium avium* complex (MAC) infection. Some of the drugs used to treat people with MAC infection, such as amikacin, azithromycin and clarithromycin, are ototoxic (Hoy, Marriott and Gottlieb, 1996).

Fungal infections such as candidiasis are very common in HIV-infected individuals and drug treatments include amphotericin B, flucytosine and ketoconazole. All these medications are associated with hearing loss, tinnitus and vertigo (Bankaitis and Schountz, 1998). Treatments for *Pneumocystis carinii* infection, such as pentamidine, TMP/SMX and primoquine, have also been associated with hearing loss.

Other sexually transmitted infections and hearing loss

None of the other sexually transmitted diseases are significantly associated with hearing loss. Some, such as *Neisseria gonorrhoeae*, the bacterium that causes gonorrhoea, can occasionally be associated with meningitis, which may result in hearing loss, but this is discussed elsewhere (Chapter 11).

Genital herpes, caused by either herpes simplex virus type 1 or type 2, causes genital ulcers and the virus can be transmitted perinatally to a newborn, causing congenital herpes or birth-acquired herpes. Intrauterine infection with herpes simplex is rare, but can occur if the mother has a primary infection. The virus is transmitted to the fetus via the placenta and causes severe disseminated disease in the infant, including brain damage and eye disease, such as inflammation of the retina, chorioretinitis and skin lesions. This form of congenital herpes is usually fatal. More usually the infection is acquired during passage of the baby through the birth canal. If ulcerative disease is present then an elective caesarean section can be performed. However, often active genital herpes infection is asymptomatic and the mother may be unaware she is infected. In this situation the baby is infected from the mother's genital secretions via the mucous membranes. Neonatal herpes has several different forms. It can produce localised or systemic disease whereby infants may develop only a localised skin infection consisting of small fluid-filled blisters or vesicles that rupture, crust over and finally heal, often leaving a mild scar behind. A second manifestation of neonatal herpes infection leads to encephalitis, an inflammation of the brain that can result in seizures and later neurological problems including hearing loss. If untreated, it may lead to death. The third type of infection is the most devastating; a disseminated herpes infection occurs involving many internal organs including the liver, lungs, kidneys and brain. There may or may not be vesicles on the skin. Hearing loss is just one of many sequelae. This type of infection is frequently fatal.

Conclusions

Hearing loss can have many causes. For this reason it is important to take an extensive history from any patient presenting with unexplained hearing loss. Previous sexually transmitted infection must be considered, in particular the possibility of an infection with syphilis and/or HIV. A recent history of foreign travel or sexual contact with an individual from an area where the prevalence of HIV and syphilis is relatively high may be indicative. Both syphilis and HIV can cause conductive hearing impairment (e.g. intra-auditory canal gumma in syphilis and chronic otitis media infection in AIDS) and sensorineural hearing loss (e.g. neurosyphilis and opportunistic cytomegalovirus infection in AIDS). However, people infected with syphilis or HIV can be asymptomatic for long periods of time. The appearance of hearing loss may occasionally be the first indication of infection.

10 OTITIS MEDIA

J.J. Gröte and P.J. Vallely

General introduction

Otitis media (OM) is the most common bacterial infection of childhood and, in developed countries, is probably second only to upper respiratory tract infections as the illness for which medical intervention is most frequently sought. The incidence of the condition is variable with geography, season and age of the cohort under study, but most studies reveal high prevalence rates; indeed, some US studies showed 90% of infants had suffered at least one episode of OM during their first two years of life (Casselbrant *et al.*, 1995; Paradise *et al.*, 1997). OM is simply defined as inflammation within the middle ear space caused by infection. However, because of the anatomical borders of this part of the skull, otitis media may be linked with complications such as meningitis, encephalitis, brain abscess, sigmoid sinus, thrombosis, facial palsy and also labyrinthitis. Thus the inner ear can be at stake in otitis media and temporary or permanent hearing loss can occur.

Pathogenesis of OM

The middle ear and mastoid cleft is lined with mucosa and is connected to the nasopharynx via the Eustachian tube (see Figure 1.1). In an infant or young child the Eustachian tube is shorter, broader and more horizontal than that found in an older child or adult. This may make it easier for a pathogen to reach the middle ear from the nasopharynx in this younger age group and is perhaps the explanation for why young children are more prone to otitis media

Infection and Hearing Impairment. Edited by V.E. Newton and P.J. Vallely
© 2006 John Wiley & Sons, Ltd

than adults. However, the Eustachian tube has different functions such as aer-
ation, pressure regulation and clearance, and it is possible that Eustachian tube
dysfunction may also contribute to development of OM in children. In the
normal ear it is mostly closed via the velopalatine muscle, to separate the
nasopharynx and the middle ear cleft. Good function of the opening/closure
mechanism of the Eustachian tube, especially the function of the velopalatine
muscle, is important as constant closure will cause underpressure in the middle
ear cleft by resorption of oxygen, which makes the middle ear prone to inflammation and infection. Efficient function of this muscle develops with age,
as does the lumen of the entrance of the Eustachian tube. In support of the
idea that dysfunction of the Eustachian tube is a risk factor for development
of OM is the fact that in children with a history of otitis media, the active
Eustachian tube function has been found to be poorer than in otologically
normal children (Bylander, 1984). In fact, disturbance of ventilation and
clearance via the Eustachian tube, in combination with an upper airway
infection, is considered by most to be the main cause for otitis media, although
OM can also occur via the ear canal if a perforation exists in the tympanic
membrane.

Also relevant to the explanation of why children are more prone to development of otitis media than adults is the fact that because of insufficient
immunological defence they are more prone to infections (Rosenfeld, 1998).
It is now widely recognised that a viral infection of the upper respiratory tract
is usually the initiating factor for OM (Darrow, Dash and Derkay, 2003;
Heikkinen and Chonmaitree, 2003). The infection causes congestion of the
nasal and nasopharyngeal mucosa, which in turn leads to congestion in the
Eustachian tube, affecting its normal function. This causes impairment of
the pressure equilibrium between the nasopharynx and the middle ear cavity,
decreased drainage of secretions from the middle ear into the nasopharynx
and reduced ciliary clearance of invading particles including bacterial
pathogens. This latter mechanism is important as the mucociliary system is one
of the airway's most important defences against inhaled or invading particles
such as bacteria and viruses (Ohashi and Nakai, 1991).

As a result, pathogens from the nasopharynx are able to gain access to the
middle ear where they multiply and cause otitis media. This is exacerbated in
young children because, although in the first few months the baby has some
immune protection from the mother, particularly if breastfeeding is continued,
it takes several years before the child develops a robust immune response of
its own. This is the main reason why after the age of seven, in general, children have fewer upper airway infections and consequently less otitis media.
Also after this age the adenoids are in regression, which helps prevent congestion. However, in children of all ages, as well as in adults, rhinosinusitis can
cause otitis media and can be the reason for recurrent otitis media. In the case
of recurrent OM an upper airway infection is not always necessary because
bacteria colonise in the mucosa of the middle ear.

Many factors can change or complicate the natural course of otitis media, such as inherited or acquired immune disturbance (e.g. hypogammaglobulinaemia, HIV) or other defence disturbances (e.g. immotile cilia syndrome). Congenital defects of the anatomy such as palatoschisis leading to Eustachian tube dysfunction will also lead to recurrent otitis media (Kubba, Pearson and Birchall, 2000). Moreover, reflux of gastric juice into the tube is easier in children because of the supine position in which children are often placed (Tasker *et al.*, 2002). Reflux might cause transient damage to the Eustachian tube and middle ear mucosa, resulting in ideal conditions for secondary bacterial colonisation (Ru and Grote, 2004).

Otitis media can be present in different clinical forms and this is often the reason for confusion and discussion. In time a distinction is made between acute and chronic otitis media (as otitis media is considered chronic if it lasts longer than 3 months). However, more important is the distinction between the different clinical presentations: acute otitis media (AOM), otitis media with effusion (OME) and chronic otitis media (COM). Chronic otitis media can be suppurative or with cholesteatoma. The different types of otitis media can lead to sequelae such as tympanic membrane perforations, resorption of middle ear ossicles, tympanosclerosis and fibrosis, and will also influence the function of the inner ear. The features of each type of OM are discussed later in the chapter.

Microbiology of otitis media

BACTERIAL CAUSES OF OTITIS MEDIA

Numerous studies have consistently identified the three major pathogens involved in AOM as *Streptococcus pneumoniae, Haemophilus influenzae* and *Moraxella catarrhalis* (Harrison, Marks and Welch, 1985; Bluestone, Stephenson and Martin, 1992; Pichichero and Pichichero, 1995; del Castillo, Garcia-Perea and Baquero-Artigao, 1996; Jacobs *et al.*, 1998; Arguedas *et al.*, 2003). Review of the literature suggests that *S. pneumoniae* is the most common cause (30–50% of cases), it is also the most virulent, being associated with more severe clinical findings, and is the organism most often involved when complications arise with OM. More than 90 pneumococcal serotypes have been identified to date, but of these six (3, 6B, 9V, 14, 19F and 23F) are most commonly associated with otitis media. *H. influenzae* is the next most commonly detected organism in most studies (15–25%) and is often associated with bilateral OM and with related eye symptoms such as otitis conjunctivitis syndrome. In contrast, *M. catarrhalis* is found less often (10–15%) and appears to be less virulent than the other organisms, but may be more commonly associated with a mixed infection.

However, in recent years evidence has emerged that the epidemiological pattern of infection has changed. In 2000, a multivalent conjugate vaccine against pneumococcus was licensed. This vaccine is immunogenic in infants, inducing a systemic and mucosal immune response and reducing nasopharyngeal carriage of the pneumococci (Eskola *et al.*, 2001). Widespread administration of this heptavalent pneumococcal conjugate vaccine resulted in an overall small decrease (6–7%) in acute otitis media resulting from any cause and a more substantial decrease (24%) in severe or frequent OM requiring insertion of tympanostomy tubes (Eskola *et al.*, 2001; Fireman *et al.*, 2003). Significantly, however, a large study of the efficacy of the vaccine from Finland noted a 34% decrease in culture-confirmed episodes of pneumococcal OM, a 57% decrease in the number of episodes of AOM due to serotypes included in the vaccine, but an overall increase of 33% in episodes caused by serotypes not included in the vaccine (Eskola *et al.*, 2001). This may be due to so-called 'replacement phenomenon', whereby the reduction of vaccine-included serotypes of *S. pneumoniae* in the nasopharynx is associated in most studies with an increase in carriage of nonvaccine serotypes of the organism (Veenhoven *et al.*, 2003; Dagan, 2004), or even of other different organisms such as *Staphylococcus aureus* (Veenhoven *et al.*, 2003; Bogaert *et al.*, 2004).

Casey and Pichichero (2004) noted an increase in the proportion of *H. influenzae* isolated from middle ear fluids from 38% in the 1995–7 time period to 57% during 2001–3, and they suggest that *H. influenzae* has replaced *S. pneumoniae* as the predominant pathogen for persistent AOM. In contrast, using data taken from the control arm of the Finnish study on AOM, Palmu *et al.* (2004) found *S. pneumoniae* was still the most common pathogen but noted an increase in the proportion of cases due to *H. influenzae* and *M. catarrhalis*, with *M. catarrhalis* isolated more often than *H. influenzae*.

As mentioned above, there has been a relatively small decrease in the overall incidence of OM following introduction of the pneumococcal vaccine and thus it seems that incidence of OM due to organisms other than *S. pneumoniae* and to nonvaccine serotypes of *S. pneumoniae* is increasing (McEllistrem *et al.*, 2003). This is likely to have important pathogenic implications for future management of OM and for vaccine implementation.

The widespread use of antibiotics for the treatment of OM has led to the development of antibiotic-resistant strains of the commonly associated organisms. Although the prevalence of antibiotic resistance appears to differ between different geographical areas, probably due to local differences in use of antibiotic treatment practices (Nielsen *et al.*, 2004; van Kempen *et al.*, 2004). The risk factors for development of resistance include prolonged, low-dose treatment with β-lactam antibiotics coupled with close contact between children, such as occurs in daycare centres. This allows development of resistance within the child and spread of resistant strains between children. *S. pneumoniae* resistance to penicillin has increased steadily over the last two decades: a recently published study by Hoberman *et al.* (2005) found that 31.5% of pneumococcal strains isolated from children with AOM undergoing tympanocentesis between 1991 and 2003 at the Children's Hospital of Pittsburgh were nonsusceptible to penicillin. There was also an increasing trend over time for isolation of nonsusceptible or resistant strains. In an earlier US study, Sutton *et al.* (2000) identified 38% of *S. pneumoniae* isolates cultured from middle ear effusions from children undergoing tympanostomy that were penicillin resistant. Similarly, *H. influenzae* and *M. catarrhalis* develop drug resistance by production of β-lactamase, an enzyme that inactivates β-lactam antibiotics. In the study by Sutton *et al.* (2000), 65% of *H. influenzae* and 100% of *M. catarrhalis* isolates were β-lactamase producers.

Most pneumococcus antibiotic resistance is found within five serotypes (and as these are the most common in children they are included in all the available pneumoccoccus vaccines). As widespread use of the vaccine has reduced the incidence of those serotypes included in the vaccine, it follows that circulation of antibiotic-resistant strains of *S. pneumoniae* has also decreased, as has the incidence of OM caused by such strains. However, as described above, this has led to an increase in the incidence of OM caused by other organisms including *H. influenzae*. Casey and Pichichero (2004) observed an increase in the frequency of *H. influenzae* producing β-lactamase, thus replacing penicillin-resistant *S. pneumoniae*. The currently available vaccine against *H. influenzae* is a conjugated type b vaccine and as virtually all OM caused by *H. influenzae* is due to nontypeable strains the vaccine is ineffective in helping to prevent OM caused by this organism. Other vaccine approaches are under development (Cripps, Otczyk and Kyd, 2005).

Although *S. pneumoniae, H. influenzae* and *M. catarrhalis* are the most common microorganisms responsible for acute otitis media, *Staphylococcus aureus* can also be the causative organism. However, *S. aureus* together with *Pseudomonas aeruginosa* and various anaerobic bacteria are more typically isolated in chronic otitis media. Chronic otitis media is often the result of polymicrobial infection with Gram-positive and -negative bacteria. Anaerobic microorganisms that can be cultured in chronic otitis media include *Fusobacterium* sp., pigmented *Prevotella*, *Bacteroides* spp. and *Porphyromonas* spp. (Brook, 1995). Many of these organisms also produce β-lactamase, leading to antibiotic resistance.

THE ROLE OF BIOFILMS

New research indicates that bacteria preferentially exist in biofilms; these are complex, surface-attached communities of bacterial cells. They probably represent an ancient prokaryotic survival strategy as the bacteria are formed into an organised structure and are able to communicate with each other in a cooperative manner, thereby conveying considerable survival advantages over bacteria existing in a planktonic state (Post *et al.*, 2004). The bacterial biofilm is a slime-like matrix composed of polysaccharides, nucleic acids and proteins, and the bacteria are organised into cellular towers composed of complex exopolysaccharide-enclosed microcolonies. Water channels run between these, allowing the exchange of nutrients and removal of waste products from the system. Each bacterium within the system has its own phenotypic character-istics and occupies a particular microenvironment. Radically different microenvironments can exist in close proximity and because of this, aerobic and anaerobic bacteria can live in the same biofilm. This effectively affords the biofilm some of the characteristics of a complex multicellular organism (Post *et al.*, 2004).

There are clearly considerable advantages to life in a biofilm; the individual bacteria are protected from fluctuations in the environment, they are afforded some protection from the host immune system as they are too large to be phagocytosed and most will be protected from attack by antibody-mediated defence mechanisms. A further interesting phenomenon is that they seem to have considerably increased resistance to antibiotics than do equivalent plank-tonic bacterial colonies. This may be due to the lower metabolic rate that exists within the biofilm, preventing the antibiotic being metabolised and reaching its active form (Brown, Allison and Gilbert, 1988). Additionally, it is known that transfer of genetic material from one organism to another can occur within a biofilm and thus transfer of resistance factors to antibiotics may take place. In addition, if the biofilm contains some β-lactamase producing bacte-ria, this enzyme can act to protect other nonresistant species (Fergie *et al.*, 2004).

The idea that biofilms may have a role in chronic OM is gaining increasing popularity. Although a causative organism can be identified in most AOM cul-tures, most COM effusions are culture negative, leading to the conclusion that OM with effusion (OME) is primarily an inflammatory process. However, when polymerase chain reaction techniques (which detect bacterial genome) are used to test effusion fluids, many organisms are detected that would be missed by traditional culture techniques (which require growth of the organ-ism). There is increasing evidence that OME is caused by an active bacterial infection in the form of a biofilm on the mucosa of the middle ear, which induces an inflammatory process resulting in an exudate. The fact that inser-tion of tympanostomy tubes is an effective treatment for OME is under-standable if the biofilm hypothesis is considered; the procedure bypasses the dysfunctional Eustachian tube and reventilates the middle ear space. This both disrupts the biofilm and restores the oxygen concentration in the middle ear, promoting the regrowth of the ciliated epithelial cells responsible for bacterial clearance and reducing the number of secretory cells present in the middle ear. This allows clearance of the biofilm and resolution of the effusion (Post *et al.*, 2004). Indeed, biofilms have been demonstrated on tympanostomy tubes in children with refractory post-tympanostomy otorrhoea (Post, 2001). Further, *H. influenzae* biofilms have been experimentally induced in the middle ear in an animal (chinchilla) model (Post, 2001). Thus although direct evidence, in the form of visualisation of a bacterial biofilm within the middle ear space, has not yet been obtained, the likelihood that they play a role in this condition is increasing.

VIRAL INVOLVEMENT IN OTITIS MEDIA

The involvement of bacterial microrganisms in AOM has been described above; however, it would appear that in most cases the initiating factor is in fact a viral infection, typically a respiratory virus infection of the upper airways. The pathogenic mechanisms underlying this have been discussed earlier and it is clear that viruses play a crucial role in the development of acute otitis media. It is important to consider the relative importance of particular viral infections as this may help in the management of disease. A study conducted in 1999 by Heikkinen, Thint and Chonmaitree determined the prevalence of a range of common respiratory viruses in the middle ear fluid taken from 456 children with AOM. They also tested nasal-wash specimens taken at the same time and looked for the presence of specific antibody in matched serum specimens. They identified a specific viral respiratory infection in 186 out of 456 (41%) cases. Of those children infected with respiratory syncytial virus (RSV), 74% also harboured this virus in middle ear fluid. Parainfluenza virus was found in the ears of 52% of children with a parainfluenza respiratory infection and influenza in 42%. Ear involvement was less commonly found with enterovirus infection (11%) or adenovirus infection (4%). This study reflects the findings in many others where rates of viral detection in the nasopharyngeal specimens of children with AOM range from 30 to 50%, with RSV, influenza, parainfluenza and adenoviruses most commonly found. In addition, human cytomegalovirus and herpes simplex virus have been identified in middle ear fluid of children with AOM (Chonmaitree et al., 1992a). However, most of these studies have been conducted using relatively insensitive culture methods and where molecular detection methods have been employed, detection rates are much higher (Heikkinen and Chonmaitree, 2003). The effect of middle ear infection with a particular virus on the outcome of AOM is largely unknown; there are a few studies that suggest that viruses are more commonly detected in cases where symptoms are prolonged or where there is treatment failure (Arola et al., 1990; Chonmaitree et al., 1992b), but this is an area that clearly warrants further investigation. However, current findings suggest that vaccination against RSV, parainfluenza and influenza may be helpful in reducing the incidence of AOM.

Any consideration of the role of viruses in otitis media would be incomplete without reference to measles virus infection. Otitis media is the most common complication of measles, occurring in 5–15% of reported measles cases in developed countries (Leach and Jensen, 2002). The symptoms of OM usually present after the typical measles rash has faded. Measles virus and its potential role in hearing loss including that in OM are discussed in Chapter 7.

Types of otitis media

ACUTE OTITIS MEDIA (AOM)

In developed countries acute otitis media is regarded in children as a self-limiting disease. Most children can overcome the infection without antibiotics and only pain medication. From recent systemic literature review and meta-analysis it can be concluded that the natural history of acute otitis media, especially in children, is very favourable. In the majority of children it will not become a fully developed bacterial infection, with *Haemophilus influenzae* or *Streptococcus pneumoniae* bacteria, but will recover after the painful inflammation phase. AOM symptoms improve within 24 hours without antibiotics in 61% of children, rising to 80% by 2 to 3 days. Suppurative complications were comparable if antibiotics were withheld or provided. The natural history of otitis media in babies and children who may have problems clearing the infection needs a different approach. Particularly if complications take place, a more aggressive approach is necessary.

In developing countries the natural course is different, leading more to purulent otitis, often with perforation and further complications. Whether the change in the natural history of otitis media in children in developed countries is only due to a better immunological status or better hygiene or a combination of both is not known. It is also possible that the disease itself and the bacteria involved are changing.

In adults, acute otitis media is rare and is often associated with chronic upper airway infections. Patients with immune deficiency are also prone to OM, especially those with HIV and patients with tumours in the nasopharynx. In these patients complications can be more severe.

In babies and children who are prone to otitis media and in adults, antibiotics still play a role. This is also true for all patients with acute otitis media and complications. The functioning of the inner ear needs to be tested and followed up in these patients.

OTITIS MEDIA WITH EFFUSION (OME)

Otitis media with effusion is the status of the middle ear cleft with fluid of variable consistence. This fluid can be water with or without air bubbles or a sticky fluid called glue.

The pathogenesis is still under discussion. Previously it was explained as the result of underpressure due to Eustachian tube dysfunction, with this underpressure resulting in inflammation and exudate (Sade, 1994; Kubba, Pearson and Birchall, 2000). An infection was excluded because bacteria could not be cultured. However, improved techniques and experiments showed that the bacteria involved in acute otitis media were also present in the effusion (Brook *et al.*, 1983; Hotomi *et al.*, 1993; Post *et al.*, 1995), and as discussed above bacterial biofilms may also be a factor.

OME is not regarded as a serious disease in the majority of cases. More than 90% of children will have a period of OME in their youth. Recent studies show that the bacterial products after acute or chronic infection, endo- and exo-toxins, stimulate the middle ear mucosa to change into secretary epithelium for clearance (Hesseling et al., 1994; Nell et al., 1999). The persistence of these products leads to an increased proliferation of the mucosa and the secretion, whereas the cilia disappear and this prevents clearance. Only in patients without clearance after 3 months does this OME become chronic and have its effect. The associated conductive loss may influence the development of the child, but this is not yet proven in long-term follow-up.

The effusion with its high concentration of bacterial products has its influence on the tympanic membrane, middle ear, ossicles and probably on the inner ear. Whether chronic OME has an increased risk for the inner ear is not yet clear. Otitis media with effusion can be regarded as part of a self-limiting disease. Chronic OME might need treatment. The only effective temporary treatment is a tympanostomy ventilation tube. Risk groups, as described in acute otitis media, need to be followed up and the long-term risks for the inner ear have to be studied. After acute otitis media a period of otitis media with effusion follows in 50% of the cases.

CHRONIC OTITIS MEDIA

For this disease there is no universally accepted system of nomenclature, but any inflammatory disease in the middle ear for a period greater than 3 months is considered to be chronic. A chronic purulent draining ear via a perforation is termed a suppurative otitis media. Another type of chronic otitis media is cholesteatoma. This disease can be present behind a closed tympanic membrane, but is mostly accompanied by a draining ear.

CHRONIC SUPPURATIVE OTITIS MEDIA

A draining ear, with purulent discharge and conductive hearing loss, is the presenting symptom in these patients. The perforation can be caused by infection, trauma, retraction pockets after infections and therapeutic interventions such as ventilation tubes. The mucosa is thickened and has a lot of goblet cells with secretion and few cilia, leading to chronicity.

Epidemiological studies are limited but specific racial groups such as Native Americans, Innuits and Aboriginals are more prone to chronic suppurative otitis media. This is also seen in Africa. Chronic suppurative otitis media in these ethnic groups is rarely associated with cholesteatoma.

Chronic otitis media present with long-standing disease leads to irreversible mucosal changes with fibrosis. A conductive hearing loss can occur via bone erosion of the ossicles. Labyrinthitis may also develop from the purulent infection of the middle ear, resulting in inner ear hearing loss.

Acute suppurative labyrinthitis occurs most often in patients with congenital labyrinthine deformations such as Mondini's deformity. This can lead to a deaf ear.

The relationship between sensorineural hearing loss and chronic otitis media remains controversial. Retrospective studies demonstrated an association, but the magnitude of hearing loss was small, ranging between 5 and 15 dB depending on the frequency tested. The conductive loss caused by COM is more important.

CHRONIC OTITIS MEDIA WITH CHOLESTEATOMA

A cholesteatoma is a cyst in the middle ear mastoid cleft lined with squamous cell epithelium filled with debris. The pathogenesis of this disease is still unknown. A minority may arise behind the closed tympanic membrane in the middle ear of the petrosal bone through congenital origin. The majority, however, come from the epithelium of the tympanic membrane. It is skin in the wrong place. The stimulus that causes the keratinocytes to proliferate and give rise to terminal differentiation is still unknown.

A middle ear with a cholesteatoma is an unsafe ear. The cholesteatoma can be dry, but can also be infected, leading to a purulent discharge caused by a mixture of Gram-positive and negative bacteria. The combination with the keratin debris gives a typical smell. A cholesteatoma can cause all the complications known in otitis media, intra- as well as extra-cerebral.

The inner ear is at risk because of the possibility of an acute labyrinthitis as a consequence of the purulent infection, but also via bone erosion and the development of a labyrinthine fistula. A conductive loss is always prominent. The therapy for a cholesteatoma is surgery and this surgery must be radical.

Relationship of otitis media with the inner ear

The different types of otitis media can have an influence on the middle ear. Labyrinthine disease is a complication. This occurs less frequently in acute otitis media, especially in children. This disease is regarded in developed countries as a self-limiting disease (Ru and Grote, 2004). Children prone to otitis media and adults are, however, at increased risk. In cases of meningitis via acute otitis media the inner ear is, of course, at risk.

In chronic otitis media, apart from chronic otitis media with effusion, labyrinthitis can occur as a complication. Acute suppurative labyrinthitis is the bacterial invasion of the labyrinth with a total loss of auditory and vestibular function. In cholesteatoma cases this mostly occurs via a labyrinth fistula.

A proposed mechanism for sensorineural hearing loss involves bacterial toxins crossing the round window membrane entering the scala tympani, causing cochlear damage (Goycoolea, 1995). Post-mortem studies of patients with a history of otitis media give evidence of a defensive action in this region.

With this explanation, high tone loss is expected. In unilateral chronic otitis media a statistically significant interaural difference was demonstrated. More studies need to be performed.

Summary

The natural history of otitis media has changed, especially in developed countries where it can often be considered as a self-limiting disease and reduced medical and surgical therapy is indicated. However, complications do still occur and the inner ear is sometimes still at risk. The situation is different in developing countries. Further research is needed to determine whether and when antibiotic therapy is helpful, what role coinfection with viruses or the presence of bacterial biofilms plays in pathogenesis and how the development and monitoring of improved vaccination strategies helps in the prevention of OM.

11 MENINGITIS AND HEARING LOSS

K.J. Mutton and E.B. Kaczmarski

Introduction

Among the estimated 120 million people worldwide with disabling hearing impairment it is thought that in 50% the loss was potentially preventable (WHO, 1998a). Infection, and the sequelae of infection, make up a substantial portion of this potentially preventable group. Among the major preventable causes of deafness are chronic ear disease due largely to chronic otitis media, central nervous system (CNS) infection (notably meningitis) and ototoxicity (a proportion of which is due to antimicrobial agents used to treat infectious diseases). A large study of children aged between 3 and 10 years in Atlanta (USA) suggested an average annual prevalence rate for moderate to severe hearing loss of 1.1 per 1000 children, with chronic otitis media responsible for 6% of serious hearing impairment and meningitis for 4% (Van Naarden, Decouflé and Caldwell, 1999). Similarly, in a retrospective survey of children in Boston (USA), 4% of cases of sensorineural hearing loss were associated with meningitis (Billings and Kenna, 1999). Reports from many parts of the world show a similar pattern, though rates due to recognised meningitis ranged from 10 to 20% in Turkey (Dereköy, 2000) and 24% in Tanzania (Minja, 1998), to 70% in Germany (Eckel et al., 1998) and 82% in Belgium (Deben et al., 2003).

Bacterial meningitis is the most important cause of potentially preventable hearing loss acquired after birth, with significant hearing loss reported in between 3.5 and 37.2% of patients in the review by Fortnum (1992). Similar wide ranges continue to be reported in more recent literature – in Alabama an overall incidence of deafness of 13.7% after meningitis (Woolley et al., 1999), 14% in Canada (Wellman, Sommer and McKenna, 2003), 14% in the

Infection and Hearing Impairment. Edited by V.E. Newton and P.J. Vallely
© 2006 John Wiley & Sons, Ltd

Netherlands (van de Beek *et al.*, 2004), 28% in India (Cherukupally and Eavey, 2004) and 32% in Vanuatu (Carroll and Carroll, 1994). Although, as Fortnum (1992) pointed out, the reports are not always comparable because of variations in sample size, methodology and case ascertainment, it does appear that the higher rates tend to occur in resource-poor countries.

After meningitis, hearing loss presents as a spectrum of degree of loss and may be unilateral or bilateral. Taking an overview of the causes of bilateral deafness in children, Das (1996) found that in Manchester (UK) bacterial meningitis was responsible for 6.5% of cases (the largest number being idiopathic, followed by genetic causes in just over 23%). Unilateral hearing loss, although not such a problem as bilateral impairment, nevertheless is an important deficit and can affect not only the ability to localise and to recognise syllables but can also result in deleterious effects on academic and behavioural performance (Bess and Tharpe, 1984). In a Finnish study looking at the aetiology of unilateral deafness Vartiainen and Karjalainen (1998) found that 7% of cases were due to bacterial meningitis, with a third having profound hearing loss (>95 dB) and two-thirds moderate loss (41–70 dB). The ratio of unilateral to bilateral deficits after meningitis is approximately 1:1 in most series. In a Dutch series on non-*Haemophilus influenzae* meningitis, 3% were unilateral and 4% bilateral (Koomen *et al.*, 2003), similar to the findings of Dodge *et al.* (1984) who reported ten cases with bilateral impairment and nine with unilateral impairment. An exception is the recent study from Hyderabad where all cases were bilateral (Cherukupally and Eavey, 2004). In that Indian study, five (18%) patients aged 2 to 10 years had a sensorineural hearing loss ranging from 50 to 90 dB, and three (10%) patients aged 2 months to 8 years had a profound hearing loss of 90 dB or greater.

Pathogenesis of hearing loss due to meningitis

The pathogenesis of hearing loss in meningitis is complex and can involve multiple sites and pathways. Hearing loss may be cochlear (the most common situation), involving particularly the hair cells, or retrocochlear, involving the auditory nerve or brain. This may include: (a) involvement of the vestibulocochlear (eighth cranial) nerve; (b) involvement of the labyrinth; and (c) damage to central auditory pathways. Damage to the inner ear involving the outer hair cells can lead to a hearing loss of around 60–70 dB, while damage to the inner hair cells, which produce most of the sensory information that is fed to the brain along the auditory nerve pathways, leads to more profound deafness (Wright, 1999).

The primary process in most cases is the appearance of suppurative labyrinthitis. The beginnings of the processes that lead to sensorineural hearing loss in acute bacterial meningitis have been well described by Merchant and Gopen (1996). In their histopathological study of temporal bones from patients who died from acute bacterial meningitis (mostly

Streptococcus pneumoniae and *H. influenzae*), suppurative labyrinthitis occurred in 49%, and in all of these cases the cochlea was affected. The degree of labyrinthitis correlated with the severity of meningeal inflammation. The distribution of inflammatory cells was confined to the perilymphatic compartment and included the scala tympani in all cases (and the perilymphatic space of the lateral semicircular canal in half). Inflammation begins near the opening of the cochlear aqueduct at the base of the cochlea and spreads towards the apex in experimental meningitis (Bhatt, Halpin and Hsu, 1991), which is consistent with the progression of hearing loss from high-frequency to low-frequency loss. The sensory structures of the cochlea including the hair cells appeared essentially normal by light microscopy (Merchant and Gopen, 1996), so the damage to hearing is presumably at the cell ultrastructural level or the biochemical level.

Ultrastructural changes in the guinea pig cochlea seen on scanning electron microscopy have been described by Winter *et al.* (1996). They showed damage to inner hair cell stereocilia and surface cratering of inner supporting cells, with more marked changes associated with pneumococcal infection than with *Escherichia coli* infection (Figure 11.1). Ultrastructural studies in the rabbit by Rappaport *et al.* (1999b) confirm that there are major changes visible by electron microscopy, with progressively more changes as hearing loss progresses, with damage to inner and outer hair cells, their afferent and efferent synapses and, in the most severe cases, the supporting cells.

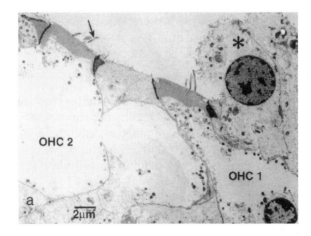

Figure 11.1. Transmission electron micrograph of the basal turn of the organ of Corti 12 hours after pneumolysin injection. The row 2 outer hair cell on the left is swollen with defects in its plasma membrane and pathological stereocilia (arrow). Mitochondria in both hair cells and neighbouring supporting cells are abnormal and vacuolated. The contents of an inner phalangeal cell are extruding through its apical surface (asterisk). (From Winter *et al.*, 1997. Reproduced by permission from the author and the American Society for Microbiology)

In the Merchant and Gopen (1996) study severe degeneration of spiral ganglion cells occurred in 12% of cases, consistent with retrocochlear damage, perhaps from a ganglionitis or perhaps from infarction of the vascular supply to the cochlea. Klein *et al.* (2003a) have also shown a decrease in numbers of spiral ganglion neurones which correlated in their experiments with the severity of hearing loss. Necrosis of spiral ganglion cells may be more important in the pathogenesis of hearing loss than was previously thought.

Similar changes to those in the rabbit model of pneumococcal meningitis (Bhatt, Halpin and Hsu, 1991) have been described in pigs infected with *Streptococcus suis*. Suppurative labyrinthitis occurs commonly in natural meningitis with *S. suis* serotype 2 (Madsen *et al.*, 2001), usually together with perineural inflammation around the vestibulocochlear nerve.

The spread of infection from the meninges to the cochlea seems likely in all animals studied. This occurs via the cochlear aqueduct and, additionally in humans, via the modiolus of the cochlea, as described by Merchant and Gopen (1996).

Labyrinthitis ossificans, the ossification of the cochlear scalae, has been regarded as a contributing factor to hearing loss after meningitis. Indeed, Hartnick *et al.* (2001) suggest that steroids may benefit hearing outcomes after meningitis by reducing the development of labyrinthitis ossificans. However, only 20–30% of temporal bones examined after meningitis have fibrosis or new bone formation present on histological examination (Keithley, Chen and Linthicum, 1998). In a Manchester cohort there was no correlation between degree of ossification and causative bacterium, age at onset of meningitis, or CSF white cell count, but those with bacteria seen in CSF by Gram staining were more likely to have ossification (Axon *et al.*, 1998). In experimental animals ossification can begin as soon as 3 weeks after intrathecal injection of pneumococci (Nabili *et al.*, 1999).

The most common bacteria causing meningitis, *H. influenzae*, *S. pneumoniae* and *Neisseria meningitidis*, are capsulated bacteria able to colonise the nasopharynx. To take one example, the meningococcus binds via pili to CD46 and other receptors on nonciliated epithelial cells; the bacteria are then engulfed by the cell but may survive in the phagocytic vacuole to cross into the bloodstream and thence the blood–brain barrier after entering the subarachnoid space, probably via the choroid plexus of the lateral ventricles (Rosenstein *et al.*, 2001). The process for pneumococcal infection is described by Meli *et al.* (2002).

The development of meningitis is driven to some extent by the release of chemically active molecules in the CNS. Disruption of the blood–brain barrier in meningitis is accompanied by generation of reactive nitrogen species and reactive oxygen species, which may combine to form the strong oxidant peroxynitrite (Beckman and Koppenol, 1996; Kastenbauer, Koedel and Pfister, 1999). The blood–brain barrier begins to break down after about 4 hours in experimental meningitis, as evidenced ultrastructurally by separation of the brain capillary endothelium tight intercellular junctions and an increase in pinocytotic vesicles – changes that become more marked with a longer duration of infection (Quagliarello, Long and Scheld, 1986). The process of disruption of the blood–brain barrier is, at least in part, driven by the actions of oxidants, particularly peroxynitrite, which reacts with a wide range of biological molecules. Nitration of tyrosine residues in proteins by peroxynitrite is enhanced by superoxide and can lead to changes in neurofilaments. Other findings include DNA single-strand breakage, inactivation of mitochondrial respiratory enzymes and initiation of lipid peroxidation (Koedel and Pfister, 1999). DNA single-strand breakage leads to activation of poly/adenosine diphosphate (ADP)-ribose synthetase, leading to depletion of its substrate NAD (nicotinamide adenine dinucleotide) and ultimately cell dysfunction and necrosis (Szabo, 1998). Kastenbauer et al. (2001) have shown that reactive oxidants such as peroxynitrite are involved in the disruption of the blood–labyrinth barrier that accompanies suppurative labyrinthitis associated with bacterial meningitis (at least in the experimental animal).

Immune responses take place in the inner ear, where the cochlea can become a target for damage by inflammatory responses (Harris and Ryan, 1995). In meningitis, immune responses and release of proinflammatory cytokines can be triggered by bacterial cell wall components and by bacterial DNA, perhaps acting initially via binding to the CD14 receptor, by stimulation of toll-like receptor-2 (TLR-2) pathways (Scheld, Koedel and Nathan, 2002). In the rabbit model of pneumococcal meningitis both steroidal and nonsteroidal anti-inflammatory agents reduce the likelihood of sensorineural hearing loss (Rappaport et al., 1999a). Other studies in animals support this idea – that by reducing the inflammatory responses due to the presence of bacteria in the subarachnoid space early in infection, meningitis sequelae can be reduced.

Inflammatory reactions are triggered, not just by bacteria but also by bacterial components. Deng, Liu and Tarkowaki (2001) have shown that bacterial DNA injected intracisternally can produce meningitis through recruitment of macrophages and release of inflammatory cytokines and chemokines and Tarlow, Comis and Osborne (1991) have shown that intracisternal injection of endotoxin from Gram-negative bacilli results in hearing impairment, which can be attenuated with steroids. There is now evidence that the inflammatory responses that occur with Gram-positive organisms such as pneumococci are driven by similar processes to those of Gram-negative bacteria. The acute phase reactant lipopolysaccharide-binding protein (LBP) which binds Gram-negative endotoxin can also bind to the glycan backbone of the pneumococcal cell wall (Weber et al., 2003) and initiate inflammatory responses through the activation of the MAPK signalling pathway, resulting in an increased release of TNF-α. In the animal, TNF-α is released from astroglial cells. Nau and Brück (2002) provide a fuller review of the ways in which these and other mechanisms operate to damage neurones in meningitis.

Matrix metalloproteinases (MMPs) are believed to contribute to mortality and neurological damage in bacterial meningitis. These endoproteases, a large family including gelatinases, collagenases and stromelysins, are secreted by monocytes and neutrophils. Certain of the MMPs are upregulated in meningitis and some, especially gelatinase B, are likely to have important roles in the breakdown of the blood–brain barrier (Kieseier et al., 1999; Meli et al., 2002).

One of the principal virulence factors of S. pneumoniae is pneumolysin, a pore-forming toxin found in all serotypes of pneumococcus and released by autolysis (Hirst et al., 2004). This acts as a TLR-2-independent immune activator (Scheld, Koedel and Nathan, 2002). Recent findings using pneumolysin-deficient pneumococcal strains suggest that pneumolysin is a much more important factor in pneumococcal meningitis than was previously thought (Wellmer, Zysk and Gerber, 2002). Pneumococci expressing pneumolysin may be better able to cross the vascular endothelium in the CNS to enter the CSF. High concentrations of pneumolysin, such as might be found late in an infection, may cause direct cellular damage, while at lower sublytic concentrations, which might be found early in an infection, there are effects including induction of apoptosis, activation of complement and induction of proinflammatory reactions in immune cells (Hirst et al., 2004). Winter et al. (1997) have also shown the importance of pneumolysin in cochlear damage and hearing loss in a guinea pig meningitis model. In their study, electron microscopy showed significant damage in the organ of Corti to the sensory hair cells and their stereocilia, the supporting cells and the nerve endings associated with the hair cells, while sensitive electrocochleographic measurements demonstrated that hearing loss was occurring at the cochlear level. Direct exposure of sensory nerve cells of the organ of Corti to pneumolysin results in a dose-dependent ototoxicity. In the experimental model, pneumolysin can be shown to reduce the compound action potential of the auditory nerve in seconds when perfused (at $10\,\mu g/50\,\mu mol$ concentration) into the guinea pig cochlea (Skinner et al., 2004). At lower concentrations a selective and earlier effect on inner hair cells is seen. Use of nonbacteriolytic bactericidal antibiotics that inhibit protein synthesis, agents such as rifampicin and clindamycin, might have benefits in reducing the amount of ototoxic pneumolysin released from pneumococci compared to treatment with bacteriolytic antibiotics such as cefotaxime and ceftriaxone.

Caspases are cellular cysteine proteases that have key roles in apoptosis and in the processing of proinflammatory cytokines (Creagh and Martin, 2001). Caspase-9 and caspase-3 have been shown to have major roles in the apoptotic cell death of aminoglycoside-affected vestibular hair cells and of auditory hair cells affected by cisplatin (van de Water et al., 2004). Pancaspase inhibitors such as z-VAD-fmk confer protection against hair cell apoptosis, at least in vitro. Of possible relevance to hearing loss in meningitis and otits media is the observation that transtympanic injection of bacterial endotoxin in the guinea pig leads to evidence of apoptosis of cells, with demonstrable activation of caspase-3, in the supporting cells of the organ of Corti and the lateral wall of the scala media (van de Watanabe *et al.*, 2001; Water *et al.*, 2004). Although no evidence of caspase-3 activation or of single-strand DNA (suggesting apoptosis) was found in sensory cells or spiral ganglion cells, electrocochleograms showed a significantly increased compound action potential threshold within 48 hours of bacterial lipopolysaccharide inoculation which could be ascribed to inner ear damage. The hair cells do not have their own blood supply but rely on diffusion of essential materials from the perilymph and endolymph; they are therefore susceptible to changes in the supporting cells and to any interference with the patterns of diffusion or changes in composition of the fluid milieu.

Bacterial meningitis

Of the causative agents of bacterial meningitis responsible for deafness in children the pneumococcus (*Streptococcus pneumoniae*) has been the most common, followed by *Haemophilus influenzae* (Deben *et al.*, 2003). The relative importance of the causative agents of bacterial meningitis is age-dependent (for example, see Figure 11.2) and has been greatly influenced in recent years by the introduction of vaccination against the major organisms associated with meningitis. Where formerly *Haemophilus influenzae* was the principal cause of meningitis in the USA, introduction of immunisation of

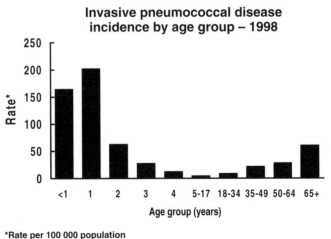

Figure 11.2. Age incidence of invasive pneumococcal disease, US. (Data from CDC, Atlanta, 2004)

infants with *H. influenzae* type b protein–polysaccharide conjugate vaccines has reduced the incidence of haemophilus meningitis by 55% and, nowadays, the pneumococcus has become the leading species (47%), followed by *Neisseria meningitidis* (25%) and *Listeria monocytogenes* (8%) (Swartz, 2004). Similarly, community-acquired meningitis in adults in the Netherlands is principally due to *S. pneumoniae* (51%), which has a particularly high risk of unfavourable outcome, and *N. meningitidis* (37%) (van de Beek *et al.*, 2004). The rate of deafness in survivors in this nation-wide Dutch series was 14%.

In resource-rich countries bacterial meningitis, formerly predominantly a disease of children, has now become more commonly a disease of adults (Schuchat *et al.*, 1997). Another trend in meningitis in adults is the increasing proportion due to nosocomial infection (Durand *et al.*, 1993).

Rates of hearing loss after meningitis are not uniform but vary with the causative organism. Thus, in a five year prospective study of children affected by meningitis when over the age of 1 month in St Louis, Missouri, Dodge *et al.* (1984) found the incidence of hearing impairment after pneumococcal meningitis to be 31%, after meningococcal meningitis 10.5% and after haemophilus meningitis 6%. In an Alabama cohort *S. pneumoniae* meningitis was followed by hearing loss in 23.8%, *H. influenzae* by 14.1% and *N. meningitidis* by 12.2% (Woolley *et al.*, 1999). This study highlights the broad range of pathogens associated with hearing loss after meningitis and includes cases due to *Staphylococcus aureus, Citrobacter diversus, Listeria monocytogenes* and β-haemolytic streptococci. Similar rates for hearing loss associated with *H. influenzae* have been reported.

There can be considerable variation in sequelae after infection with different serogroups of one bacterial species. Thus, Mayatepek *et al.* (1993) found that nonserogroup B meningococcal meningitis was associated with hearing loss in over 26% of cases, whereas serogroup B meningococcal meningitis was followed by hearing impairment in just over 3%. Nonserogroup B infections were also more likely to be associated with complement deficiencies (Mayatepek *et al.*, 1993).

The epidemiology of meningitis has been transformed in recent years by the introduction of vaccination against *H. influenzae* type b and *N. meningitidis* type C. Cases of these infections have declined in countries where vaccination has been introduced (Figure 11.3), and as a result deafness from these causes has also fallen. In the Alabama study (Woolley *et al.*, 1999) *H. influenzae* type b infection was responsible for 25 cases of deafness in children before vaccination was introduced in 1990 but for no cases after 1991, and the overall rate of haemophilus meningitis dropped by over 90%. Overall reduction in haemophilus type b meningitis in Denmark has fallen by 97–99% since the introduction of conjugate vaccine in 1993 (Hviid and Melbye, 2004).

Meningococcal serogroup C conjugate vaccine has reduced serogroup C meningitis by over 80% in the vaccinated groups in the UK (Trotter, Ramsay and Kaczmarski, 2002) and even in unvaccinated groups there appears to be

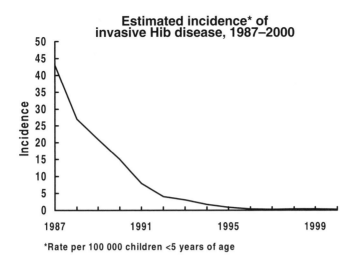

Figure 11.3. Efficacy of vaccination in reducing *Haemophilus influenzae* type b (Hib) disease, US. (Data from CDC, Atlanta, 2004)

a reduction in disease through a herd immunity effect (Balmer, Borrow and Miller, 2002). Introduction of pneumococcal conjugate vaccine into childhood immunisation schedules can be expected to have a similar effect on the incidence of invasive pneumococcal disease (Shafinoori *et al.*, 2005). Serogroup A *N. meningitidis* has been the principal causative agent of epidemic meningococcal meningitis in sub-Saharan Africa, with the greatest number of cases occurring in the so-called 'meningitis belt' between Senegal in the west and Ethiopia in the east. In addition there is a high rate of endemic disease from *N. meningitidis*, *S. pneumoniae* and *H. influenzae*, and a rise in sporadic cases of meningococcal infection often precedes epidemics (WHO, 2000a). Epidemics occur every 8–15 years and last for two to three dry seasons. Overall mortality is between 5 and 10%. Although all age groups are affected (WHO, 1998b), the majority of cases occur in those between 5 and 10 years (exceptionally in the Ghana epidemic of 1997 (Hodgson *et al.*, 2001), the mean age was 24 years, with the highest incidence, 34.5% of cases, in the 10–19 years group). Follow-up studies of survivors of the 1997 Ghana epidemic found hearing loss in 6%, with severe deficits in 1.6% (Hodgson *et al.*, 2001), while an earlier study had found profound hearing loss in 3.9% (Smith *et al.*, 1988).

The epidemiology of meningococcal disease has shown changes in recent years, examples being the increased role of *N. meningitidis* serogroup X in outbreaks in Niger and the predominance of W135 in infections acquired at the Hajj in 2000 (Karima *et al.*, 2003; Lingappa *et al.*, 2003). Over recent years *N. meningitidis* serogroup W135 has come to predominate over serogroup A in some African countries, with over 70% of meningococcal meningitis in Burkina Faso being due to W135 (Taha *et al.*, 2002; Parent du Chatelet *et al.*, 2005) Information is lacking on the rate of hearing loss after infection with serogroups such as W135 and should be further studied, not least because (as Greenwood pointed out in his 1998 Manson Lecture (Greenwood, 1999)) the implications of deafness in resource-poor countries where specialist services are lacking are far worse than in developed countries.

The relative importance of *Listeria monocytogenes* in community-acquired meningitis has risen. Hearing loss, however, seems to be surprisingly uncommonly reported after *Listeria* meningitis, given the high rate (32%) of neurological deficits associated with this condition (Mylonakis, Hohmann and Calderwood, 1998). This may be a reflection of the high death rate in this disease which, in turn, is associated with the increased likelihood that the patient is at the extremes of age or is immunocompromised.

The effects on hearing after meningitis are similar in adults. In a series of 87 adult patients from Munich who had pneumococcal meningitis the rate of hearing loss was 19.5% in all patients and 25.8% in those who survived (Kastenbauer and Pfister, 2003). This is probably an underestimate as hearing loss was detected only in the surviving patients, who were tested by audiometry on suspicion of hearing loss after recovery from the critical phase of the infection. Hearing loss was symmetrical in 11 of the 17 affected. Using the criteria set out by Dodge *et al.* (1984) who defined hearing loss as mild if 30–55 dB, moderate 55–70 dB, severe 70–90 dB and profound >90 dB, the findings were mild hearing loss in six patients, moderate in two, severe in one and profound in two. The incidence of hearing loss was particularly striking among the nine surviving splenectomised patients reported in this series, four of whom had bilateral hearing loss, two mild and two profound.

BACTERIAL MENINGITIS IN THE NEONATE

A range of conditions, of which meningitis is one, can lead to sensorineural hearing loss around the time of birth (Newton, 2001). The neonate has a relatively high risk of bacterial meningitis. The incidence of neonatal meningitis, i.e. meningitis occurring in the first 28 days of life, is 0.1 to 0.4 per 1000 live births and the rates of significant neurological sequelae are high (Stevens *et al.*, 2003). The epidemiology of neonatal bacterial infection has been changing over the last 20 years, with the incidence of meningitis as a complication of early-onset sepsis declining from around 25 to 30% to around 3 to 10% (Edwards and Baker, 2002).

Early-onset meningitis occurs within one week of birth as a result of transmission of infection from the mother and in developed countries is principally due to group B streptococcus (*Streptococcus agalactiae*), *Escherichia coli* and *Listeria monocytogenes* (Dawson, Emerson and Burns, 1999; Heath, Nik Yusoff and Baker, 2003).

Late-onset meningitis also includes cases due to *E. coli* and other Gram-negative bacilli, as well as Gram-positive bacteria such as coagulase negative staphylococci (associated with intraventricular haemorrhage in very low birthweight babies, a foreign body such as a ventriculoperitoneal shunt or post-neurosurgical intervention) (Heath, Nik Yusoff and Baker, 2003).

The pattern of infectious agents in early onset meningitis may be different in less developed countries with a greater preponderance of Gram-negative bacilli and less group B streptococcal disease (Kuruvilla *et al.*, 1999). However, this pattern is not universal in developing countries (Kuruvilla *et al.* 1999), and in Western countries group B streptococcal disease may be declining (Andersen, Christensen and Hertel, 2004). In the US, the decline in neonatal sepsis and meningitis due to group B streptococci from 1.7 per 1000 live births in 1993 to 0.6 per 1000 by 1998 has been ascribed to the introduction of intrapartum chemoprophylaxis against group B streptococci (Schrag *et al.*, 2000). US guidance on prevention of group B streptococcal disease was revised in 2002 (Anon, 2002). Group B streptococci remain susceptible to penicillin and ampicillin (Morales *et al.*, 1999; Biedenbach, Stephen and Jones, 2003; Fluegge *et al.*, 2004) but resistance to erythromycin and clindamycin has increased to the extent that local susceptibility patterns need to be assessed before using these drugs for prophylaxis or therapy. Fluegge *et al.* (2004) found 10% of isolates to be resistant to erythromycin and almost 6% to clindamycin, but in Canada erythromycin resistance rates have risen to over 13% (de Azavedo *et al.*, 2001) and in France erythromycin resistance exceeds 21% (De Mouy *et al.*, 2001).

An extensive study from Dallas, Texas, puts the importance of bacterial meningitis due to Gram-negative rods into perspective. Over a 21 year period, 98 cases of meningitis due to Gram-negative rods, mainly Enterobacteriaceae, were seen, which amounted to 3.6% of all the meningitis cases diagnosed in neonates, infants and children. The median onset of meningitis was 10 days (Unhanand *et al.*, 1993) and the commonest organisms were *E. coli* (53% of infections), *Klebsiella* and *Enterobacter* spp. (16% together), *Citrobacter* and *Salmonella* spp. (each 9%). Of the survivors 61% had long-term sequelae, with hearing loss noted in 17%.

In a case control study assessing the long-term outcomes of a cohort of survivors of neonatal meningitis in England and Wales, 3.6% (4 out of 111) were found to have moderate to severe hearing loss (Stevens *et al.*, 2003), although as formal testing was not undertaken this might be an underestimate, particularly for mild impairment. Of the three cases with documented positive bacteriology one had severe bilateral sensorineural deafness due to *E. coli*, one had severe unilateral deafness due to a Gram-negative bacillus other than *E. coli* and one had moderate unilateral hearing loss due to *Listeria* sp. (Stevens *et al.*, 2003).

Deafness has also been described after neonatal meningitis due to group B streptococcus (Wald *et al.*, 1986). In this large series from Pittsburgh, 9.3% of survivors (5 out of 54) were reported as having deafness. Those who died or recovered with neurological deficits were more likely to be male and were more likely to have had seizures. There was also a suggestion of earlier onset of infection (a median of 11 days of age at onset versus 23 days for those without neurological sequelae) and lower CSF cell counts at diagnosis. Hearing loss is clearly an important consequence of neonatal meningitis, although reported rates vary widely and reflect retrospective analysis of data. Aside from the organisms outlined above it should not be forgotten that neonatal infections also occur with *S. pneumoniae*, *H. influenzae* and *N. meningitidis*, albeit at relatively low rates. The annual incidence of neonatal meningococcal disease in the US, to take one example, is estimated to be 9 per 100000 (Shepard, Rosenstein and Fischer, 2003).

The development of subdural effusion during the course of meningitis in infants does not correlate with an increased risk of hearing loss on long-term (median 5.5 years) follow-up (Snedeker *et al.*, 1990).

Other bacterial infections associated with hearing loss

Hearing loss due to treponemal infection is discussed in Chapter 9 of this volume.

Streptococcus suis is well known as a CNS pathogen in pigs. In humans, meningitis due to *S. suis* has been described principally in people working in the pig industry or associated with domestic or wild pigs (Arends and Zanen, 1988; Robertson and Blackmore, 1989). Hearing loss occurs in over 50% of survivors in *S. suis* meningitis and appears early (Kay, Cheng and Tse, 1995; Donsakul, Dejthevaporn and Witoonpanich, 2003). Vestibular dysfunction is also described after *S. suis* meningitis by Rinne *et al.* (1998), affecting two butchers and a farmer.

Central nervous system involvement in *Borrelia burgdorferi* infection (Lyme disease) is not uncommon, occurring in about 10% of untreated cases (Hengge *et al.*, 2003), often after a long latent period. In chronic Lyme disease, sometimes called post-treatment Lyme disease syndrome (PTLDS), moderate bilateral hearing loss was reported by 1.5% of patients in the study of Moscatello *et al.* (1991), while in a series of 27 patients with chronic neurological symptoms thought to be associated with chronic Lyme disease, Logigian, Kaplan and Steere (1990) reported that 15% of this group had evidence of hearing loss and 7% had tinnitus. Shotland *et al.* (2003) performed an audiometry study in 18 patients with PTLDS and found a hearing abnormality in 44% (8 out of 18) at one or more test frequencies. However, these were subtle abnormalities – all less than 20 dB loss and, therefore, not regarded as clinically relevant (WHO, 1980). The majority (78%) had unilateral hearing loss. Perhaps more striking than hearing loss was the demonstration of intolerance of loud sounds. *Bartonella henselae*, the agent of cat-scratch fever, can cause very similar meningitis to that of Lyme disease. Although it can co-infect with *B. burgdorferi* (Podsiadly, Chmielewski and Tylewska-Wierzbanowska, 2003) it has not been reported as causing hearing loss.

Brucellosis involves the CNS in 5 to 10% of cases (Lulu *et al.*, 1988), with CNS involvement, neurobrucellosis, occurring in both acute and chronic infection. Sensorineural hearing loss is well described in neurobrucellosis, particularly in endemic areas (Thomas *et al.*, 1993; Bodur *et al.*, 2003; Al-Sous *et al.*, 2004). In a case report from Turkey of a young woman with chronic neurobrucellosis with a suprasellar granuloma, the bilateral sensorineural hearing loss failed to respond to treatment although the other manifestations of the disease, including visual loss, resolved (Çiftçi, Erden and Akyar, 1998). A case report from Hull (UK) clearly demonstrates severe hearing loss in association with lymphocytic meningitis due to *Brucella melitensis* (Clarke, Ray and Abdelhadi, 1999), with hearing loss progressing to a profound bilateral high-tone sensorineural hearing loss after a recurrence of symptoms.

Chlamydial infections have been reported to cause meningitis and other neurological syndromes on occasions (Korman, Turnidge and Grayson, 1997). Most cases of meningitis have been associated with evidence of *C. pneumoniae* infection although the link between the CNS infection and the organism has usually been made only on serological grounds (Anton, Otegui and Alonso, 2000). Hearing loss has been noted in association with *C. trachomatis* conjunctivitis, but this is due to otitis media (Gow, Ostler and Schachter, 1974). Sudden sensorineural hearing loss coincident with *C. psittaci* pneumonia has been reported (Brewis and McFerran, 1997) and, in a recent Polish abstract, Dunne *et al.* (2004) suggest that there may be a significant role for *C. pneumoniae* as a cause of sudden sensorineural hearing loss.

Hearing loss associated with *Mycoplasma pneumoniae* infection appears to be uncommon and was not specifically discussed in the recent review by Waites and Talkington (2004). Involvement of the central nervous system, mainly encephalitis, occurs in about 1 in 1000 mycoplasma cases (Koskiniemi, 1993) and can occur in the absence of respiratory symptoms (Bitnun *et al.*, 2001). Although neurological sequelae were seen in 64% of cases of probable childhood mycoplasma encephalitis described by Bitnun *et al.* (2001) hearing loss was not documented. Occasional cases of sensorineural hearing loss with *M. pneumoniae* infection that are described, however, are usually unilateral (Okada *et al.*, 1996; Schönweiler, Held and Schönweiler, 2001). The German case described by Schönweiler, Held and Schönweiler (2001) was believed to have outer hair cell dysfunction. Hearing loss associated with otitis media due to *M. pneumoniae* is also believed to be uncommon, given that the detection of *M. pneumoniae* in middle ear fluid is rare in childhood acute otitis media (Roberts, 1980; Block, 1999). Sensorineural hearing loss, often reversible, has been described in bullous myringitis, but only a minority of these cases has been shown to be associated with *M. pneumoniae* infection (Wetmore and Abramson, 1979; Feinmesser *et al.*, 1980; Roberts, 1980; Hariri, 1990), even using PCR detection (Kotikoski, Kleemola and Palmu, 2004).

Tuberculosis is extremely important in world terms, with the global incidence rate estimated to be growing at 1.1% per year. There were an estimated 8.8 million new cases in 2002 (WHO, 2004a). The incidence in England and Wales is also increasing, with overall incidence (2003) around 12.7 per 100000 (Health Protection Agency, 2004a). In London this has reached 40.6 per 100000, a level above that defined by WHO as of 'high prevalence' (Atkinson et al., 2002). The rates reflect immigration patterns, for among UK-born individuals the rate is 4.1 per 100000 compared to 90 per 100000 in those born outside the UK (Health Protection Agency, 2004a). Tuberculous meningitis or miliary spread occurs in 15–20% of children within the two years after primary infection (Carroll, Clark and Cant, 2001). As there is no sign of respiratory disease in about 35% of cases of extrapulmonary tuberculosis (Kumar et al., 1997; Paganini et al., 2000) treatment for tuberculous meningitis should always be started on suspicion, even in the absence of chest radiograph support. Tuberculous meningitis is more common in HIV-infected individuals (Berenguer et al., 1992) and the risk in HIV-infected children is higher as immunity wanes (Carroll, Clark and Cant, 2001). Outcomes are generally worse in those with HIV infection (Topley et al., 1998).

Reported rates of deafness after tuberculous meningitis vary widely. An estimate of the risk of hearing loss in survivors in the developed world can be gathered from a cohort of children in California receiving antituberculous therapy (mostly with adjunctive steroids) (Saitoh et al., 2005). When assessed at one year 35% of survivors had severe neurological deficits and, of these, 25% had severe hearing loss. Mild hearing loss was seen in 13% of those with moderate neurological sequelae. This is in contrast to the surprising report of no cases of deafness in a cohort of mainly poor South African children of whom only 20% remained functionally normal after recovery from the infection (Schoeman et al., 2002). Abnormal brainstem auditory evoked responses (BAER) were found in 24% of Turkish children with tuberculous meningitis tested before treatment was begun (Topcu et al., 2002), so there is certainly potential for deafness even allowing for the reversibility of BAER changes in some patients. Unilateral deafness of sudden onset together with fever and night sweats has recently been described as the presenting features of a case of tuberculosis in London (Kotnis and Simo, 2001).

BCG vaccination programmes are advisable in countries with high rates of tuberculosis, where WHO recommends BCG for all infants including those born to HIV-infected mothers (Moss, Clements and Halsey, 2003). Although the efficacy of BCG at preventing pulmonary disease in adults is debatable, vaccination does seem to be effective in reducing the risk of tuberculous meningitis and miliary spread in children. Contacts of tuberculosis cases should be given chemoprophylaxis to prevent infection, as otherwise 40–50% of infants and 15% of older children will develop the disease within two years of the contact (Shingadia and Novelli, 2003).

Rare cases of meningitis and hearing loss may be associated with tuberculous osteomyelitis of the temporal bone (Kearns *et al.*, 1985). Similar lesions in actinomycosis can also cause deafness (Sobol, Samadi and Wetmore, 2004).

Definitive diagnosis of tuberculous meningitis depends upon CSF examination, but treatment should be begun on suspicion. Direct examination of CSF for acid-fast bacilli should be undertaken, but the yield is variable, as low as 10–20% in most series. *Mycobacterium tuberculosis* can take up to eight weeks to grow on solid media. Substantial reduction in the time taken for culture, together with improved diagnostic yields, have been achieved in recent years by the use of liquid cultures and radiometric and fluorescence-based detection systems (Brunello, Favari and Fontana, 1999). Use of *M. tuberculosis* PCR on CSF has given some improvement in the diagnostic repertoire, largely because of the speed with which a result can be obtained. Specificity is high but sensitivity relatively low in the range of 40–60% (Thwaites *et al.*, 2000; Pai *et al.*, 2003).

Treatment of tuberculous meningitis should commence with a two month intensive course of isoniazid, rifampicin and pyrazinamide, plus ethambutol (or streptomycin or ethionamide) as the fourth drug, followed by a continuation period with rifampicin and isoniazid of four to eight months (Donald and Schoeman, 2004) or until 12 months (Joint Tuberculosis Committee of the British Thoracic Society, 1998). The use of adjunctive steroids is also desirable for more severe disease.

For tuberculous meningitis addition of steroids accelerates resolution of tuberculous cerebral lesions and may reduce mortality and give better outcomes in survivors in terms of intellect, but there is no significant beneficial effect on intracranial pressure, basal ganglia infarcts, hemiparesis or quadriplegia, blindness or deafness (Schoeman *et al.*, 1997). In a Vietnamese study of more than 500 patients aged over 14 years with tuberculous meningitis (Thwaites *et al.*, 2004) steroid administration generally offered a survival benefit regardless of the severity of the disease (the difference did not reach significance in a subgroup of HIV positive patients not receiving antiretrovirals). However, there was not a reduction in neurological sequelae or in rates of hearing loss. Tuberculous meningitis due to drug-resistant *M. tuberculosis* is an increasing problem in some parts of the world. Outcome tends to be poor because of delays in initiating appropriate therapy while awaiting susceptibility test results and the lesser efficacy of second-line drugs in treatment. Of 350 cases of tuberculous meningitis seen in Kwazulu-Natal, 8.6% were resistant to rifampicin and isoniazid at least, and the mortality among these was approximately 57% (Patel *et al.*, 2004).

Ototoxic drugs and meningitis

Drug-induced ototoxicity is discussed in Chapter 13 of this volume. It has been particularly important in those treated for tuberculosis, including tuberculous meningitis, with ototoxicity described for several drugs no longer in common use in developed countries – streptomycin, kanamycin and capreomycin (Holderness, 1987). The aminoglycoside antibiotic gentamicin is ototoxic and is used for the treatment of sepsis due to Gram-negative bacilli as well as in the treatment of meningitis due to Gram-negative bacilli, particularly in neonates. While there may be no entirely safe regimen for gentamicin ototoxicity (Black, Pesznecker and Stallings, 2004) the risk to neonates may be somewhat less than in older patients (Aust, 2001).

Meningitis associated with otitis media

A proportion of cases of meningitis are due to ear infection, although this is much less of a problem compared to the pre-antibiotic era. In their 20 year study from North Carolina Baptist Hospital, Gower and McGuirt (1983) described 100 cases of central nervous system disease complicating middle ear disease. Most (85 of the 100) were in patients under 20 years of age. Meningitis was the commonest complication, occurring in 76 cases, 63 acute and 13 chronic, with an overall death rate of 12% (Gower and McGuirt, 1983). A more recent report, an 18 year study from Paris, describes 79 patients with bacterial meningitis associated with ear infection (Barry et al., 1999). Among these, 32 had acute otitis media, 29 chronic otitis media (16 with cholesteatoma) and 18 had cerebrospinal fluid (CSF) leaks from a variety of causes including surgery and gunshot injury to the temporal bone. S. pneumoniae was the most common single organism isolated from CSF or blood culture in cases associated with acute otitis media (22 cases, 69%) and chronic otitis media without cholesteatoma (5 cases, 42%), and CSF leakage. Gram-negative bacteria and anaerobes were common in the group with cholesteatomatous chronic otitis media, where Proteus mirabilis was found in three cases (18%), S. pneumoniae in two (12%) and anaerobic bacteria, principally Bacteroides fragilis, in 24%.

The correlation between cultures from the otological focus of infection and the CSF isolate is poor and cannot be regarded as a useful guide to the likely organism causing meningitis. Gram-negative bacilli (mainly P. mirabilis and P. aeruginosa) are much more common in ear swabs than in CSF. Only eight otological samples grew the same organism as the CSF (17%). Broad-spectrum antibiotic cover is needed, particularly in those with cholesteatoma. The subject of hearing loss and otitis media is discussed in Chapter 10 of this volume.

Fungal meningitis

As many as 27% of cases of meningitis due to Cryptococcus neoformans result in hearing loss (Low, 2002), with most cases occurring in individuals with AIDS (Kwartler et al., 1991). Vestibular dysfunction is also common but sometimes reversible (Hughes *et al.*, 1997). Histological findings vary among reported cases, with some showing both cochlear and vestibular nerve and end-organ damage, and others showing involvement of spiral ganglion cells and cochlear nerves with sparing of the organ of Corti and the vestibular nerves and end-organs (Harada, Sando and Myers, 1979). The diagnosis of cryptococcosis should be considered early in 'at risk' individuals and appropriate testing carried out (Portegies *et al.*, 2004). The diagnosis may be made by visualisation of the encapsulated yeast cells in cerebrospinal fluid using the India ink method, followed by culture of the organism, but should also employ cryptococcal antigen detection on CSF (Barenfanger, Lawhorn and Drake, 2004) and/or serum (Yeo and Wong, 2002). Cryptococcal PCR testing might also be considered (Rappelli *et al.*, 1998; Paschoal *et al.*, 2004). The preferred treatment for cryptococcal meningitis is combination amphotericin B and flucytosine, followed by fluconazole maintenance therapy (Saag *et al.*, 2000).

Meningitis due to parasites

The rat lungworm, *Angiostrongylus cantonensis*, is a causative agent of meningitis in South-East Asia and the Pacific Islands as a result of ingestion of infective larvae from a range of sources including snails, slugs, prawns and contaminated water and vegetables (Alicata, 1991). The infection is increasingly recognised in the Caribbean (Lindo *et al.*, 2002). The meningitis is characterised by a predominance of eosinophils in the CSF and eosinophilia in the peripheral blood, although this is not always seen at the time of initial presentation (Slom *et al.*, 2002). Sensorineural deafness associated with angiostrongyliasis has been reported in a single case from Thailand (Chotmongkol, Yimtae and Intapan, 2004). The degree of hearing loss improved in this case after administration of steroids, and was presumably due to an inflammatory reaction to worm components. Antihelminthic agents are best avoided as they may aggravate the condition.

Deafness has not been noted in the much rarer cases of eosinophilic meningitis due to *Gnathostoma spinigerum* and *Baylisascaris procyonis* (Lo Re and Gluckman, 2003). Hearing loss was noted in a case of eosinophilic meningitis caused by *Toxocara canis* (Vidal, Sztajnbok and Seguro, 2003). Neurocysticercosis, infection of the CNS by *Taenia solium*, may occasionally present with hearing loss due to compression of the eighth cranial nerve by cysts (Revuelta *et al.*, 2003; Jarupant *et al.*, 2004). Surgical removal of cystic material and antihelminth treatment with albendazole are indicated.

Viral meningitis

Hearing loss due to viral meningitis is much less important than that due to bacterial meningitis. Deafness associated with mumps is well recognised and is described fully in Chapter 6 of this volume. In general, hearing loss associated with mumps without symptomatic CNS involvement is uncommon, and even where there is evidence of mumps meningoencephalitis the reported rates of hearing loss vary substantially, from no cases of hearing loss in 50 mumps cases (Azimi, Cramlett and Haynes, 1969) to 3.5% of 79 cases in Israel (Garty, Danon and Nitzen, 1985). A recent Turkish audiology study comparing hearing in mumps cases with and without meningoencephalitis suggests that there is detectable hearing loss in those with meningoencephalitis (relative to those without CNS involvement), although this was not necessarily of clinical significance (Kanra *et al.*, 2002).

Varicella-zoster virus (VZV) meningitis has been reported as a cause of hearing loss in a single case report. In the case described by Schwab and Ryan (2004), the diagnosis of VZV meningitis was confirmed by positive VZV PCR on CSF. Mild to moderate unilateral sensorineural hearing loss was demonstrable at a 6 week hearing evaluation, but this had resolved by two years.

Hearing loss associated with herpes simplex (HSV) meningitis is rarely reported in the literature. Most HSV meningitis is caused by HSV type 2, but among the 27 cases of HSV type 2 meningitis reported in a Swedish series (Bergström *et al.*, 1990) there was just a single case of hearing impairment. Hearing loss is not a feature of recurrent herpes simplex type 2 meningitis (Dylewski and Bekhor, 2004). Rabinstein *et al.* (2001) report a case of sudden-onset bilateral hearing loss associated with HSV type 1 stomatitis which showed changes on gadolinium-enhanced MR scanning suggestive of an inflammatory neuritis involving the seventh and eighth cranial nerves (Saraf-Lavi and Sklar, 2001). A similar condition with hearing loss and marked structural changes in the cochlea can be produced in guinea pigs by inoculation of herpes simplex virus into the perilymph (Stokroos, Albers and Schirm, 1998), adding some weight to the idea that herpes virus infections (either primary or reactivation of latent virus) may be important in the syndrome of sudden sensorineural hearing loss.

Most cases of viral meningitis are caused by enteroviruses. Acute enteroviral meningitis is generally not thought to be linked to significant hearing loss (Bergman *et al.*, 1987; Baker *et al.*, 1996; Bernit *et al.*, 2004) and there appears to be no risk of hearing loss after enteroviral meningitis in the neonate (Bergman *et al.*, 1987; Baker *et al.*, 1996).

In the Munich study by Nowaks, Boehmer and Fuchs (2003) of aseptic meningitis due to a range of causes, hearing loss was not noted, although only five patients were tested using auditory-evoked potentials. An abstract from the Japanese literature reports bilateral deafness in an agammaglobulinaemic patient with chronic enteroviral meningitis (Ito *et al.*, 1996). In a more recent case report, Schattner *et al.* (2003) describe the sudden onset of severe bilateral hearing loss and tinnitus in association with enteroviral meningitis (the virus involved was shown by CSF PCR and stool culture to be echovirus type 4), while a recent German study suggests that enterovirus infection (as demonstrated by detection of enterovirus RNA in serum by nested PCR) can be found in as many as 40% of cases of sudden deafness (Mentel *et al.*, 2004).

Paralytic poliomyelitis due to either polio virus or nonpolio virus enteroviruses is associated with hearing loss, but the relationship between this syndrome and the meningitis caused by poliomyelitis is unclear. A number of cases suggest that the hearing loss may be due to a direct effect on the cochlear neurones (Bachor and Karmody, 2001). In their study of over 400 patients involved in the 1949 poliomyelitis outbreak in Massachusetts, Weinstein *et al.* (1952) found that in bulbar poliomyelitis the eighth cranial nerve was involved in 0.9% of cases, the least involvement of any of the cranial nerves across the whole age spectrum. All cases of eighth nerve involvement, however, were confined to the 16 to 30 years age group.

Hearing loss does not seem to have been reported in studies of meningitis and meningoencephalitis due to West Nile virus in the US or the Middle East (Klein *et al.*, 2002; Petersen and Marfin, 2002; Watson *et al.*, 2005).

Noninfectious causes of meningitis

One important syndrome in the differential diagnosis of hearing loss associated with infection is the Vogt–Koyanagi–Harada syndrome. This is an autoimmune disorder in which there is acute inflammation of melanocyte-containing tissues, including skin, uvea, inner ear and meninges. It presents classically with aseptic meningitis, sensorineural deafness, uveitis, vitiligo and diffuse hair loss (Read, 2002) and is treated with steroids or other immunosuppressive agents. Although initially steroid-responsive, the deafness may persist (Iwata *et al.*, 2002). Carcinomatous meningitis has also been described as causing bilateral deafness (Zeller *et al.*, 2002).

Nonsteroidal anti-inflammatory agents are occasionally associated with aseptic meningitis. Bilateral hearing loss has occurred in this condition (Davison and Marion, 1998).

Chronic pachymeningitis is a rare condition characterised by chronic inflammatory thickening of the dura mater. Many cases are idiopathic but recognised causes, often treatable, include autoimmune disease such as rheumatoid disease, malignancy and infections including tuberculosis and syphilis. Occasional cases of deafness associated with this condition have been described (Oghalai *et al.*, 2004). Diagnosis is best achieved by gadolinium-enhanced magnetic resonance (MR) scanning, and treatment is directed to the underlying cause. Parney, Johnson and Allen (1997) suggest that there may be a case for a trial of antituberculous therapy in some apparently idiopathic cases.

Time course of hearing loss in meningitis

Hearing loss begins to occur early in acute bacterial meningitis, in some cases within 48 hours of the onset of the infection as measured by brainstem auditory evoked potentials (BAEP) (Kaplan *et al.*, 1984; Vienny *et al.*, 1984). In the rat model of meningitis-associated hearing loss, after meningitis following inoculation of 10^5 to 10^7 colony-forming units of *Streptococcus pneumoniae* into the subarachnoid space, serial auditory brainstem evoked potentials show hearing loss developing 12 to 15 hours postinoculation, progressing to complete hearing loss in almost all animals by 24 hours (Kesser *et al.*, 1999). Similarly, in the rabbit inoculated intracisternally with *S. pneumoniae*, auditory evoked potentials show hearing loss beginning 12 hours after infection (Bhatt *et al.*, 1993).

There is an initial phase in the first two weeks in which recovery or progression may occur. Richardson *et al.* (1997a) found that about 10% of children had reversible hearing loss, with an initial phase of resolution within 48 hours in 69% of these (Richardson *et al.*, 1997a). It is possible that early treatment with appropriate antibiotics can reduce the risk of progression although this is not proven. Some early hearing loss may be a transient phenomenon seen in serious illness other than meningitis (Davey *et al.*, 1983) and a number of studies cited by Wright (1999) failed to show a relationship between duration of symptoms and deafness (Wright, 1999). On the other hand, duration of symptoms was found to be a risk factor for hearing loss in the more recent study by Koomen *et al.* (2003).

Woolley *et al.* (1999) found that among 59 children with postmeningitis deafness 78% had stable hearing loss and 22% progressive or fluctuating deficit. Stabilisation occurred between 3 months and 6 years, but in only 2 of 13 children was there long-term improvement of hearing. Hearing loss can show initial recovery: Wellman, Sommer and McKenna (2003) reported that although 32.3% of postmeningitic children initially had abnormal BAEP, permanent sensorineural hearing loss was found in 13.9%, findings similar to those of Guiscafre *et al.* (1984) where an initial 25% had abnormalities on BAEP early after pyogenic bacterial meningitis, with these persisting at 6 months in 8%. In one study 5 of 51 children had persistent BAEP abnormalities after the first two weeks from the onset of meningitis and all of these children had persistent hearing loss while 11 had transient BAEP abnormalities (Kaplan *et al.*, 1984). The prognostic value of BAEP in this context comes from the fact that there were no late cases of unexpected deafness and little in the way of significant late recovery. Persistence correlates with initial severity.

After the early phase, true sensorineural hearing impairment does not resolve (Dodge *et al.*, 1984) and over the years may progress in as many as half (Hugosson *et al.*, 1997). Impairment that resolves after bacterial meningitis is for the most part coincidental conductive hearing loss (Richardson *et al.*, 1997a).

Predictors of hearing loss

Hearing loss is said to be more likely with more severe meningitis, more prolonged fever, fits and low CSF glucose (Yogev, 2002). Bhatt *et al.* (1993)

reported that in an animal model, a high white cell count, high protein and high lactate levels in CSF were predictors of progressive meningitis and hearing loss, but not all studies confirm this and certainly in the human the situation is not clear. The most robust biochemical parameter seen over a majority of studies is reduced CSF glucose (Table 11.1). In a recent review from Texas of children who had hearing loss after bacterial meningitis, only elevated CSF protein, decreased CSF glucose and coexisting cranial neuropathies were predictive of hearing loss (Kutz *et al.*, 2003).

The association of a low CSF glucose level with sensorineural hearing loss is perhaps best seen in the retrospective British study of Eisenhut, Meehan and Batchelor (2003). In this study, which compared CSF glucose levels in 47 cases (patients with sensorineural hearing loss after meningitis) with levels in 145 controls (patients with meningitis without hearing loss), the mean glucose level was 1.3 mmol/L in cases and 2.5 mmol/L in controls, indicating a significant difference. Subgroup analysis showed that low CSF glucose correlated with sensorineural hearing loss in meningitis due to *S. pneumoniae* and *H. influenzae*, but not *N. meningitidis*. In the Alabama study (Woolley *et al.*, 1999), low CSF glucose level correlated with increased risk of hearing impairment; additional risk factors were evidence of raised intracranial pressure on a CT scan, male sex and *S. pneumoniae* as the aetiological agent.

Similar risk factors were identified more recently by Koomen *et al.* (2003) who were able to select five high-risk criteria that identified a group that included all cases of hearing loss after meningitis not caused by *H. influenzae*. The criteria were duration of symptoms of over 2 days before admission,

Table 11.1. Typical CSF findings in meningitis

Condition	Opening pressure	White cell count	Protein	Glucose
Normal	50–200 mm of water	<5 cells/µl (lymphocytes)	1.5–5 g/L	2.5–4.5 mmol/L (60% of serum level)
Bacterial meningitis	Raised	500–10 000 cells (predominantly polymorphs)	Raised >10–50 g/L	Low <2.2 mmol/L
Tuberculous meningitis	Raised	50–500 cells (predominantly lymphocytes)	Raised >10–300 g/L	Low <2.5 mmol/L
Viral meningitis	Raised	5–1000 cells (predominantly lymphocytes, can be polymorph predominance early)	Raised 5–10 g/L	Normal

absence of petechiae, low CSF glucose level, *S. pneumoniae* as the aetiological agent and ataxia. Using a scoring system based on these criteria, 62% of patients required auditory screening to identify all cases of hearing loss.

Where initial screening in the acute phase of meningitis is done by BAEP, patients with normal results do not go on to develop hearing loss (Kaplan *et al.*, 1984; Vienny *et al.*, 1984; Richardson *et al.*, 1998).

Diagnosis and management of bacterial meningitis

Traditionally the clinical diagnosis of meningitis is confirmed by the CSF findings and by bacterial culture of CSF and blood. Typical CSF findings are outlined in Table 11.1. It must be noted, however, that it is not uncommon for CSF to be normal early in infection; 8% of cases of meningococcal meningitis in the study from Gloucestershire reported by Wylie *et al.* (1997) fell into this category. In recent years in developed countries use of lumbar puncture has declined because of concerns about cerebral herniation (Kneen, Solomon and Appleton, 2002), but ideally CSF should be collected to establish the diagnosis if there is no evidence of incipient herniation, abnormal posturing, tonic seizures or obvious meningococcal disease (Wylie *et al.*, 1997; Kneen, Solomon and Appleton, 2002).

Failure to obtain CSF for culture can make it difficult to give optimal antibiotic therapy in the absence of antimicrobial susceptibility test results and can lead to unnecessarily prolonged treatment if the clinical and laboratory findings cannot exclude bacterial meningitis (Kanegaye, Soliemanzadeh and Bradley, 2001). Collection of CSF is especially important in diagnosing meningitis in low birth weight infants, where one-third of those with meningitis have negative blood cultures (Stoll *et al.*, 2004). The decline in CSF testing has led to a need for sensitive assays on other samples such as nasal swabs and blood. Real-time PCR using whole blood gives excellent sensitivity in the diagnosis of meningococcal (Hackett *et al.*, 2002a) and pneumococcal disease (van Haeften *et al.*, 2003) and should always be undertaken when these diagnoses are suspected, particularly if CSF has not been collected.

Quantitation of bacterial load in blood by culture has been reported as predicting meningitis in pneumococcal and haemophilus sepsis (Sullivan, LaScolea and Neter, 1982) and meningococcal DNA levels correlate with severity of disease (Hackett *et al.*, 2002b), but there is no information as to whether this has any predictive value for hearing loss. Molecular detection methods can be used to detect several relevant pathogens simultaneously (Corless *et al.*, 2001). Antigen detection methods for pneumococcus, haemophilus and group B streptococcus are widely available but are probably of no more value than Gram staining of CSF (Finlay, Witherow and Rudd, 1995), except for partially treated cases, although, recently, ultrasonication has been shown to enhance the sensitivity of agglutination reactions (Ellis and Sobanski, 2000). The use of the ultrasound-enhanced latex immunoagglutination test (USELAT) for detection of meningococcal antigen from CSF and plasma offers markedly improved sensitivity over conventional agglutination methods and is a satisfactory typing assay (Gray *et al.*, 1999; Sobanski *et al.*, 2002), but overall performance is still inferior to PCR (Gray *et al.*, 1999; Porritt, Mercer and Munro, 2003). Further information on diagnosis is to be found in Chapter 14 of this volume.

Antibiotics should be started on suspicion of meningitis, as soon as possible after the onset of symptoms. Initial treatment of bacterial meningitis should cover infections due to *H. influenzae*, *N. meningitidis* and *S. pneumoniae*; thus a third-generation cephalosporin such as cefotaxime or ceftriaxone is generally recommended (Begg *et al.*, 1999; Heyderman *et al.*, 2003). The addition of ampicillin should also be considered to cover *Listeria monocytogenes* in the elderly. US guidance is similar and is set out in an excellent guideline from IDSA (Tunkel *et al.*, 2004). Adjunctive dexamethasone is recommended for pneumococcal meningitis in adults (Tunkel *et al.*, 2004). The treatment regimen can then be adjusted to take account of positive laboratory findings and sensitivity test results if available. Treatment of proven *Listeria* meningitis should be continued for 15–21 days, with ampicillin 2 g × 4 hourly recommended, plus adjunctive gentamicin for the first week (Mylonakis, Hohmann and Calderwood, 1998).

Vancomycin (probably together with rifampicin) should be added if there is a possibility of a penicillin-resistant pneumococcus being involved (Cohen, 2003; Tunkel *et al.*, 2004). Management of pneumococcal infection is becoming more difficult with increasing antibiotic resistance in these organisms. Penicillin resistance in *S. pneumoniae* had reached 7% of isolates in England and Wales by the year 2000 (CDSC, 2000) while resistance to erythromycin had reached 15%. In global terms these are relatively low rates. In France, 51% of strains isolated from children have reduced susceptibility to penicillin with a high level of resistance in 15%. In Spain, penicillin resistance appeared early, with 6% of CSF isolates penicillin-resistant in 1979 and an overall rate of reduced susceptibility to penicillin of 39.4% of the strains causing systemic infection in the 1990–6 period (Fenoll *et al.*, 1998). Among cases of pneumococcal meningitis recorded in the Rhone-Alpes region of France in 1999, 48.6% of isolates were penicillin-resistant (Chomarat *et al.*, 2002), although mortality was higher among infections with penicillin-susceptible strains (six of seven deaths). Recent US data from Pottumarthy *et al.* (2005) report that 32% of strains overall are penicillin-resistant but that there are wide geographic variations. They also point out (Pottumarthy *et al.*, 2005) that resistance is substantially lower in isolates from blood than in isolates from noninvasive infections or carriage.

Similar differences in sensitivity were reported in the first Asian Network for Surveillance of Resistant Pathogens (ANSORP) study (Song *et al.*, 1999). Penicillin resistance has reached very high rates in Asia, but again there is marked geographic variation. In the second ANSORP study (Lee *et al.*, 2001) less than 10% of strains from Taiwanese children were found to be fully sensitive to penicillin, with intermediate susceptibility in 43.5% and high-level resistance in 47.8%. Other countries surveyed included South Korea (54.5% intermediate, 31.3% high-level resistance), Vietnam (58.2%, 12.2%) and Sri Lanka (70.6%, 5.9%), yet India had only 12.8% with intermediate resistance and none with high-level resistance and in the Philippines only 2.1% of strains showed reduced susceptibility to penicillin (Lee *et al.*, 2001).

In the neonate, treatment with antibiotics should be begun on suspicion as presenting features of neonatal meningitis may not always be localising. General features of sepsis include fever (present in about 60%), lethargy, poor feeding, vomiting and jaundice. Respiratory distress may also be present. Irritability, loss of tone, altered conscious level and especially seizures (occurring in over 40% of cases) signal CNS infection. Neck stiffness is uncommon in the neonate, and bulging of the fontanelle is less common in premature babies than in term babies (Klein, 2001). Consideration should be given to covering *Listeria*, group B streptococcus infection and meningitis due to Gram-negative bacteria in the neonate.

Meningitis is a notifiable disease in many countries, allowing a public health response. Contacts of cases of meningococcal meningitis should always be offered chemoprophylaxis as soon as possible (up to 28 days from the exposure), with rifampicin, ciprofloxacin or ceftriaxone, depending on age. In addition, vaccination should be offered if the infecting strain is of serogroup A, C, W135 or Y. The index case should also be given rifampicin or ciprofloxacin to eradicate pharyngeal carriage of *N. meningitidis* if ceftriaxone has not been given for treatment (Public Health Laboratory Service, Public Health Medicine Environmental Group, Scottish Centre for Infection and Environmental Health, 2002). For haemophilus meningitis, chemoprophylaxis with rifampicin is recommended for household contacts under the age of 5 years (British National Formulary, 2004). Prophylaxis is not currently recommended for contacts of sporadic cases of pneumococcal meningitis. However, where there is a cluster of epidemiologically linked cases of pneumococcal infection, chemoprophylaxis with rifampicin may be considered together with appropriate vaccination.

USE OF ADJUNCTIVE THERAPIES IN
THE TREATMENT OF MENINGITIS

Mortality and morbidity remain high in bacterial meningitis, particularly pneumococcal meningitis (Kastenbauer and Pfister, 2003), even when the bacteria involved are highly susceptible to antibiotics. The factors that lead to neurological damage involve a complex interaction between the effects of bacterial invasion and host responses, summarised diagrammatically in an editorial by Davis and Greenlee (2003). It is these host responses that lead to the release of damaging molecules including cytokines, chemokines and reactive oxygen and nitrite radicals, against which therapies adjunctive to antibiotics are aimed. It should be noted that different strategies may be required for different infections, as different bacteria can produce different effects on meningeal cells (Fowler *et al.*, 2004).

Steroids

The use of steroids as adjunctive therapy to antibiotics in the management of meningitis appears to be beneficial in a number of studies, at least in the outcome of meningitis due to *S. pneumoniae* and *H. influenzae* presenting early (Chaudhuri, 2004). As much of the morbidity in bacterial meningitis, including sensorineural hearing loss, is believed to be due to vigorous host inflammatory responses against the bacteria there is a theoretical appeal in dampening these responses (Townsend and Scheld, 1993), particularly as the initiation of bactericidal antibiotic therapy increases the inflammatory response because of increased release of bacterial components.

In the experimental animal, both steroids and nonsteroidal anti-inflammatory agents can be shown to minimise or prevent sensorineural deafness as a result of bacterial meningitis (Rappaport *et al.*, 1999a), with dexamethasone given 10 minutes before ampicillin being particularly effective. On overall meta-analysis it seems that the outcome for hearing does benefit from steroid use (van de Beek *et al.*, 2003), but there are variations among clinical studies regarding the benefits of steroids for both hearing and for neurological damage in general. This may depend on the age of the patient, other underlying problems and the organism involved. In the European Dexamethasone in Adulthood Bacterial Meningitis study, dexamethasone (10 mg given prior to, or with the first dose of, antibiotic, then 6 hourly for 4 days) significantly lowered mortality from pneumococcal meningitis, but not from meningococcal meningitis (de Gans and van de Beek, 2002). The reduced mortality from pneumococcal infection was due to a lessening of systemic complications, particularly cardiorespiratory failure (van de Beek and de Gans, 2004a).

Although there was no evidence of any benefit of dexamethasone in the frequency of neurological sequelae or hearing (de Gans and van de Beek, 2002; van de Beek and de Gans, 2004b), it could be argued that this reflected the higher number of severely ill patients who survived and could therefore be evaluated. A meta-analysis of studies in children suggested that risk of severe hearing loss was reduced if steroids were given in *Haemophilus influenzae* meningitis. There was also some benefit in pneumococcal meningitis if steroids were given before or at the time of the first dose of antibiotic (McIntyre *et al.*, 1997). Steroid administration for two days is probably optimal, with no additional benefit in outcome but increased risk of gastrointestinal bleeding after two days (McIntyre *et al.*, 1997).

Studies in developing countries, on the other hand, have not consistently shown benefits from the use of dexamethasone as an adjunctive therapy to antibiotics. On the one hand, a study in Costa Rican infants and children found that among survivors of meningitis followed up after 15 months, 14% of those who received dexamethasone before cefotaxime therapy was commenced had neurological or auditory sequelae, compared with 38% of those who received cefotaxime alone (Odio *et al.*, 1991). On the other hand, in a double-blind study of 598 children with bacterial meningitis treated in Malawi, the number of deaths was the same with or without dexamethasone given for two days at the start of therapy, and the overall rate of sequelae including deafness was identical in each arm of the study at 28% (Molyneux *et al.*, 2002). The principal bacteria involved were *S. pneumoniae* (40%), *H. influenzae* type b (28%), *N. meningitidis* (11%) and *Salmonella* spp. (13%); no significant improvement in outcome could be shown within any of these aetiological groups. In the report of Ciana *et al.* (1995) from Mozambique, use of steroids significantly reduced early mortality from bacterial meningitis, but did not show a significant benefit in overall mortality or neurological outcome. Similarly, in a Pakistani study (Qazi *et al.*, 1996) there was no benefit of steroids on either mortality or morbidity. Mortality in the adjunctive dexamethasone group was 25% compared with 12% in the placebo arm. Of survivors, 42% of the dexamethasone group had hearing impairment, compared to 30% in the placebo group. In summary, it appears that steroids may be of little or no benefit in resource-poor settings, particularly where there are additional underlying problems such as malnutrition and HIV infection, or where patients present for treatment late.

Further studies on outcomes with steroid use in meningitis are needed, particularly assessing the effects on learning following the recent study by Leib *et al.* (2003). In their infant rat model of pneumococcal meningitis there was increased neuronal apoptosis in the dentate gyrus of the hippocampus when antibiotics were combined with dexamethasone, and the rats were significantly less able to learn in a water maze, a test of spatial learning. Similar findings were previously described in the rabbit by Zysk *et al.* (1996).

Other adjunctive therapies

There are no current recommendations for use of adjunctive therapies other than corticosteroids. However, a number of approaches suggest themselves from what is known about the pathogenesis of meningitis and causes of hearing loss, and many studies have been done in the research setting. If the concepts of the role of reactive nitrogen and oxygen moieties in pathogenesis are important, then adjunctive treatment with antioxidants might be expected to attenuate hearing loss. This indeed is the case in experimental pneumococcal meningitis, where in the rat model treatment with the antibiotic ceftriaxone together with the antioxidants Mn(III)tetrakis(4-benzoic acid)-porphyrin, a catalyst of peroxynitrite decomposition, and *N*-acetyl-L-cysteine, which supports endogenous antioxidant responses by increasing glutathione concentrations as well as being a free-radical scavenger, significantly reduces early and long-term hearing loss (Klein *et al.*, 2003b). Histological changes are reduced and the integrity of the blood–labyrinth barrier is protected by antioxidants.

Nonsteroidal anti-inflammatory agents were given to rabbits with experimental pneumococcal meningitis by Tuomanen *et al.* (1987) in the hope of blocking the production of some arachidonate metabolites induced in response to bacterial cell wall components. The lipoxygenase inhibitor nordihydroguaiaretic acid did not reduce the inflammatory response in CSF significantly but cyclooxygenase inhibitors did. Of the cyclooxygenase inhibitors tested, oxindanac was more effective than diclofenac and indomethacin. Bacterial killing in animals treated with ampicillin plus oxindanac remained effective in spite of the reduced inflammatory response. Rappaport *et al.* (1999a) showed that adjunctive therapy with the nonsteroidal anti-inflammatory ketorolac was of benefit in reducing hearing loss in the rabbit model, although the effect was less than that of dexamethasone.

The tetracycline antibiotic doxycycline is an inhibitor of MMPs and when given with ceftriaxone in pneumococcal meningitis in rats confers benefits in survival and cerebral cortex damage without influencing CSF bacterial counts (Meli *et al.*, 2003). There is much interest in the tetracycline antibiotic minocycline as a neuroprotective agent in a variety of conditions (reviewed by Zemke and Majid, 2004). Like doxycycline, minocycline is a lipophilic molecule that penetrates well into brain. Minocycline appears to have a protective effect for hair cells *in vitro* against aminoglycoside-induced apoptotic damage. The mechanisms involved may be of some relevance to the meningitis situation. Minocycline inhibits caspase-3 activity as well as inhibiting the p38 MAP kinase pathway, preventing the release of cytochrome *c* (which activates caspases) and inhibiting inducible nitric oxide synthetases (Corbacella *et al.*, 2004; Wei *et al.*, 2005). It is also an MMP inhibitor and an inhibitor of inducible nitric oxide synthase in activated microglial cells, as well as inhibiting phosphorylation of p38 MAPK. This leads to diminished release of proinflammatory cytokines from microglia exposed to lipopolysaccharide. In addition, as shown by Kremlev, Roberts and Palmer (2004), there is inhibition of expression of proinflammatory chemokine receptors at the cell surface.

Brain-derived neurotrophic factor (BDNF) is an endogenous neurotrophin that may have a protective effect in meningitis. External BDNF confers protection against neuronal apoptosis in rat models of pneumococcal meningitis and group B streptococcal meningitis. It inhibits caspase-3 dependent (apoptotic) and caspase-3 independent (pyknotic) cell death, the latter probably by interfering with translocation of an apoptosis-inducing factor to the cell nucleus (Bifrare *et al.*, 2005).

Rifampicin inhibits release of pneumolysin in pneumococcal meningitis (see the section on pathogenesis) and also has the effect of reducing the release of teichoic and liopoteichoic acids and bacterial DNA. Mortality in experimentally infected mice is reduced (Nau *et al.*, 1999). In the rabbit pneumococcal meningitis model described by Böttcher *et al.* (2000) production of reactive oxygen radicals and proinflammatory compounds is reduced by rifampicin. Although the high rate of resistance to rifampicin precludes its use alone in therapy of pneumococcal disease, pretreatment of meningitis with rifampicin before commencing a β-lactam drug such as ceftriaxone might be of benefit. Clinical trials of such an approach have not been reported.

Melatonin, a secretory product of the pineal gland, acts as a broad spectrum antioxidant that can scavenge oxygen and nitrogen species including peroxynitrite. It is well tolerated in humans and crosses the blood–brain barrier. As well as improving outcomes in experimental pneumococcal meningitis, melatonin-treated animals show preservation of hippocampal dental gyrus neurones (Gerber *et al.*, 2005).

Cochlear implantation and meningitis

Significant improvement may occur in many cases of postmeningitis deafness with conventional amplification (Brookhouser and Auslander, 1989), sometimes after a considerable delay. For those who do not show significant benefit from hearing aid amplification, cochlear implantation is widely used, with a tendency to place the implant early, particularly in children (Gates and Miyamato, 2003). One of the principal factors in successful speech perception and speech production after cochlear implantation is the age at which deafness occurred. Speech perception after cochlear implantation has been shown to be significantly better in children with meningitis-associated hearing loss acquired after the age of two years than in those with hearing loss resulting from meningitis under the age of two or those with congenital deafness (Mitchell *et al.*, 2000). In the same study there was a trend towards better speech production in the group with deafness acquired after the age of two years, but this did not reach statistical significance.

Retrocochlear damage might be greater in younger children (Harada *et al.*, 1988) and the ability to process auditory signals from implants might be poorer after early hearing loss due to meningitis, in association with other evidence of persisting neurological problems as evidenced by lower IQ scores (Taylor *et al.*, 1984). This would appear to be supported by the lack of correlation between numbers of surviving spiral ganglion cells and word recognition after cochlear implantation (Khan *et al.*, 2005).

Early cochlear implantation at 7 to 12 months of age is advocated in some centres for meningitis-induced hearing loss to allow full insertion before ossification occurs (James and Papsin, 2004). Defining the extent of ossification after meningitis is important in determining the ability to insert a cochlear implant, and since ossification is believed to be progressive, and sometimes rapid (Dodds, Tyszkiewicz and Ramsden, 1997), earlier implantation may offer a better chance of finding a patent cochlea (Jackler *et al.*, 1987; Axon *et al.*, 1998). Assessment of the presence and degree of ossification can be made by

CT scan (Johnson *et al.*, 1995; Axon *et al.*, 1998). CT scanning may, however, be inaccurate within 6 months of meningitis, and MR scanning may offer earlier accurate estimates (Axon *et al.*, 1998).

Although early implantation may have a benefit in maintenance of vocabulary scores (El-Hakim *et al.*, 2001a), there is benefit in older age groups as well (El-Hakim *et al.*, 2001b). Auditory performance after cochlear implantation is generally satisfactory in those with postmeningitis deafness, although the possibility that the oxidative stress caused by the actual implantation of the device causes further neuronal loss and hair cell damage has been raised (Scarpidis *et al.*, 2003). Higher initial stimulation levels are often required in the postmeningitis group and, particularly in those with labyrinthitis ossificans, progressively increasing levels of stimulation may be needed over time (Eshragi *et al.*, 2004).

The most serious risk from cochlear implants is believed to be that of meningitis due to infection spreading from the middle ear to the inner ear and thence to the meninges. The implant potentially presents a relatively large area of 'dead space' material, which like all implanted devices can serve as a focus for infection (reviewed by Clark, 2003). Introduction of a fascia graft allows a sheath to develop around the implant which provides protection against infection both mechanically, through the development of mucus-secreting cells, and by allowing mobilisation of polymorphs around the sheath and of lymphocytes between the sheath and the electrode (Clark, 2003). Cochlear implantation is nowadays regarded as a relatively safe procedure and meningitis after it has been regarded as uncommon. In the recently reported series of 300 consecutive children treated in Nottingham no major surgical complications were reported within the first week after implantation and overall there was only a 2.3% rate of what were regarded as later major surgical complications (Bhatia *et al.*, 2004). Although a number of reported complications had the potential to cause bacterial meningitis, e.g. there were three CSF leaks from suture holes, one dural tear and several flap infections, early recognition of the problem and prompt intervention with antibiotics and surgery should successfully resolve most of these complications. No cases of meningitis after the procedure were seen in this paediatric series (Bhatia *et al.*, 2004), nor in the Manchester series of 240 adult cochlear implant operations (Green *et al.*, 2004), and only a single case of meningitis was noted in the review by Hoffman and Cohen (1995) of over 1900 paediatric implants.

After an apparent increase in reports to the US Food and Drug Administration (FDA) of meningitis after cochlear implantation in 2002, a major investigation was undertaken by the Centers for Disease Control and Prevention (CDC). The CDC study looked at children who had received a cochlear implant at age 6 years or under between 1997 and 2002. From 4262 implants there were 26 children who had confirmed bacterial meningitis. A case control study showed that those children with all types of cochlear implants were at greater risk than other children for meningitis; that the principal cause of postimplant meningitis was pneumococcal as the incidence of meningitis caused by *S. pneumoniae* was 138.2 cases per 100 000 person-years, more than 30 times the incidence in the general US population of the same age; that children with implants who had inner ear malformations and CSF leaks were at increased risk; and that children with implants that had a positioner were more likely to contract meningitis (Reefhuis *et al.*, 2003). No cases were caused by *N. meningitidis*. The manufacturer of the implants with a positioner (a small Silastic wedge inserted next to the electrode to facilitate transmission of the electrical signal by pushing the electrode against the medial wall of the cochlea) withdrew the product from the market in July 2002. An additional six cases of meningitis, five of which were associated with implants with a positioner, were reported after the study had been completed (Reefhuis *et al.*, 2003); all were due to *S. pneumoniae*. Up until May 2003, the FDA had learned of 118 cases of meningitis associated with cochlear implants worldwide, with 55 of these in the US. Cases in the US had onsets ranging from less than 1 day to over 6 years after the procedure; 32 cases occurred within one year of implantation (FDA, 2003). Of the 69 cases with positive CSF culture results, 46 grew *S. pneumoniae* (66.7%), 9 *H. influenzae* types b and non-b (13%), 4 *Escherichia coli* (5.8%), 3 *Streptococcus viridans* (4.3%), 4 staphylococci and 4 others (FDA, 2003).

As noted earlier, prompt recognition and treatment of infective complications of cochlear implantation is critical. Preventive measures against infection can also be employed. Although a published audit cast doubt on the need for routine perioperative antibiotic prophylaxis for cochlear implantation (Robinson and Chopra, 1989), intraoperative antibiotic prophylaxis is commonly given. In Nottingham, cephradine, one dose at induction, then two further doses within the first 24 hours after the procedure, has been given (Bhatia *et al.*, 2004). Short-course antibiotic prophylaxis such as this was associated with fewer complications than longer courses in a retrospective review of infection rates in Kilmarnock (Basavaraj *et al.*, 2004). In this Scottish study the antibiotics used for prophylaxis were cefuroxime or coamoxiclav.

The organism most likely to cause postimplant meningitis is *S. pneumoniae*. For this reason most authorities recommend pneumococcal vaccination for patients undergoing cochlear implant surgery, preferably begun at least two weeks before surgery. In England and Wales, the UK Department of Health recommends pneumococcal vaccination to all individuals who have cochlear implants. Recommended vaccines and dose schedules are found in the on-line Department of Health 'Green Book' publication. For those under 5 years of age the current recommendation is for 7-valent conjugate vaccine, together with 23-valent pneumococcal vaccine after the age of two years to broaden the serotype coverage. For children over 5 years and for adults, 23-valent vaccine should be offered (Anon, 1996a). US guidance is similar (Anon, 2003). Additional vaccination against *Haemophilus influenzae* type b (Hib) in individuals over 5 years of age is not specifically recommended after cochlear implantation (there is no data suggesting increased risk) and neither is there a need for additional vaccination against *N. meningitidis* in the cochlear implant population in the absence of some other risk factor for meningococcal infection.

Meningococcal and Hib vaccines should be given as part of a universal vaccination strategy, with conjugate Hib vaccine (usually as a component of a multivalent vaccine) being indicated for infants and children from 2 months to 10 years of age (Anon, 1996b) and meningococcal C conjugate vaccine indicated for infants (Anon, 1996c).

Follow-up after meningitis

Because damage occurs early all children who have had bacterial meningitis should have a brainstem auditory-evoked response test (ABR) or pure-tone audiometry before discharge from hospital to check for hearing loss. Clinical audiometric assessment remains important in addition to ABR. Use of otoacoustic emission (OAE) screening before the patient with meningitis leaves hospital may allow even higher assessment rates (Richardson *et al.*, 1998). Few cases of postmeningitic hearing loss (those few with retrocochlear damage) would be missed by OAE screening. The efficacy of using otoacoustic emissions (OAEs) for screening for hearing loss is debated; a loss of some 30 dB, or the presence of fluid in the middle ear, is required before OAEs are absent. Although Fortnum, Farnsworth and Davis (1993) reported that OAEs gave results in less than 55% of patients, other workers have felt that this simple technique can be used successfully as a screening test postmeningitis in the 48 hours before discharge from hospital. According to Richardson *et al.* (1998) OAEs have satisfactory characteristics for a screening test, with a sensitivity of 100% compared to ABR, a specificity of 91%, a negative predictive value of 100% and a positive predictive value of 44%. Hall and Penn (2002) and Hickson (2002) provide useful overviews of methods of testing for hearing loss in childhood. If not actually tested before discharge audiometric evaluation should be offered soon after discharge from hospital. Testing rates of over 80% within six weeks of discharge have been achieved in some centres by developing local standards of care involving referral for audiometry before discharge from hospital and checking against public health notifications of meningitis cases (Wilson, Roberts and Stephens, 2003).

Vestibular damage can also result from meningitis and may develop independently of hearing loss (Rahko *et al.*, 1984), so tests of vestibular function, which might include electronystagmography, should also be considered in evaluating patients after meningitis. Some 11% of cases of the uncommon condition of bilateral vestibular failure are due to bacterial meningitis. Of the five cases with a confirmed bacterial cause described by Rinne *et al.* (1998), three were due to *S. suis*, one to *N. meningitidis* and one to *S. pneumoniae*.

Vestibular function should also be tested in the postmeningitis hearing-impaired child (Angeli, 2003) and neuropsychological assessment is also advocated by some authors (Hugosson *et al.*, 1997).

Conclusions

This chapter has dealt with a primary event of meningitis resulting in hearing loss as a sequela of the infection. The clinician should always bear in mind that on rare occasions the association of hearing loss and meningitis may not be due to cochlear damage following bacterial infection but rather the reverse. An underlying abnormality such as a congenital labyrinthine fistula (Phelps, King and Michaels, 1994) may lead to deafness and a CSF leak that is likely to lead to meningitis as a secondary event.

Hearing loss follows meningitis in 5–30% of cases, particularly after pneumococcal infection. Hearing loss after nonbacterial meningitis is rare. The epidemiology of postmeningitis hearing loss has changed substantially in recent years, with successful vaccination programmes in developed countries against *H. influenzae* type b and *N. meningitidis* serogroup C, and the introduction of wider immunisation against *S. pneumoniae* is likely to lead to a further dramatic reduction in cases. In sub-Saharan Africa implementation of vaccination programmes against *N. meningitidis* serogroup A will lead to significantly less hearing loss from that cause while leaving the greater impact of pneumococcal meningitis largely untouched. The burden of hearing impairment following meningitis can be expected to decline further in the future as additional vaccination programmes reduce infections due to pneumococci and meningococci in developed countries as they have done with *H. influenzae*. Such initiitatives must be made available to resource poor countries as well as to the developed world. The single initiative that will have the greatest benefit in the near future in global terms is the Meningitis Vaccine Project, a partnership of the WHO and the Programme for Appropriate Technology in Health, which aims to introduce vaccination against *N. meningitidis* serogroup A in Africa with a vaccine costing less than $US 1 per dose. Careful monitoring will be required to recognise and to react to changes in the epidemiology of bacterial meningitis produced by the vaccination programme.

The pathogenesis of hearing loss is complex, although the most common lesion is cochlear. The principal antecedent is suppurative labyrinthitis with breakdown of the blood–labyrinth barrier. This leads to detrimental changes in the inner ear due to alterations in the biochemical environment, direct damage to hair cells and indirect damage through immunological and proinflammatory responses. There may be an early stage at which damage is reversible but once established sensorineural hearing loss does not resolve. Antibiotics sterilise CSF rapidly, but adjunctive therapies such as steroids and antioxidant compounds may have beneficial effects in reducing neuronal damage and hearing loss. Use of antibiotics increasingly requires knowledge of local resistance patterns among bacterial pathogens. Studies in humans of novel adjunctive therapies, especially drugs already used in man such as minocycline and melatonin, are warranted.

A strategy for arranging screening of patients for hearing loss and balance disturbance after meningitis should be in place at all centres managing meningitis. It might be possible to reduce the number of individuals requiring follow-up by using 'high-risk' criteria to identify those at risk of hearing loss. However, screening should be undertaken soon after recovery from infection to allow early intervention, including cochlear implantation, before cochlear ossification occurs.

Exciting findings regarding the capacity of differentiated hair cells to divide, the identification of stem cells in mouse vestibular organs that have the potential to differentiate into hair cells and the demonstration that supporting cells in the mature guinea pig cochlea can be induced to become hair cells by transfection with the gene for the Math-1 transcription factor (see the overview by Taylor and Forge, 2005) may be the beginnings of a journey that will lead ultimately to the ability to repair cochlear hearing loss with replacement hair cells.

12 INFECTIOUS DISEASES AND HEARING IN THE TROPICS

R. Hinchcliffe and S. Prasansuk

Introduction

TROPICAL MEDICINE

In the UK, Patrick Manson (1844–1922) is widely regarded as the father of tropical medicine. When he became Medical Adviser to the Colonial Office, he saw the need for special training. In 1898 he persuaded the Secretary of State for the Colonies to establish Schools of Tropical Medicine in both Liverpool and London in 1898 to educate doctors in tropical diseases. In the same year he published his textbook on tropical medicine (Manson, 1898). The Portuguese, of course, will remind us that the first textbook on tropical medicine was by Garcia d'Orta in 1563.

In his Foreword to the first edition of the US military's *Manual of Tropical Medicine*, the Surgeon General (Kirk, 1945) pointed out that it is difficult to separate the scope of tropical medicine from the wide field of general medicine. Moreover, tropical medicine is an arbitrary term since there is no sudden change in the nature and prevalence of diseases as one crosses the Tropic of Cancer in moving north from the Equator or the Tropic of Capricorn in moving south. It has become increasingly clear that what one should be talking about is 'geographical' medicine, which is reflected in the titles of textbooks on the subject, e.g. *Tropical and Geographical Medicine* (Warren and Mahmoud, 1984). 'Geography' is a multifactorial concept, involving climate, culture, ethnic factors and religion (Mann, 1966) as well as 'dirt, squalor and bad hygiene' (Platt, 1972) and topography (Balls *et al.*, 2004). One is, therefore, not surprised that the pattern and extent of hearing impairments in the tropics are influenced by what might be termed microgeographical conditions

Infection and Hearing Impairment. Edited by V.E. Newton and P.J. Vallely
© 2006 John Wiley & Sons, Ltd

(McPherson and Holborow, 1988). These concepts were already emerging in Britain in the 19th century as, for example, when doctors began to consider the effects of climate (Tylecote, 1880) and geography (Haviland, 1879) on health and disease.

The picture of tropical medicine – of geographical medicine – is not static. This is clear from the rapidly changing scene with the emergence of HIV/ AIDS and some other infectious diseases. Moreover, the increasing availability and speed of transportation between all parts of the World is reflected in the global spread of tropical infectious diseases. For example, France (Menard et al., 2003), Germany (Jelinek et al., 2002), the Netherlands (de Vries, Keret and Kortbeek, 2001) and the UK (Moore et al., 2003) have all reported gnathostomiasis being introduced into their countries from Thailand and other south-eastern Asian countries. Angiostrongylosis was brought back to Australia by a soldier after only six weeks service in Vanuatu (Fernando, Fernando and Leong, 2001). During 2000, four cases of fatal Lassa fever were imported from Africa to Europe (Schmitz et al., 2002). Two patients seen in Great Britain in 1971 were retrospectively diagnosed as having had Lassa fever (Gilles and Kent, 1976) and the importation of malaria into nontropical countries is a continuing problem (Cooper et al., 1982; Emond et al., 1982).

INFECTIOUS DISEASES

What Guthrie (1945) referred to as the 'dawn of scientific medicine' – the 19th century – was characterised by an increasing number of publications on the infectious diseases. In the clinical arena, Jenner (1849) clearly distinguished between relapsing fever, typhoid fever and typhus. In their 1847 book *Om Spedalskhed*, the Norwegians Danielssen and Beck gave, for the first time, a picture of leprosy based on clinical observations and post-mortem findings.

The 19th century also witnessed a number of seminal bacteriological and parasitological publications that are relevant to this chapter. For example, Sir Richard Owen (1836) reported a new species of parasitic worm, *Gnathostoma spinigerum*, which many years later was shown to be responsible for the gnathostomiasis that is endemic in Thailand and neighbouring tropical countries. In 1880, while serving in the French Army in Algeria, Charles Laveran recognised the malarial parasite in human blood and received the Nobel Prize for this work. Laveran was one of many doctors and scientists who received the award in the 19th century for work on identifying the cause of various infectious diseases (Liljestrand, 1962).

Resulting in part from Owen's discovery of *G. spinigerum* and the eventual elucidation of its life cycle by Daengsvang (1968) and others, there has been the increasing recognition that there is a group of infectious diseases, the zoonoses, that are worthy of separate study (Palmer, Soulsby and Simpson, 1998). Zoonoses are defined as diseases and infections that are transmitted naturally between vertebrate animals and man (WHO, 1959).

A more recent development in the understanding of the infectious diseases, especially of those cited in this chapter, has been the application of mathematics to their epidemicity and transmissibility. This has been both in respect of general analyses (Anderson and May, 1991) and of specific diseases, e.g. malaria (Aron and May, 1982). The importance of the infectious diseases in causing disorders of hearing was also documented in the 19th century by, for example, Roosa (1880), McBride (1882, 1884) and Schwartze (1892).

Tropical infections and their effect on hearing

VIRAL INFECTIONS

Lassa fever

As Howard (1998) points out, the Lassa virus made a dramatic appearance in Nigeria in 1969 as a lethal and highly transmissible disease. In a story akin to science fiction, doctors were first made aware of the threat by a nurse from the United States who contracted the disease in that year while working in a mission in the north-eastern town of Lassa (hence the name). When the nurse's condition continued to deteriorate she was flown to a hospital in Jos, where she died the following day. While she was in hospital she was cared for by two other nurses from the US. One of these became ill after an eight day incubation period. She also died (after an illness lasting eleven days). The head nurse of the hospital who had cared for the second nurse and assisted at the postmortem of the first nurse also became ill one week after the death of the second nurse. This third nurse was evacuated to the US in the first class cabin of a commercial aircraft with two attendants and screened from the economy class passengers only by a curtain. After a severe illness she slowly recovered under intensive care. A virus, subsequently termed the Lassa virus, was isolated from her blood by Yale Arborvirus Unit. One of the virologists also became ill but recovered following an immune plasma transfusion donated by the surviving nurse.

The virus is transmitted by the respiratory route and by direct contact with contaminated materials. Persistent complement-fixing antibodies have been demonstrated in patients who had recovered from the disease. The causative agent, a member of the arenavirus group, is known to be enzootic in rodents, particularly the Natal rat *Praomys natalensis*. *Praomys natalensis* is the most common rat in Africa. It digs into houses and eats everything, just as rats and mice do in the rest of the world. In some countries, e.g. Sweden, it has been adopted as a pet.

It was realised that Lassa fever constituted a disease of public health importance in several countries of Africa, especially West Africa (Fabiyi, 1976). Lassa fever has an insidious onset and is initially difficult to diagnose. It has 'nonspecific' clinical symptoms which have been confused with those of yellow fever and typhoid. It is highly contagious and was initially thought to have a high mortality rate. However, it is now recognised that in some areas of West Africa, infection with the virus may not be fatal as often as believed, or indeed may not always cause severe or clinically recognisable disease.

The US National Center for Infectious Diseases (NCID) investigated the epidemiology and clinical presentation of Lassa fever in the West African state of Guinea, where Lassa fever is barely recognised (Bausch *et al.*, 2001). A surveillance system was established and suspected cases were enrolled at five Guinean hospitals. The patients were examined clinically. Blood was taken for enzyme-linked immunosorbent assay testing and isolation of Lassa virus. Lassa fever was confirmed in 22 (7%) of 311 suspected cases. Another 43 (14%) had Lassa IgG antibodies, indicating past exposure. Both sexes and a wide variety of age and ethnic groups were affected. The disease was more frequently found, and the IgG seroprevalence generally higher, in the southeastern forest region. In some areas, there were significant discrepancies between the incidence of Lassa fever and the prevalence of antibody. Clinical presentations between those with Lassa fever and other febrile illnesses were essentially indistinguishable. Clinical predictors of a poor outcome were noted, but again were not specific for Lassa fever. Case fatality rates for those with Lassa fever and non-Lassa febrile illnesses were 18 and 15% respectively. Seasonal fluctuation in the incidence of Lassa fever was noted, but occurred similarly with non-Lassa febrile illnesses. The findings indicated that Lassa virus infection was widespread in certain areas of Guinea, but difficult to distinguish clinically.

The virus is considered to have a marked nosocomial propensity. Fisher-Hoch and his colleagues (1995) investigated two hospital outbreaks of Lassa fever in southern central Nigeria. Among 34 people with Lassa fever, including 20 patients, six nurses, two surgeons, one physician, and the son of a patient, there were 22 deaths (65% fatality rate). Staff had been infected during emergency surgery and while caring for nosocomially infected patients. Apart from doctors and nurses, UN peacekeepers in West Africa are also at risk of contracting Lassa fever (ter Meulen *et al.*, 2001).

In cases of fever of uncertain origin, Lassa virus infection should be considered not only in patients in West Africa but also in those returning from that area to other parts of the world. Of particular consideration should be those who present only with fever and neurological signs. Gunther and his colleagues (2001) report the case of a Nigerian patient who presented with fever, disorientation and seizures. Lassa virus was found in the cerebrospinal fluid (CSF) but not in the serum.

An effective, safe vaccine against Lassa virus can and should be made. Its evaluation for human populations is a matter of humanitarian priority (Fisher-Hoch *et al.*, 2000).

Lassa fever has been implicated in hearing loss. A prospective audiometric evaluation of 69 hospitalised febrile patients in Sierra Leone demonstrated a sensorineural hearing loss in 14 (29%) of 49 confirmed cases of Lassa fever and in 0 of 20 febrile controls. A sensorineural loss was present in 9 (17.6%) of 51 people who had evidence of previous Lassa virus infection. Of 32 local residents who had previously sustained a sudden hearing loss 26 had antibody titres to Lassa virus of 1:16 or greater, compared with 6 of 32 matched controls with titres at this level. Lassa fever is associated with an incidence of SNHL that considerably exceeds that previously reported with any other postnatally acquired infection. It accounts for a prevalence of virus-related hearing impairment in the Eastern Province of Sierra Leone that is greater than that reported from anywhere else in the world (Cummins *et al.*, 1990).

BACTERIAL INFECTIONS

Typhus

Typhus refers to a group of infectious diseases that are caused by rickettsial organisms and result in an acute febrile illness (Woodward and Osterman, 1984). Arthropod vectors transmit the causative agent to humans. The principal diseases of this group are epidemic typhus, its recrudescent form known as Brill–Zinser disease, together with murine typhus and scrub typhus. Epidemic typhus is the prototypical infection of the typhus group of diseases. The pathophysiology of this illness is representative of the entire category. The arthropod vector of epidemic typhus is the body louse (*Pediculus corporis*). This is the only vector of the typhus group in which humans are the usual host. *Rickettsia prowazekii*, the aetiologic agent of typhus, lives in the alimentary tract of the louse. A *Rickettsia*-harbouring louse bites a human to take a blood meal and defecates as it eats. It causes a pruritic reaction on the host's skin and when the host scratches the site, the lice are crushed. *Rickettsia*-laden excrement is inoculated into the bite wound, and these organisms then travel to the bloodstream. A rickettsaemia develops, and *Rickettsia* parasitise the endothelial cells of the small arterial, venous and capillary vessels. The organisms proliferate and cause endothelial cellular enlargement with resultant multiorgan vasculitis. This process may cause thrombosis. Small nodules may develop from the deposition of leucocytes, macrophages and platelets. Gangrene of the distal portions of the extremities, the nose, ear lobes and genitalia, may occur as a result of thrombosis of the supplying blood vessels. This vasculitic process may also result in loss of intravascular colloid with subsequent hypovolaemia and decreased tissue perfusion and, possibly, organ failure. Loss of electrolytes is common.

Clinically, typhus is characterised by fever of abrupt onset, with the temperature rising to 39–41 °C. A relative bradycardia is associated with the fever. The headache of typhus is also of abrupt onset and unremitting. Between the fourth and seventh day, a macular, maculopapular or petechial rash appears typically on the trunk and in the axilla before spreading to involve the rest of the body, except for the face, palms and soles. A regional lymphadenopathy develops. Deafness and/or tinnitus are reported as being less common symptoms of typhus. The vasculitic process may lead to CNS dysfunction, which may range from mental dullness to coma, multiorgan system failure and death. Several months may pass before survivors recover completely from fatigue and malaise.

Epidemic typhus occurs in Africa, Central and South America, northern China and certain regions of the Himalayas. Overcrowding leads to close personal contact and the spread of the arthropod vector among individuals. Lack of personal hygiene, such as infrequent bathing and changing of clothes, provides a hospitable environment for the body lice.

The incubation period for the typhus group of fevers is around 12 days. Prior infection with *R. typhi* provides subsequent and long-lasting immunity to reinfection by that organism. However, some people may have a recrudescence of the typhus (Brill–Zinsser disease). After a patient is treated with antibiotics and the disease has seemingly been cured, *Rickettsia* may linger in the body tissues. Months, years or even decades after treatment, organisms may reemerge and cause a recurrence of the typhus. The presentation of Brill–Zinsser disease is less severe and the mortality is much lower than that for epidemic typhus. Risk factors that may predispose a person to recrudescence include malnutrition and improper or incomplete antibiotic therapy. Brill–Zinsser disease occurs in around 15% of those with a history of the primary epidemic typhus.

Scrub typhus is caused by *Orientia tsutsugamushi* (formerly *Rickettsia tsutsugamushi*) via the mite, *Leptotrombidium akamushi*, and, possibly, *Leptotrombidium deliense*. The life cycle of the mite involves four stages of development but only the larval stage (chigger) requires a blood meal and is infectious to humans and other mammals. Once the mite is infected it acts as a reservoir for the organism. Humans are accidental hosts in scrub typhus. Mice, rats and larger mammals are the usual hosts. Scrub typhus occurs in northern Australia, the Indian subcontinent and the western Pacific region. Many cases of scrub typhus remain undiagnosed because of the nonspecific manifestations and the lack of laboratory diagnostic testing in endemic areas. However, a report on scrub typhus in Malaysia gave the incidence as 3% per month. Multiple infections in the same individual may occur because of a lack of cross-immunity among the various strains of *O. tsutsugamushi*.

The mortality rate for untreated epidemic typhus cases may be as low as 20% for healthy individuals but as high as 60% for elderly or debilitated individuals. Since the advent of widely available antibiotic treatment, mortality rates have fallen to about 3–4%. The mortality rate for treated patients with murine typhus is 1–4% and is almost 0% for scrub typhus.

In the 19th century, Hartmann examined 130 patients who were convalescing from typhus for signs of hearing impairment. Excluding six patients whose external meati were occluded by wax, 36 had ear disease. The lesions recorded were:

Catarrh of the Eustachian tubes and tympana	14
Acute otitis media with intact membrane	4
Acute otitis media with perforation	9
Increase of previous tinnitus and deafness	3
Return of a healed otorrhoea	1
Tinnitus without objective signs	2
Disease of the labyrinth	3

In his 19th century textbook on *The Diseases of the Ear*, Toynbee (1868) reported a case of 'partial deafness following an attack of typhus fever':

> Miss A.M., aged 16, saw me on March 1st, 1851. Eleven years previously she had an attack of typhus fever, and during the illness became so deaf as not to be able to hear the human voice. After the symptoms of fever had disappeared, the power of hearing slowly returned, until she was able to hear when loudly spoken to close to the head. There was no appearance of disease in either ear.

At the beginning of the 20th century, Wittmaack (1907) reported that degeneration of the nerve of hearing was the pathological basis for impairment of hearing resulting from typhus.

Diphtheria

The first unmistakable description of diphtheria was given by Aretaeus nearly two thousand years ago. The first clear and complete description in the English language was by Home in 1765. More than one hundred years later, Klebs (1883) first described the causative organism, *Corynebacterium diphtheriae* (Norman, 1991). Man is the only significant reservoir for the organism.

The toxic-appearing child with a bull-neck and an asymmetric, adherent, grey pharyngeal membrane which bleeds on removal presents no diagnostic problem (Halsey and Smith, 1984). The report on a large series of diphtheria cases half a century ago (Naiditch and Bower, 1954) provides useful clinical information. A complicating polyneuritis is not uncommon. Should this occur in the usual faucial diphtheria, it begins with a palatal paralysis 10 to 14 days after the onset of the illness. Neurological complications are thought to occur more commonly in the tropics.

That the disease can result in hearing loss has been well described in the older literature; e.g. McBride (1882, 1884) had the following to say about diphtheria (page 176):

> This disease may involve the external or middle ear, and probably also the labyrinth. Diphtheritic inflammation of the meatus is characterized, according to Gruber, by the formation of a false membrane in the canal, and by the fearful unremitting pain which accompanies it. It is a rare affection but has also been observed by others. Burnett describes a variety of otitis, which often results from

diphtheria, as follows: 'In children, there is often found at the termination of an attack of diphtheria, inflammation of the external ear. This rapidly extends, in some cases directly to the bone of the canal, and backwards to the mastoid process. Pain is not a prominent symptom in these inflammations which follow diphtheria, and this fact will readily distinguish them from the truly diphtheritic form of external otitis, in which the peculiar false membrane is found in the auditory canal. The form of disease now referred to is one arising from the broken-down condition of the little patient rather than a form of the disease already described as the diphtheritic. In the former case the pain is not great, the swelling is considerable, and the tendency to attack bone is marked. Fluctuation is soon felt over the mastoid region, and after evacuation of pus, the bone beneath is felt denuded, and in some cases crumbling.' Acute otitis media, which may and often does become chronic, is a common accompaniment of diphtheria. In this disease – as in scarlatina and variola – the labyrinth may be attacked. Wendt found that in a large proportion of cases the cartilaginous portion of the Eustachian tube was filled or lined by false membrane, while in one case only was he able to trace the diphtheritic process into the tympanum. . . . The occurrence of deafness due to post-diphtheritic paralysis is mentioned by writers of medicine, but has not yet attracted the attention of specialists.

The first accounts of the histopathological basis for the hearing loss in diphtheria were provided by Moos and Steinbrügge (1883). The report was based on the examination of six temporal bones of three children who had died of the disease.

Typhoid fever

Typhoid fever is caused by the bacterium *Salmonella typhi*, transmitted principally via contaminated drinking water but also by eating contaminated food or direct contact with an infected individual. The disease has thus been virtually eliminated in developed regions with treated water supplies but is still seen in developing countries where water supplies may become contaminated with faecal matter containing the organism. Richens (1996) has provided a useful general account of typhoid from the historical perspective in Cox's *Illustrated History of Tropical Diseases* (1996).

McBride (1884) had the following to say on typhoid: 'During the course of this disease the ear is not unfrequently attacked.' He then refers to a number of German authorities (Hoffmann, Moos, Politzer and Schwartze) (page 178):

According to Schwartze, deafness occurring in the course of typhoid may be due to – (1) suppuration of the middle ear, (2) pharyngeal catarrh extending towards the tympanum by way of the Eustachian tubes, or (3) central nervous disorders. Moos has demonstrated – *post mortem* – in several cases a cellular infiltration of the membranous labyrinth. Politzer found ecchymosis in the labyrinth in two cases, and Schwartze congestion of the cochlea in one instance.

Thus even in the 19th century there was a body of evidence showing that typhoid fever could result in both conductive and sensorineural hearing losses.

Thirty years ago sensorineural hearing loss complicating typhoid fever was being reported from India where a study showed almost 18% incidence of post-enteric sensorineural deafness, proving that *Salmonella* infection can produce otoneurotoxicity (Kakar, 1974). The vestibulocochlear damage seen in typhoid fever was described in more detail by Escajadillo and colleagues (1982).

Tuberculosis

Many countries in Africa, including Malawi (Kang'ombe *et al.*, 2004), Mozambique (MacArthur *et al.*, 2001) and Zambia (Mwaba *et al.*, 2003), are in the midst of a tuberculosis (TB) epidemic, with no signs of it abating. This explosion of tuberculosis is directly attributable to the HIV/AIDS pandemic as well as the associated breakdown of TB services. At one major hospital in Malawi 77% of TB patients were HIV positive. After seven years, only 17% of these patients were alive. HIV positive patients had higher death rates than HIV negative patients. Increased resistance to isoniazid and streptomycin was also reported (MacArthur *et al.*, 2001).

To accentuate these problems the severity of the disease process, e.g. in pulmonary tuberculosis cases, was found to be associated with the extent of malnutrition, as reflected by BMI and body composition studies using bioelectrical impedance analysis (Van Lettow *et al.*, 2004). Against this backdrop one would expect that such tropical countries would be more likely to have hearing impairments due to tuberculous aural and vestibulocochlear (meningitic or nonmeningitic) disease.

Sensorineural hearing losses due to tuberculous meningitis have been covered in Chapter 11. However, independently of tuberculous meningitis, tuberculosis *per se* may have a direct effect on the ear, either the middle ear or the internal ear.

Tympanic tuberculosis

Tuberculous otitis media is described by Michaels (1987) as:

> ... an unusual form of chronic otitis media, which is generally associated with active pulmonary tuberculosis. In the initial stages multiple perforations of the tympanic membrane develop. Granulations in the middle ear are pale and profuse and complications, especially involvement of the facial nerve, are more frequent than in the commoner form of chronic otitis media. Culture of the middle ear tissue may produce tubercle bacilli. Histological examination shows tuberculoid granulation tissue composed of epithelioid cells, Langhaus giant cells and areas of

caseation situated in the middle ear mucosa. There is much bone destruction. Acid-fast bacilli are found with difficulty.

Michaels had recently examined the sections from:

> . . . two remarkable cases of tuberculous otitis media. Both cases were otherwise healthy adult males with no evidence of tuberculosis of lung or other internal organ. In each case there was sclerosis of the temporal bone. Vast numbers of acid fast bacilli were present in the granulomas. They were confirmed as *Mycobacterium tuberculosis hominis* by culture.

Leprosy

Over half a million cases of leprosy are still detected each year. The clinical course of the disease is variable, ranging from the finding of a small macule with no symptoms and doubtful impairment of sensation, to widespread infiltration, plaques or nodules, often with involvement of numerous peripheral nerves, leading to loss of sensation and muscular weakness. In the words of McDougall (1996):

> Leprosy is not infrequently defined as a chronic communicable disease mainly attacking the nerves and skin, but the truth of the matter is that it is a complex disease, the proper definition of which calls for attention not only to its bacterial aetiology, but also to the variable immunological responses in individuals, the frequent occurrence of nerve damage, leading to loss of sensation and paralysis, and a range of social, psychological and economic factors, all of which have far reaching implications for the patient with leprosy and the operation of control programmes.

In their 1847 book *Om Spedalskhed*, the Norwegians Danielssen and Beck gave, for the first time, a picture of leprosy based on clinical observations and post-mortem findings. They distinguished leprosy from Norwegian scabies, psoriasis, scurvy and syphilis. Moreover, they realised that there were two main forms of the disease, i.e. the tuberculoid and the lepromatous forms. It was left to the Norwegian physician and bacteriologist Hansen to demonstrate the infective aetiology in 1873. Leprosy is now endemic throughout the tropics and occurs particularly in areas with poor socioeconomic conditions (McDougall, 1996).

WHO (1998c) recognises six types of leprosy. The three commonest are indeterminate leprosy (IL), tuberculoid leprosy (TL) and lepromatous leprosy (LL). IL is the earliest lesion of leprosy and may heal or progress to one of the other types. It presents as a hypopigmented dry macule, a few centimetres in diameter, which may be erythematous in white skin. There may be hypoaesthesia. The macule may be mistaken for psoriasis or tinea. In most cases spontaneous healing occurs, depending on the immunity. TL affects skin and peripheral nerves. The nerves commonly involved are the lateral popliteal, posterior tibial, greater auricular, median, radial and ulnar. The combination of a thickened nerve with peripheral nerve lesions differentiates leprosy from other neurological conditions. LL has a very extensive clinical presentation, involving the skin, peripheral sensory nerves, eyes, the cartilage of the nose, the liver, the testis, kidneys and bone, principally that of the nasal and zygomatic process, as well as the joints of the fingers. Induration of skin of the face and earlobes produces the characteristic leonine facies. Loss of eyelids on the lateral aspect characterises madarosis. Innumerable bacilli are found in the skin and in the bloodstream. The patient has no established immunity. The condition is fatal if untreated (Fernando, Fernando and Leong, 2001).

Shehata and his colleagues (1970) reported vestibulocochlear nerve involvement in leprosy. Singh and his colleagues (1984) investigated the auditory and vestibular function of 125 cases of lepromatous leprosy as well as 26 cases of tuberculoid leprosy. Impaired hearing was detected in 52% and vestibular hypofunction in 7.2% of the lepromatous cases. Conductive hearing loss was attributed to 'Eustachian tube catarrh secondary to atrophic rhinitis associated with the disease'. The sensorineural hearing loss and vestibular hypofunction were attributed to a labyrinthine lesion 'probably due to an ENL [erythema nodosum leprosum: an acute type of lepromatous reaction with generalised systemic involvement characterised by deep, tender subcutaneous nodules of the face, arms and thighs; apparent in untreated leprosy patients] reaction'. Vestibulococlear nerve involvement was considered to be unlikely. Damage to hearing was not observed in any of the tuberculoid cases.

PROTOZOAN INFECTIONS

Malaria

Malaria (Bruce-Chwatt, 1988; McGregor, 1996; Fernando, Fernando and Leong, 2001) is the infection caused by protozoa of the genus *Plasmodium*. Four species of this genus affect humans, i.e. *P. falciparum*, *P. malariae*, *P. ovale* and *P. vivax*.

In his book *Airs, Waters and Places*, the first book written on medical geography, Hippocrates described the association of splenic enlargement and poor health with the drinking of water from marshy places (McGregor, 1996). He can thus be considered to be the first malariologist (Russell, 1955).

The discovery of the insecticide DDT in 1942 and its effectivness against the malaria parasite made the ideal of global eradication of malaria seem possible, and throughout the 1950s and 1960s efforts were made to do this. However, although these efforts appeared successful initially the complete eradication of malaria was not achieved in many countries. The reasons for this are numerous and include development of resistance by the organism, but failure to implement the control measures effectively for social, economic and political reasons also played a role. Since this time, malaria incidence has increased steadily and current estimates suggest there are 350–500 million clinical episodes of malaria each year (Korenromp, 2004), with 1 million deaths occurring in Africa, mostly in children (WHO, 2003). In the year 2000 some 42% of hospital diagnoses and 32% of hospital deaths in one tropical African country (Tanzania) were attributed to malaria (Ministry of Health, 2002). These figures are considered to be typical for those African countries where malaria is endemic (WHO, 2003).

Cerebral malaria

Malaria can affect the nervous system in a number of ways (Osuntokun, 1983). *Plasmodium falciparum* remains one of the most common causes of central nervous system infection worldwide. In falciparum malaria, 10% of all admissions to hospital and 80% of deaths are due to CNS involvement. Yet CNS disturbances are fairly common in malaria. They could be due not only to severe *P. falciparum* infection but also to high-grade fever or to antimalarial medication. Focal neurological deficits, neck rigidity, photophobia, papilloedema and neurological sequelae are very rare in falciparum malaria and such a picture would therefore suggest other possibilities. Patients with cerebral malaria may show nonspecific electroencephalographic abnormalities. The CT scan of the brain is usually normal.

For a diagnosis of cerebral malaria (CM), the following criteria should be met: (a) deep, unarousable coma, which should persist for more than 30 minutes after a generalised convulsion (to exclude transient postictal coma); (b) exclusion of other encephalopathies; (c) confirmation of *P. falciparum* infection: asexual forms of this parasite must be demonstrated in a peripheral blood or bone marrow smear during life or in a brain smear after death.

Recently, differences between the pathophysiology of cerebral malaria in African children and nonimmune adults have been discovered, new syndromes occurring after malaria infection described and mechanisms for the pathogenesis proposed (Newton and Warrell, 1998).

The basic underlying defect in cerebral malaria seems to be clogging of the cerebral microcirculation by the parasitised red cells. These cells develop knobs on their surface and develop increased cytoadherent properties, as a result of which they tend to adhere to the endothelium of capillaries and venules. This results in sequestration of the parasites in these deeper blood vessels. An electron microscopic study of 65 patients who died of severe malaria in Thailand and Vietnam showed that sequestration of parasitised red blood cells (PRBCs) in cerebral microvessels was significantly higher in the brains of patients with CM compared with those with noncerebral malaria (NCM) in all parts of the brain. The degree of sequestration of *P. falciparum*-infected erythrocytes in cerebral microvessels was quantitatively associated with pre-mortem coma (Pongponratn *et al.*, 2003).

Clinically, abnormal retinal vessels unique to cerebral malaria have been shown to be associated with a poor outcome in African children. The retinal vessels in children with cerebral malaria contain many parasitised red blood cells; these cells tended to cluster at the periphery of vessels or, in the case of capillaries, to fill the vessel. Those with late-stage parasites had markedly reduced amounts of haemoglobin. The pattern of dehaemoglobinisation corresponds to the pattern of clinically abnormal vessels. The sequestration of late-stage parasitised red blood cells with reduced amounts of haemoglobin accounts for the unique white and pale orange retinal vessels seen in cerebral malaria. Clinical examination of these 'marked' vessels offers a method to monitor a basic pathophysiological process of cerebral malaria *in vivo* (Lewallen *et al.*, 2000).

The clinical diagnosis of cerebral malaria in *Plasmodium falciparum*-endemic regions is strengthened by the post-mortem demonstration of cerebral sequestration. Sequestered parasites in a cytological preparation of a supraorbital brain sample, obtained after death, can be studied by use of standard thin blood-film staining. When confirmation by a post-mortem examination is not possible, this procedure is a reliable surrogate for the histological study of tissue (Milner *et al.*, 2005).

Cerebral malaria carries a mortality of around 20% in adults and 15% in children. Residual deficits are unusual in adults (<3%). About 10% of the children (particularly those with recurrent hypoglycaemia, severe anaemia, repeated seizures and deep coma) who survive cerebral malaria may have persistent neurological deficits. Cerebral malaria may be the primary cause of sudden death in nonimmunised persons during or after travelling in endemic areas of Africa (Yapo Ette *et al.*, 2002).

Hearing disorders in malaria

Attributable to antimalarial medication

Quinine, which is derived from the bark of the cinchona tree, was introduced to Europe by the Jesuits. It became the first and only antimalarial drug until the synthesis of such substances. However, excessive doses of quinine can lead to 'cinchonism'. This is a condition that is characterised by ringing in the ears, hearing impairment, blurred vision, nausea and abdominal upset. In severe cases, it may even lead to circulatory collapse, kidney failure and coma. Acute quinine toxicity may present as acute bilateral blindness, as well as the classic symptoms of cinchonism, including nausea, vomiting and tinnitus. Two cases showed prolongation of the Q-T interval on the ECG. Serum quinine levels of 5.3 and 13 mg/L were measured (Wolf, Otten and Spadafora, 1992).

The adverse effects of quinine were sufficiently a problem to have been investigated by Wittmaack (1904, 1919, 1936) in a series of experimental studies. Subsequent studies on experimental animals (Permin, 1957; Hennebert, 1959) produced some conflicting information.

Chloroquine, an antimalarial that has had widespread use, was developed as a synthetic analogue of quinine. There have been a number of reports of its ototoxicity (Matz and Naunton, 1968; Dwivedi and Mehra, 1978; Mukherjee, 1979; Obiako, 1985; Hadi, Nuwayhid and Hasbini, 1996). Mukherjee's case report concerned a 6 year old girl suffering from severe cochlear-vestibular dysfunction following a series of chloroquine phosphate injections. 'Prompt institution of therapy with steroids and vaso-dilators helped to restore the hearing to a serviceable (socially acceptable) level.' However, experimental studies with the drug on the guinea pig failed to demonstrate permanent damage to the hair cells of the cochlea (Sykes, 1984).

Attributable to cerebral malaria

A London otologist who visited a typical tropical country, Malawi, some 30 years ago had the following to say: 'Like General Drummond, I have encountered a considerable number of young children who have lost virtually all their hearing after feverish illnesses often accompanied by coma but not apparently by ear infection. Some of them may be viral encephalitis as General Drummond suggested; others are regarded as cases of cerebral malaria and this has been proved in a few cases' (Salmon, 1974).

Holding and Snow (2001) suggest that malaria in general, let alone cerebral malaria, in childhood is likely to have effects on general cognitive and behavioural development. It is therefore a matter of conjecture as to whether or not the survivors of cerebral malaria will also have central auditory processing difficulties.

METAZOAN INFECTIONS

Among the metazoa, members of both the nematodes (roundworms) and the cestodes (flatworms) are parasites of man. The nematodes *Angiostrongylus cantonensis* and *Gnathostoma spinigerum* are endemic in Thailand and other parts of South-East Asia. In that same region of the world, eosinophilic meningitis is also endemic. Extensive studies in Thailand in the 1960s indicated that the eosinophilic meningitis was almost invariably due to invasion of the CNS by *Angiostrongylus cantonensis* or *Gnathostoma spinigerum* – so much so that the term 'eosinophilic meningitis' has become synonymous with angiostrongylosis or gnathostomiasis. Moreover, it was also recognised that there are broadly two types of eosinophilic meningitis, i.e. eosinophilic meningoencephalitis (Tangchai, Nai and Beaver, 1967) and eosinophilic myeloencephalitis (Punyagupta *et al.*, 1968; Bunnag, Comer and Punyagupta, 1970), which were due to *Angiostrongylus cantonensis* and *Gnathostoma spinigerum* respectively (Sorasuchart, Khunadorn and Edmeads, 1968; Nye *et al.*, 1970). Perhaps the largest series of eosinophilic meningitis cases was reported from Thailand by Punyagupta, Juttijudata and Bunnag (1975).

In practice, considerable variability in this dichotomous classification is observed. For example, in a review of the neurological findings in 24 patients with nervous system gnathostomiasis, Boongird and his colleagues (1977) noted that the commonest presenting features were radiculomyelitis or radiculomyelitis terminating with encephalitis. A primary encephalitic form was noted in two patients. A severe radiculomyeloencephalitic form of angiostrongylosis affecting infants was reported by Graber and his colleagues (1999) from the island of Mayotte (one of the Comoro group of islands in the Indian Ocean).

More recent reviews of eosinophilic meningitis (Hughes, Magret and Fishbain, 2003; Lo Re and Gluckman, 2003) have pointed out that other infections as well as noninfectious conditions may also be associated with the condition (Ismail and Arsura, 1993; Woods and Englund, 1993; Chan *et al.*, 2004).

Angiostrongylosis

Two species of *Angiostrongylus* infect man, i.e. *A. cantonensis* and *A. costaricensis*. The latter, as its name implies, is found in Costa Rica. It is responsible for abdominal angiostrongylosis. *A. cantonensis* is responsible for cerebral angiostrongylosis (sometimes referred to as angiostrongyliasis, but see Kassai *et al.*, 1988).

When discovered in 1944 the rat lungworm, *Angiostrongylus cantonensis*, was thought to be a parasite of rodents only. It was subsequently found in a teenager's brain in Taiwan. Since then *A. cantonensis* infections of man have been reported from Australia (Heaton and Gutteridge, 1980; Senanayake *et al.*, 2003), Jamaica (Lindo *et al.*, 2002, 2004), Mayotte (Graber *et al.*, 1999), Réunion (Badiaga *et al.*, 1993), the tropical Pacific region (Porciv and Brindles, 1984), Tahiti (Thobois *et al.*, 1996), Thailand (Tangchai, Nye and Beauer, 1967), the US and other countries.

The life cycle of *A. cantonensis* (Fernando, Fernando and Leong, 2001) requires that the definitive host be a terrestrial mammal and the intermediate host an invertebrate. The definitive hosts for *A. cantonensis* are usually rodents from the genus *Rattus*, particularly *R. norvegicus* and *R. rattus*. The main intermediate hosts are slugs and snails, e.g. *Achatina fulica* and *Ampullarium canaliculatus*, from which one child in Taiwan appears to have become infected when rearing them as pets (Wan and Weng, 2004). Other children, even those living outside the tropics, have become infected after swallowing a raw snail 'on a dare'. Paratenic hosts, i.e. those in which no further development occurs, include anything that eats the molluscs. Some main ones include terrestrial planarians and crabs, freshwater shrimp and frogs, toads, marine

fish and sea snakes. The Division of Parasitic Diseases of the Centers for
Disease Control and Prevention (a component of the US Department of
Health and Human Services) maintains an information source on angiostrongylosis   at   http://www.cdc.gov/ncidod/dpd/parasites/angiostrongylus/
factsht_angiostrongylus.htm (accessed 2 June 2005).

Chotmongkol and his colleagues (2004) reported the case of a 59 year
old woman who presented with chronic headache, neck stiffness and left-
sided hearing loss. The diagnosis of angiostrongylus eosinophilic meningitis
was made. The patient and her hearing improved after treatment with
prednisolone. Angiostrongylus eosinophilic meningitis associated with
sensorineural hearing loss had not previously been reported.

Gnathostomiasis

Long before its role in the causation of eosinophilic meningitis was recognised,
gnathostomiasis was known to be endemic in Thailand. The first case was that
of a Bangkok woman whose breast abscess was incised in 1889. The organism
that was recovered from the abscess was subsequently identified as *Gnathostoma spinigerum*. Over the past 80 years, clinical forms of gnathostomiasis,
other than the commoner cutaneous type and including some with neurological complications, have come to be recognised. Over a 5 year period (1940–5),
528 cases were recorded from one hospital (Siriraj Medical School Hospital)
alone (Chitanondh, 1963).

Cases of gnathostomiasis have now been reported from Australia (Heydon,
1929), Cambodia and Indonesia (Margono, Idris and Brodjonegoro, 1978),
Israel (Witenberg, Jacoby and Stechelmacher, 1950), Japan (Ishida *et al.*, 2003),
Korea (Nawa, 1991), Mexico (Puente *et al.*, 2002), Myanmar (Nomura *et al.*,
2000), Peru (Chappuis, Farinelli and Loutan, 2001), the Philippines (Fernando,
Fernando and Leong, 2001), Sri Lanka (Samarasinghe, Perera and Ratnasena,
2002), Taiwan (Nawa, 1991), Vietnam (Fernando, Fernando and Leong, 2001)
and Zambia (Hale, Blumberg and Frean, 2003).

Until the early 1980s, all gnathostomiasis cases found in major endemic
areas in Asia were due to *G. spinigerum*. Subsequently, *G. doloresi* and *G.
hispidum* were incriminated (Nawa, 1991) and, later, *G. malaysiae* (Nomura
et al., 2000) and *G. nipponicum* (Ishida *et al.*, 2003).

Gnathostomiasis is a zoonosis. As its life cycle (Daengsvang, 1968; Rojas-
Molina *et al.*, 1999) indicates, humans acquire the disease by eating the second
intermediate hosts (as uncooked food) of the third-stage larvae (L3) of
Gnathostoma spp. These second intermediate hosts have themselves acquired
the infection by ingesting the freshwater copepod, *Cyclops*. This first intermediate host ingests the first-stage larvae of *Gnathostoma* spp., which enables
it to be transformed into the second- and then third-stage larvae. Ordinarily,
the cat and the dog constitute the definitive (final) host.

In South-East Asia the second intermediate host that is eaten by humans is one or other of various species of freshwater fish. The raw flesh of *Ophicephalus striatus* is considered a delicacy by Thai women. Sliced raw *O. argus*, *O. tadiamus*, *Cyprinus auratus* (the crucian carp) and *Acanthogobrus hasta* (goby) constitute the 'sashimi' of Japan. The raw carp (*Cyprinus carpio*) is the basis for 'naniura' in Indonesia. The largemouth bass (*Micropterus salmoides*) has also been incriminated in Japan (Ishida *et al.*, 2003), as have swamp eels (*Monopterus alba*) purchased from Klong Toey market, the largest market in Bangkok (Saksirisampant *et al.*, 2002).

The University of London and Mahidol University have provided a useful review of the subject of gnathostomiasis (Moore *et al.*, 2003). Some 30 years ago we reported an unusual case of gnathostomiasis (Prasansuk, 1974; Prasansuk and Hinchcliffe, 1975). A 23 year old man from Nakhon Ratchasima had been admitted to Mahidol University's Siriraj Hospital in Bangkok with a right facial palsy of two weeks' duration. About one month previously the patient had experienced vertigo and headache of sudden onset. These symptoms were accompanied by vomiting and pains in the right lower limb. Shortly afterwards he had lost consciousness for a few minutes. On regaining consciousness he noticed that the headache was worse and he had difficulty hearing on his right side. In addition there was weakness and numbness of the right lower limb. Two weeks after the onset the patient noticed the facial weakness along with 'swelling' of the right eye. He denied having eaten uncooked foods. The examination on admission revealed proptosis of the right eye and a partial infranuclear facial palsy on that side. There was a right external rectus palsy together with a right-sided hemifacial hypalgesia, hearing loss and absent corneal reflex. The conjunctiva of the right eye was markedly injected. Fundoscopy showed bilateral congested retinal veins but normal optic discs. There were no signs of meningeal irritation.

Otoscopic examination showed the right tympanic membrane to be imperforate and mobile but hyperaemic. Audiometric examination showed a moderate sensorineural hearing loss on the right. There was a small conductive component and evidence for abnormal auditory adaptation, but no indication of a cochlear lesion on short increment sensitivity index (SISI) testing. No spontaneous or positional nystagmus was observed but the caloric test showed impairment of vestibular nerve function on the right side.

Important negative findings emerged from the investigations. There were no subcutaneous nodules. A Venereal Disease Research Laboratory (VDRL) test was negative. Radiological examination of the skull showed no abnormality. The cerebrospinal fluid was under normal pressure and contained no cells, let alone eosinophils. Eosinophilic meningitis was therefore excluded on the basis that there was neither meningism nor eosinophiloracchia.

Nearly two months after admission to hospital, the patient developed an exacerbation of both his right earache and his tinnitus. He said it was as though something were biting inside his ear. These two symptoms persisted for about two hours, at the end of which time a drop of blood and a worm was discharged from the right external acoustic meatus. This was identified as *Gnathostoma spinigerum*. It was postulated that the pathological basis for this man's symptoms was a mild combined dural venous thrombosis involving the cavernous, inferior petrosal and basilar sinuses.

If such a patient were admitted with these symptoms today we would not have had to wait until the organism made its appearance to provide the correct diagnosis. The University's Helminthology Department is now able to do serologic testing for gnathostomiasis (the presence on immunoblot of the specific 24 kDa band diagnostic of *Gnathostoma* infection). Moreover, MRI is now being used in Thailand for the assessment of gnathostomiasis cases (Sawanyawisuth *et al.*, 2004). As Sawanyawisuth and his colleagues point out, serology is the criterion standard for diagnosing gnathostomiasis, whereas MR imaging represents a complementary tool for assessing severity and extent of disease. Furthermore, effective treatment for gnathostomiasis is now available – albendazole and ivermectin (Nontasut *et al.*, 2000; Chappuis, Farinelli and Loutan, 2001; Germann *et al.*, 2003).

Even longer delays than this case have been experienced between initial symptoms and diagnosis. A five year delay in another case was attributed to the absence of eosinophilia (Slevogt, Grobusch and Suttorp, 2003).

The man from Nakhon Ratchasima reflected one of the conclusions from an analysis of neurognathostomiasis cases in Thailand (Boongird *et al.*, 1977) and at the same time provided an exception to another. One of the conclusions was that 'No single area of the nervous system was inaccessible to the highly invasive gnathostome larva'. Another conclusion was that 'Multiple cranial nerve palsies were usually bad prognostic signs'. However, this merely reflects the uniqueness of the individual (Medawar, 1961) – the importance of the single case history (Vandenbroucke, 1999).

Sparganosis

Sparganosis is found throughout the world, but is most common in Eastern Asia. Human infection is not common. It is a disease that is associated with the development of 'spargana', or cysts, in subcutaneous connective tissue and superficial muscles. The lesion is nodular, develops slowly and can be found on any part of the body. The sparganum may be itchy, inflamed and painful. The subcutaneous lesion resembles a lipoma, fibroma or sebaceous cyst. These spargana are stages in the life cycle of a tapeworm. The cycle requires two intermediate hosts. The first is a copepod (planktonic crustacean) which ingests embryos that develop from the tapeworm's eggs when they reach the water with the faeces of dogs or cats (the worm's normal host). The infected copepod is then ingested by one of many vertebrates, including amphibians, reptiles, birds, fish, small mammals (rodents and insectivores), nonhuman primates and pigs. Humans can contract the disease by ingesting infected first-intermediate hosts (e.g. infected copepods in drinking water) or infected second-intermediate hosts (e.g. raw or undercooked amphibians, mammals or reptiles).

Once in the human host the spargana can migrate to virtually any part of the body and grow to be quite large. The pathology associated with sparganosis depends on the number and size of spargana and the organs involved. Infections consisting of one or two spargana in the deep muscles might cause no overt symptoms and go undiagnosed. Infections in the eye can result in blindness, while infections of subdermal tissues can result in painful 'lumps' that might be misdiagnosed as cancer.

It is almost impossible to identify spargana to species, so it is unclear how many or which species of pseudophyllidean cestodes will infect humans. There are no specific treatments but the spargana may be removed surgically. The Queensland Government provides information on sparganosis at http://www.dpi.qld.gov.au/health/3928.html (accessed 02 June 2005).

Kittiponghansa and his colleagues (1988) reported on a Thai patient with ocular sparganosis who also had a hearing loss. A subconjunctival mass lesion had been produced by a larva of *Spirometra* sp. The parasite was removed intact and alive with complete preservation of the patient's vision. It was thought that the mode of infection was probably through consumption of contaminated drinking water.

Other factors affecting hearing loss in the tropics

It is generally said that, in the tropics, the same patient will be labelled with a number of diagnoses. There will therefore always be questions as to which, if any, of various general medical conditions might be responsible for a person's hearing loss. For example, HIV/AIDS is pandemic in parts of the tropics and a substantial number of these patients have a sensorineural hearing loss (Soucek and Michaels, 1996). The presence of a noninfective general medical condition can also confound any attribution, e.g. the widespread sickle cell anaemia, which can also cause a hearing loss (Tsibulevskaya, Obwrra and Aluoch, 1996).

Further, even in the poorest and most diseased tropical countries enough of their inhabitants are living long enough to be troubled by the effect of ageing processes on the auditory system, whether we call it 'presbyacusis' or something else. For example, 23% of the hearing aid fittings at the Ang Duong Hospital in Phnom Penh (Cambodia) were for presbyacusis (Vaughan, personal communication, 2004). 'Ageing hearing loss' was the most common cause (29%) of sensorineural hearing losses uncovered by a large survey of the general population in Vietnam (Huynh, 2000). The ageing factor therefore needs to be considered in all attributions of hearing loss, even in the tropics.

However, a diagnosis of 'presbyacusis' still raises the question of cause. It is likely that much of this type of hearing loss is attributable to undiagnosed cases of familial or genetic-related hearing loss (Lowell and Paparella, 1977). Indeed, here as elsewhere, the most commonly misdiagnosed high-tone hearing loss in adults is progressive genetic hearing loss (van Camp, 1996).

Summary

In the Ormerod–Shillingford Report (1961) on *Deafness in Africa* we read:

> KENYA: the otologists . . . were very much aware of the many cases of deafness following a febrile illness which might consist only of a day or two of pyrexia or might include convulsions or coma for a number of days. On recovery the child was profoundly depressed, often totally deaf, and had lost the ability to speak, and did not regain either hearing or the power of speech unless retrained. It was agreed that this must be due to a virus.

Ormerod did not visit Malawi but a few years later Sir Alexander Drummond (1968) conducted an epidemiological study there. Drummond reported:

> Malawi has causes of deafness such as ARBOR virus infections which at present are not in Britain. . . . Post-natal virus infections . . . patients in the Lilongwe district who, following a high fever and severe illness, developed deafness without infection of the middle ear . . . some five miles away at the Likuni Mission Hospital an African child, aged three years was seen. His condition was described as post-aseptic meningitis. No organisms were found in his cerebro-spinal fluid. The boy was totally deaf with normal eardrums. He had no interest in his mother or in his surroundings but occupied himself by repeatedly putting his right hand five or six times through a metal band and then biting the band twice. This type of repetitive action was noticed in Malaya in patients who were convalescent following virus infections and is a post-encephalitic syndrome.

Audiograms of ten cases attributed to virus infection – measles in two – were presented. Malawi was also visited by a London otologist, Salmon (1974). He said:

> Like General Drummond, I have encountered a considerable number of young children who have lost virtually all their hearing after feverish illnesses often accompanied by coma but not apparently by ear infection. Some of them may be viral encephalitis as General Drummond suggested; others are regarded as cases of cerebral malaria and this has been proved in a few cases. It is certainly true that in some cases the result is a sort of autistic picture with a child failing to respond not only to sound stimuli but to other stimuli also. Perhaps, as was suggested to me yesterday, some of these cases are not deaf.

These observations remain timely and illustrate the need not only for more and continuing epidemiological studies concerning the causes of hearing loss in the tropical regions but also for case histories and pathological studies, including histopathological examinations of temporal bones of affected individuals. Only by these methods can one construct the mechanism-based medicine that the clinician uses to diagnose and manage a disorder. Indeed, a single case history, even those recorded many years ago, can help the clinician diagnose the cause of a disorder of hearing which perhaps rarely complicates a common or rare infectious disease.

13 OTOTOXIC DRUGS

R. Taylor and A. Forge

Introduction

Ototoxic agents are those that damage the end-organs of hearing (in the cochlea) and balance (in the vestibular system) of the inner ear. Agents that cause hearing impairment or balance dysfunction through effects on the respective neural pathways and centres are not considered in this chapter. A diverse range of therapeutically useful drugs and some environmental agents have been reported to be ototoxic (Table 13.1). The adverse effects of these agents vary between relatively minor reversible deficits to permanent functional impairment, although for some of the agents listed in Table 13.1 the evidence for ototoxicity is limited; sometimes it derives from individual case reports, where other confounding factors may have contributed to the observed effect, and there are no confirmatory experimental studies in animals. Hearing loss is the common ototoxic effect of the agents listed (cochleotoxicity), but many affect the vestibular system as well. There are few agents known to be exclusively vestibulotoxic, although in humans, with some aminoglycosides balance dysfunction is the primary ototoxic symptom with relatively little hearing impairment (e.g. streptomycin), but with others, hearing loss is the predominant side-effect (e.g. neomycin). The reasons for this difference in vulnerability between the cochlea and the vestibular organs to different aminoglycosides are not known, and the differential susceptibility varies with species. This has sometimes led to difficulties in choosing appropriate animal models for toxicity testing (Forge and Harpur, 2000; Forge and Schacht, 2000). Histologically, the inner ear is composed of sensory epithelia, ion-transporting epithelia that maintain the environment in which the sensory cells function and nonspecialised epithelia, as well as neurones and connec-

Infection and Hearing Impairment. Edited by V.E. Newton and P.J. Vallely
© 2006 John Wiley & Sons, Ltd

Table 13.1. Compounds known to be or reported to be implicated in ototoxicity

Classification	Compounds	Usual effects
Aminoglycoside antibiotics	Amikacin, dibekacin, dihydrostreptomycin, framycetin, gentamicin, kanamycin, neomycin, netilmicin, ribostamycin, sisomicin, streptomycin, tobramycin	Permanent hearing loss (progressive; high to low frequencies) Vestibular dysfunction
Macrolide antibiotics	Erythromycin, azithromycin, clarithromycin	Temporary hearing loss
Other antibiotics	Ampicillin, capreomycin, chloramphenicol, colistin (polymyxin E), minocycline, polymyxin B, rifampicin, vancomycin, viomycin	See text
Antitumour agents	cis-Platinum, carboplatin antinomycin, bleomycin, nitrogen mustards (e.g. mustine), misonidazole	Permanent hearing loss
Anti-inflammatory agents	Salicylate (aspirin)	Temporary hearing loss
	Fenoprofen, ibuprofen, indomethacin, naproxen, phenylbutazone	
Antimalarials	Quinine, chloroquine	Temporary hearing loss
Loop diuretics	Bumetanide, ethacrynic acid, frusemide (furosemide), piretanide	Temporary hearing loss
Iron chelators	Desferrioxamine	See text
Beta-blockers	Practolol, propranolol	
Contraceptives	Medroxyprogesterone	
Industrial chemicals	Trimethyltin, toluene, trichloroethylene, styrene, xylene	Permanent hearing loss

tive tissue. Broadly, ototoxic agents may act on the sensory epithelia, the ion-transporting epithelia or both, and the varying symptomatology of different ototoxic agents reflects their site and mode of action. While some of these (e.g. loop diuretics) are not directly relevant to infection, their inclusion will show the range of ototoxic side-effects that might be expected.

Distribution of ototoxins to the inner ear

The complete enclosure of the inner ear structures within the bone means that they are not exposed directly to potentially damaging environmental agents. Access to the perilymphatic compartment of the inner ear is possible from the middle ear cavity via the membrane covering the round window at the base of the cochlea. Potentially bacterial toxins associated with middle ear infections as well as ototoxic drugs may enter the inner ear in this way, although this is rare for the former. Access to perilymph via the cochlear aqueduct from the cerebrospinal fluid (CSF) is also possible and this may also be a route of entry for bacterial toxins, such as those associated with meningitis, and perhaps bacteria themselves (Figure 13.1). Usually, however, ototoxic agents reach the inner ear predominantly through the blood supply. There are, however, restrictions on the entry of agents to the fluids of the inner ear. Analysis of the composition of perilymph (Wangemann and Schacht, 1996) reveals that it is not simply an ultrafiltrate of blood plasma, nor does it derive from CSF. Further-

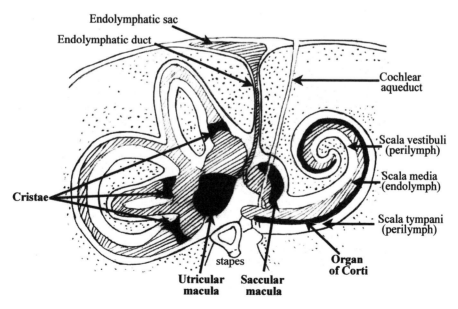

Figure 13.1. Diagrammatic representation of the human inner ear. Shading marks the endolymphatic spaces

more, the composition of perilymph in scala vestibuli differs from that in scala tympani. This indicates that perilymph is produced and circulated locally and that there is a so-called 'blood–perilymph' barrier. Glucose entry, for example, requires facilitated diffusion through glucose transporters (Wangemann and Schacht, 1996). This may limit access of potentially damaging agents to the peri-lymphatic compartment. However, if entry to perilymph is gained, there is direct access to the lateral membranes of the hair cells, to their synaptic regions and to the nerve fibres.

Effects and actions of ototoxic drugs

Ototoxic agents differ in their effects in the inner ear. Some primarily cause death of the hair cells and lead to permanent hearing loss (permanent 'thresh-old shifts', PTS: an increase in the minimum sound pressure level necessary to elicit a response) and/or vestibular dysfunction. Aminoglycoside antibiotics and *cis*-platinum fall into this category. Others, such as quinine and salicylate, predominantly produce temporary impairment of hair cell function (tem-porary threshold shifts, TTS) which is often accompanied by tinnitus (the perception of sound in the absence of an auditory signal). A third group, exemplified by the 'loop' diuretics and erythromycin, have acute effects in the stria vascularis, resulting in temporary hearing loss. The occurrence and extent of ototoxicity are to some extent dependent upon the dosing regime but are compounded by the status of the patient receiving the drug and multiple drug regimes. Malnourishment may increase sensitivity, as may stress produced by infection. Drug interactions can also result in much greater damage than would be expected from single drug regimes. A particular example is the inter-action between loop diuretics and aminoglycosides, which produces a devas-tating, rapid, profound permanent hearing loss. A number of ototoxic agents, including aminoglycosides, polypeptide antibiotics and antineoplastics, are also nephrotoxic so that possible damage to the kidney may result in reduced drug clearance and higher serum levels potentially increasing the risk to the inner ear. In addition, certain genetic factors may predispose to ototoxin-related damage. Individuals under similar conditions and with similar drug-dosing regimes differ in their sensitivity to ototoxic side-effects. Some of the mutations associated with such predisposition to drug-induced hearing loss have been identified, such as the 'A1555G' mutation in a mitochondrial gene that results in enhanced sensitivity to aminoglycosides (see below). For these reasons it is not always possible to predict a likely effect following adminis-tration of a potentially ototoxic drug.

AMINOGLYCOSIDE ANTIBIOTICS

The aminoglycoside antibiotics constitute the clinically most important group of ototoxic agents (see Forge and Schacht, 2000, for a detailed review). Their ototoxic effects are the most widely studied and illustrate several features more generally applicable to understanding ototoxicity and particularly for other agents, most notably *cis*-platinum whose effects resemble aminoglycosides in many ways.

Aminoglycosides cause death of hair cells in the cochlea and vestibular system and thus irreversible hearing loss and/or balance dysfunction. Although all aminoglycosides are potentially both cochleotoxic and vestibulotoxic, the different aminoglycosides exhibit differences in their toxic potential and organ preference. Experimental studies in animals (Lodhi *et al.*, 1980) and in *ex vivo* cultures of the organ of Corti (Kotecha and Richardson, 1994) have indicated that neomycin is the most toxic, gentamicin, kanamycin and tobramycin less so, and amikacin and netilmicin least toxic, but such differential toxicity may not apply in a clinical setting. Streptomycin and gentamicin are considered more vestibulotoxic than cochleotoxic to humans, whereas amikacin and neomycin are primarily cochleotoxic in the human inner ear. The reasons for such preferences are not known, but it is not related to any site-specific uptake mechanism or drug levels in the tissues (Forge and Schacht, 2000).

The effects of aminoglycosides usually become manifest only after days or weeks of parenteral treatment. Single systemic administrations are not normally damaging to the inner ear. The severity of the effects increase progressively with time, continuing after drug administration has been stopped, although, insidiously, in some cases, hearing impairment may not even begin until after treatment has ceased. The initial effect in the cochlea is a hearing loss confined to the high frequencies (Fausti *et al.*, 1984), indicating hair cell damage in the most basal region of the cochlea (Figure 13.2) The hearing loss then continues progressively to include successively lower frequencies, indicating a spread of the damage to hair cells apicalwards along the organ of Corti spiral, and involving frequencies in the human speech range to cause a permanent communication disability. Although single systemic administrations of aminoglycosides are usually not damaging, topical application of a single dose of the drug to the middle ear cavity can almost immediately initiate the progressive damage observed after chronic systemic treatment (Wersäll, Lundquist and Björkroth, 1969; Forge, Li and Nevill, 1988). This might suggest that the use of ear-drop preparations that frequently contain an aminoglycoside is contra-indicated, but usually the tympanic membrane acts as a barrier to entry to the middle ear space. Topical application of gentamicin to the middle ear cavity is, however, sometimes used therapeutically to ablate vestibular hair cells in cases of severe unilateral Ménière's disease.

A bilateral depression in hearing sensitivity of more than 10 dB at one or more frequencies is regarded as an initial indication of hearing impairment (Wright, 1998), but because accurate pure-tone audiometry, requiring a high-quality soundproof room, is difficult for assessing sick patients, a loss of 20 dB at two or more adjacent test frequencies is accepted as a hearing loss. However, most 'routine' audiometry covers the frequency range only from

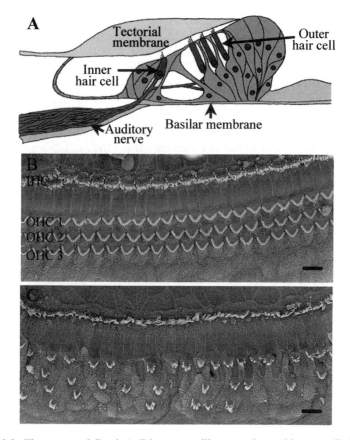

Figure 13.2. The organ of Corti. A. Diagram to illustrate the architecture. B. Scanning electron microscope (SEM) image of the surface of the organ of Corti (mouse); tectorial membrane removed to reveal the apical (endolymph-facing) surface, the reticular lamina. IHC = inner hair cells; OHC = outer hair cells. Each hair cell displays a bundle of stereocilia, organised in a W-shape on each OHC and a wide curve on IHCs. The surfaces of supporting cells intervene between each hair cell. Scale bar: 10 μm. C. Early stage of aminoglycoside-induced hair cell loss; SEM of the mouse organ of Corti. The remaining outer hair cells are scattered along the organ of Corti, some showing signs of ongoing degeneration. The locations from which hair cells have been lost are filled by expansion of the apical surfaces of supporting cells. Inner hair cells are unaffected at this stage. Scale bar: 10 μm

about 8 kHz downwards, but in the average person the high-frequency limit is about 16–18 kHz. Thus, unless high-frequency audiometry is used in patients receiving aminoglycosides, the initial ototoxic effects of the drug will be missed. Vestibular damage from systemic aminoglycoside administration results in severe unsteadiness, which becomes worse in the dark. Perception of unreal movement, usually elicited by head motion, can also occur. Objective clinical assessment is, however, difficult and limited. Rotational testing assesses only certain aspects of the vestibular system; caloric irrigation in conjunction with electronystagmography is unsuited for testing bilateral effects expected of aminoglycoside-induced dysfunctions, and dynamic posturography requires specialised equipment (Wright, 1998).

Aminoglycosides enter perilymph rapidly, within minutes of systemic administration, but perilymph levels are usually about one-tenth those in serum. However, clearance from perilymph is delayed and the drug persists in the inner ear long after it has been cleared from the bloodstream. The half-life of aminoglycoside in the inner ear has been estimated as more than 30 days (Tran Ba Huy, Bernard and Schacht, 1986), whereas half-life in serum is approximately 3–5 hours. Aminoglycosides also enter endolymph, though the entry to scala media is delayed relative to that in perilymph. The entry to endolymph coupled with persistence in perilymph may account for the delayed and progressive effects of aminoglycosides. Several pieces of evidence from a range of experimental models suggest that aminoglycosides affect hair cells through access from their endolymphatic (apical) surface. The delayed responses and progressive effects may result from slowly increasing endolymphatic concentrations of the drug to critical levels that can cause damage.

The primary effect of aminoglycoside is death of hair cells that occurs in a distinct pattern. In the organ of Corti, in line with the pattern of hearing loss, loss of hair cells occurs first in the basal coil and spreads apicalwards with time and with increasing dosage, and outer hair cells (OHCs) are more sensitive than inner hair cells (IHCs). OHCs in the first (innermost) row are those initially affected, followed by those in the second and then third row. IHCs do not usually appear to die until all the OHCs in their immediate vicinity are lost. Following the loss of IHCs, the spiral ganglion neurones that innervate them begin to die, because these require both trophic factors supplied by the IHC and continuing stimulation for their survival. The death of each hair cell is accompanied by expansion of the supporting cells around them to close the lesion and effect tissue repair. Supporting cells are not usually affected by aminoglycosides (or other ototoxins).

In the vestibular system, the cristae appear more sensitive and show greater hair cell loss than the utricular maculae, and the saccule generally shows less hair cell loss than the utricle (Lindemann, 1969; Forge, Li and Nevill 1988). Hair cells at the crest of the saddle-shaped cristae are lost initially, with the damage progressing down the skirts towards the periphery with time and increasing drug dosage. In the utricle, and when it occurs in the saccule, hair cell loss is first apparent in an anatomically defined strip along the middle of the sensory patch, the striola, then progressing outwards towards the peripheries. Unlike the organ of Corti, where lost hair cells are not replaced, there is some evidence for regeneration of hair cells in the mammalian utricle (Forge et al., 1993; Lopez et al., 1997; Forge, Li and Nevill, 1988), but the extent to which this occurs is limited and only a proportion of the lost hair cells may be replaced by new ones (Forge, Li and Nevill, 1988). Regeneration of hair cells is extensive and can lead to complete recovery of damaged sensory epithelia in birds and other nonmammalian vertebrates (Stone, Oesterle and Rubel, 1998; Cotanche, 1999; Smolders, 1999).

There is considerable evidence that aminoglycoside causes death of hair cells both in the cochlea and vestibular system following entry into the cell, and inducing apoptosis (Forge and Li, 2000; Forge and Schacht, 2000), a programme of biochemical events that lead to cell death. Apoptosis results from a cascade of biochemical reactions triggered in the cell and thus it is potentially possible to rescue cells that would otherwise die by inhibiting the initial triggering event or intervening in the subsequent biochemical pathways. One known initiator of the apoptotic cascade is free radicals. Free radicals are compounds with an unpaired electron, rendering them able to oxidise various other cellular molecules, resulting in structural changes and functional inactivation. Activation of degradative enzymes then ensues. Outer hair cells have been shown to be sensitive to free radical damage and there is a differential sensitivity that matches the vulnerability to aminoglycosides (and several other agents that cause hair cell death including *cis*-platinum) (Sha *et al.*, 2001). OHCs in the basal coil of the organ of Corti are more vulnerable to free radicals than those at the cochlear apex and IHCs are more resistant than OHCs. It has also been found that aminoglycosides can chelate (bind) iron (Fe^{3+}), the iron–aminoglycoside complex becoming a source of free radicals, and that the iron–aminoglycoside complex may be an initiator of the hair cell death (see Forge and Schacht, 2000, for a review). Understanding of the occurrence of apoptosis and how it may be triggered is leading to investigation of procedures for preventing aminoglycoside-induced damage (Forge and Schacht, 2000; Rybak and Kelly, 2003). Co-administration of iron chelators with an aminoglycoside, to prevent formation of the aminoglycoside–Fe^{3+} complex, or of free-radical scavengers, to 'mop up' generated free radicals, have proved capable of attenuating ototoxicity in animal models (Song, Anderson and Schacht, 1997). Interestingly, salicylate (aspirin), which has both iron chelating and free-radical scavenging properties and is known to be able to enter cochlear perliymph rapidly and thus to be available in the right place to be effective, has been shown to ameliorate hair cell loss and hearing impairment when co-administered with aminoglycoside in animal models (Sha and Schacht, 1999). Alternative therapies are directed towards interfering with the biochemical pathways that lead to cell death, in particular inhibiting those enzymes, the caspases, that are specifically activated when programmed cell death is triggered (Forge and Li, 2000; Pirvola *et al.*, 2000; Rybak and Kelly, 2003). Such therapies may have a wider value since apoptosis is now thought to be the common mechanism of hair cell death in a variety of conditions including that related to noise exposure and with ageing.

Cells naturally possess free radical scavenging systems but it is when these are overwhelmed or depressed that damage occurs. The stresses of infection or poor nutrition may deplete natural scavenging systems. Glutathione is a primary cellular antioxidant and part of the defence against free radicals. Animals fed a less than optimal diet show enhanced susceptibility to aminoglycoside ototoxicity, but dietary supplementation of glutathione will reduce the magnitude of the toxicity (Garetz, Altschuler and Schacht, 1994; Lautermann, McLaren and Schacht, 1995). Thus, attention to proper nutrition may enhance resistance to aminoglycosides. Conversely, poor nutrition may be one factor underlying the higher incidence of aminoglycoside ototoxicity in developing countries compared with the West.

A predisposition to aminoglycoside ototoxicity is also conferred by the A1555G mutation (an adenosine-to-guanosine substitution at base position 1555) in the gene for the mitochrondrial ribosomal-RNA. This mutation sometimes results in profound hearing loss after only a single parenteral injection, rather than the usual situation where hearing loss occurs only after chronic administration. The presence of this mutation in the mitochondrial chromosome was identified through a maternal inheritance pattern. It has been found in Chinese, Arab–Israeli, Japanese and North American families (Prezant et al., 1993; Usami et al., 1998). A carrier rate of 17% of those developing aminoglycoside-induced hearing loss has been estimated. This implies that a family history of aminoglycoside-induced hearing loss should be determined for any prospective patient for aminoglycoside treatment.

Aminoglycosides may also present a problem in two other 'at risk' groups, those with tuberculosis and cystic fibrosis patients. Aminoglycosides were first developed for use against tuberculosis and with the current resurgence in the incidence of tuberculosis, coupled with the emergence of multiple-drug resistant strains of the tubercle bacillus, aminoglycosides are now increasingly part of combination drug treatment programmes against this disease. However, there is evidence that maybe as many as 80% of patients who receive aminoglycosides chronically to treat tuberculosis develop ototoxic side-effects. Cystic fibrosis patients also receive regular, continuing treatment with aminoglycosides to combat pneumonia. The incidence of hearing loss in these patients has been recorded as 16% (Mulherin et al., 1991), although this may be an underestimation because the earliest changes in auditory sensitivity may not have been detected by the methods used; more sensitive measures using OAEs to examine OHC activity suggest a much higher figure (Mulheran and Degg, 1997).

One further consideration is that aminoglycoside antibiotics can cross the placenta. Thus there is a potential to cause deafness in the fetus. Studies of development in animals have suggested a 'critical period' in development, when sensitivity to the ototoxic agent is greatest at around the time of the onset of auditory function during development. The existence and timing of a critical period in humans has not been identified but, based on anatomical findings comparing development of the human inner ear with that of experimental animals, it has been estimated that a critical period for the human cochlea may be present in about the 18th to 20th week of gestation. An ototoxic action of aminoglycosides during intrauterine life of human embryos has been reported (Rasmussen, 1969). Thus, the administration of aminoglycoside to women during early pregnancy should be made with caution.

Although the primary site of action of aminoglycosides is upon hair cells, studies in experimental animals have indicated that in addition they may damage the stria vascularis, causing a permanent decrease in strial thickness probably by inducing death of the marginal cells (Forge, Wright and Davies, 1987). Initially this appears to have little effect on strial function; EP (endocochlear potential) is maintained at normal levels for some time, possibly because the stria has some 'structural redundancy', enabling it to accommodate damage while sustaining function. However, after a period of some weeks, a decrease in EP is noted. These effects in the stria may have two consequences. Firstly, a decline in EP may increase the extent of hearing loss, especially into those locations along the cochlea where hair cell loss is incomplete and scattered, thus resulting in hearing impairment over a greater frequency range than might otherwise be the case. Secondly, the stria vascularis compromised by aminoglycoside-induced damage yet still able to maintain normal function may be less able to withstand a subsequent unrelated challenged and becomes incapable of maintaining EP, resulting in a severe, perhaps sudden, hearing loss.

ANTINEOPLASTICS: cis-PLATINUM AND CARBOPLATIN

The effects of cis-diamminedichloroplatinum II (cisplatin) are similar to those of aminoglycosides. Chronic systemic treatment leads to a permanent hearing loss, which is relatively slow in onset and progressive, beginning with the highest frequencies. This corresponds to loss of OHCs initiated in the basal coil and progressing into the more apical regions (Laurell and Bagger-Sjoback, 1991). Inner hair cells appear to be less vulnerable (Kaltenbach et al., 1997). Vestibular dysfunctions due to death of vestibular hair cells may also occur (Wright and Schaefer, 1982). The incidence of hearing loss may be higher than many clinical reports suggest because high-frequency audiometry is not usually used to monitor patients on long-term therapy (Garetz and Schacht, 1996). Short-term administration may produce only transient hearing loss that may result from entry of the drug to endolymph and blockage of the transduction channels. Injection of cis-platinum into scala media in animals results in threshold shifts in neural responses (McAlpine and Johnstone, 1990). This is unlikely to account for the hair cell death as IHCs as well as OHCs would be affected by inhibition of the transduction apparatus. Independently, and in addition to effects on hair cells, cis-platinum also causes the death of marginal cells in the stria vascularis resulting in strial atrophy (Laurell and Engstrom, 1989). Carboplatin (cis-diammine-1,1-cyclobutane dicarboxylate platinum II) also causes a progressive hearing loss, beginning at the highest frequencies after prolonged administration but usually only at the highest doses used clinically and it is generally regarded as less ototoxic than *cis*-platinum (van der Hulst, Dreschler and Urbanus, 1988; Macdonald *et al.*, 1994; Simon *et al.*, 2002). High-dose treatment of experimental animals produces a progressive base-to-apex gradient in hair cell loss with both inner and outer hair cells damaged (Saito *et al.*, 1989), although in the chinchilla, in particular, moderate dosing produces, unusually, a loss of only the inner hair cells. Outer hair cells are affected, beginning in the basal coil only at higher dosing levels (Hofstetter *et al.*, 1997). The basis for this unusual pattern of damage is not known.

Hair cell death due to *cis*-platinum toxicity is apoptotic, probably triggered by excess free radicals, though the basis for the presence of excess free radicals in the hair cells is probably different from that with aminoglycosides. *Cis*-platinum may suppress natural free-radical scavengers such as glutathione and other antioxidant systems in hair cells (Ravi, Somani and Rybak, 1995; Rybak, Ravi and Somani, 1995; Rybak and Kelly, 2003). Consequently certain antioxidants including *d*-methionine and salicylate have proved to be effective in animal models and organotypic cultures in protecting cochlear hair cells from *cis*-platinum induced damage and without compromising the antitumour activity of the drug (reviewed in Rybak and Kelly, 2003). Likewise, carboplatin ototoxicity appears to be related to induced oxidative stress and reduced glutathione activity (Henderson *et al.*, 1999; Husain *et al.*, 2001). Various antioxidants, including sodium thiosulfate, have been tested as a means to ameliorate its effects (Neuwelt *et al.*, 1996; Rybak and Kelly, 2003).

QUININE

Therapeutic doses of ca. 200–300 mg per day are reported to have ototoxic side-effects in ca. 20% of patients receiving the drug causing threshold shifts at all frequencies almost equally, indicating effects along the entire cochlear spiral, as well as tinnitus. Vertigo may also occur, indicating effects in the vestibular system. Such effects, however, are usually entirely reversible, disappearing within a few days of withdrawal of the drug (Tange *et al.*, 1997). There are reports of occasional cases of permanent hearing loss as a consequence of quinine administration, but there are no well-controlled studies to confirm this.

The magnitude of the threshold shift produced by quinine is directly related to the serum concentration (Alvan *et al.*, 1991). Experimental studies in animals have shown that quinine enters perilymph rapidly (Alvan *et al.*, 1991) and produces decreases in CM (cochlear microphonic) and CAP (cochlear action potential), the extent of which are related to the perilymphatic concentration of the drug (Puel, Bobbin and Fallon, 1990). OAEs are also affected in humans, providing not only a sensitive means to assess the ototoxic effects but also suggesting an effect on the activity of OHCs. Quinine has been shown to cause vaso-constriction in the cochlear vasculature but EP is unaffected following administration of the drug and thus its effects on hair cell-related evoked responses are not secondary to effects in the stria vascularis and decline in EP, but are most likely due to direct effects in the outer hair cells. This is supported by electron microscopy of the organ of Corti in quinine-treated animals, which show reversible morphological damage exclusively in OHCs. However, at the lowest effective concentrations quinine does not affect OHC responses, OAE or CM, but produces a reversible elevation in threshold for the CAP, which derives from stimulation of IHCs, without affecting neural tuning (Mulheran, 1999; Zheng *et al.*, 2001). Tuning derives from the activity of OHCs that produces amplification. This suggests that the initial site of action of quinine may be on the IHC, synaptic transmission at the base of IHCs or/and upon the spiral ganglion neurones themselves, with OHCs affected as well only at higher concentrations.

Thus the ototoxicity of quinine is related to its ability to cross the blood–perilymph barrier freely, becoming distributed throughout the perilymph along the entire cochlea and gaining access to the neurones and OHCs that are affected through a site of action accessed via their baso-lateral membranes. However, the actual site and mechanism of action in the OHC has not yet been conclusively demonstrated.

SALICYLATE

Like quinine, salicylates produce tinnitus and threshold shifts at all frequencies. The shifts are usually no more than ca. 40–60 dB and almost equal across the frequency range or somewhat greater at higher frequencies. These symptoms are completely reversible within 1–3 days following withdrawal of the drug, and usually develop only at the high dosage levels used in treating rheumatoid arthritis, 2–5 g/day (Garetz and Schacht, 1996). Again like quinine, salicylate enters perilymph rapidly after systemic administration, peak levels in perilymph being reached 1–2 hours after injection. The concentration in perilymph is linearly related to the serum concentration (Jastreboff *et al.*, 1986; Boettcher, Bancroft and Salvi, 1990), and deterioration of the CAP threshold is linearly related to perilymph salicylate concentration. Thus, the degree of threshold shift is quantitatively related to salicylate plasma concentration.

Experimental studies in animals have shown that salicylate inhibits CM responses and CAP only at low stimulus intensities; responses to stimuli above ca. 60 dB appear to be unaffected. The tuning of responses of individual nerves to their characteristic frequency is also lost. In addition, otoacoustic emissions, which derive from the active responses of OHCs, are reversibly suppressed in humans (Long, Tubis and Jones, 1986; Martin *et al.*, 1988) and animals (Stypulkowski, 1990; Kujawa, Fallon and Bobbin, 1992). These findings suggest effects on OHCs and inhibition of the activity that produces signal amplification in the cochlea. Salicylates have been shown to cause constrictions of the cochlear capillaries, possibly associated with their interactions with prostaglandins. Potentially this could produce ischaemia and thereby affect the activity of the stria vascularis to reduce the driving potential for the cochlear amplifier. However, EP is unaffected following salicylate administration (Puel *et al.*, 1989; Stypulkowski, 1990) and effects of salicylates on cochlear vasculature are not considered to be a significant factor in their ototoxicity. Rather, OHCs appear to be the primary target of salicylate following its entry into the perilymph and access to a site of action on the baso-lateral membrane. It has been shown that salicylates inhibit electrically driven motile responses of isolated OHCs that *in vivo* are thought to underlie the cochlear amplification mechanism (Shehata, Brownell and Dieler, 1991; Tunstall, Gale and Ashmore, 1995). This electromotile response is driven by 'motor' proteins packed into the baso-lateral plasma membrane of the OHC (Dallos and Fakler, 2002). This protein, named 'prestin' (Zheng *et al.*, 2000), is unique to OHCs and there is evidence that reversible interactions with anions produces conformational changes in prestin that result in the reversible electrically driven changes in OHC length (Oliver *et al.*, 2001). Salicylate, an anion, appears able to interact with prestin and block the electromotile response (Oliver *et al.*, 2001).

LOOP DIURETICS

All loop diuretics, i.e. those diuretics whose principal site of action is in the ascending limb of the loop of Henle, are ototoxic. This group includes ethacrynic acid, frusemide (furosemide), bumetanide and piretanide. They produce a transient hearing loss across most of the frequency range, and sometimes dizziness and vertigo, usually following intravenous administration of large doses. Impaired renal function may enhance the risk of diuretic-induced effects. The effects are rapid in onset, within minutes or hours, and persist for some hours, but are usually completely resolved within one day if the drug is discontinued. Although there have been cases of permanent hearing loss reported, this seems to be unusual and repeated diuretic administration does not appear to cause permanent damage to the inner ear.

Histological studies of the temporal bones from patients who have died while on diuretic treatment (Matz, 1976; Arnold, Nadol and Weidauer, 1981) have shown extensive oedema and swelling of the stria vascularis. Experimental studies on animals have confirmed the stria as the principal site of action and that diuretics produce a rapid reversible decline in EP. In experimental studies using high doses of the drug, EP is seen to decline within seconds of intravenous injection or minutes following intraperitoneal injection, falling from the usual +80 mV to ca. negative values as low as −40 mV (Pike and Bosher, 1980; Forge, 1981; Lee and Harpur, 1985). The rate of decline and the level of suppression are dependent upon the dose of drug administered (Rybak, Whitworth and Scott, 1991). The EP then recovers over a period of a few hours but takes several hours to return to normal levels after a single administration. In parallel with the decline in EP an extensive oedema occurs; the extracellular spaces become grossly enlarged and the strial thickness almost doubles. This oedema is reversible, resolving within about two to four hours, prior to complete recovery of EP (Pike and Bosher, 1980; Forge, 1981). The decline in EP correlates with suppression of CM and CAP (Forge and Brown, 1982) and of otoacoustic emissions, a finding that provides evidence that EP is the power that drives the active mechanical responses of the organ of Corti in response to sound (Ruggero and Rich, 1991). This illustrates the importance of EP maintenance to the cochlear amplification mechanism and why damage to the stria will cause hearing impairment.

The occurrence of oedema indicates that diuretics inhibit ion-transporting processes in the stria vascularis; the accumulation of ions in the extracellular spaces, confined by the tight junction sealing between basal cells and those between marginal cells, resulting in osmotic uptake of fluid. The rapid onset of their effects suggests that the diuretics gain direct access to their site of action through entry from the strial vasculature and thus to the baso-lateral membranes of the marginal cells. In the kidney, diuretics act on an Na–K–Cl co-transporter. A similar co-transporter is localised in the baso-lateral membrane of the marginal cells (Ikeda et $al.$, 1997) and diuretics have been shown to interact with this co-transporter in preparations of strial marginal cells and vestibular dark cells (Marcus and Marcus, 1989; Wangemann, Liu and Marcus, 1995). It is thought, therefore, that the diuretics reversibly inhibit the action of an electroneutral Na–K–Cl co-transporter, in the baso-lateral membranes of strial marginal cells and vestibular dark cells leading to inhibition of ion transport. In the stria vascularis, this results in accumulation of ions in the extracellular spaces and inhibition of the electrogenic K^+ transport mechanisms by which EP is maintained (Wangemann, 2002).

Although the ototoxic effects of the loop diuretics when administered alone may not appear relevant in the present context of infections and the ear, when administration of a loop diuretic is combined with various other known ototoxic agents, in particular aminoglycosides, a quite dramatic effect is produced. As pointed out, single injections of diuretic have no effect on hair cells and single systemic administration of an aminoglycoside also do not normally affect hair cells. However, with administration of single doses of the two drugs within a short period of a few hours of each other, a permanent profound hearing loss develops rapidly and there is extensive loss of hair cells (West, Brummett and Himes, 1973; Brummett, 1981). In experimental studies in animals, complete loss of all outer hair cells along the entire cochlear spiral may occur within two days of a combined treatment protocol. The basis for this interaction is not yet known, but it is likely that diuretics may markedly increase the penetration of aminoglycoside into endolymph (Tran Ba Huy et $al.$, 1983). A similar interaction occurs between diuretics and cis-platinum.

MACROLIDE ANTIBIOTICS

Erythromycin and the newer macrolide antibiotics azithromycin and clarithromycin produce generally transient threshold shifts, tinnitus and vertigo (Brummett, 1993a) that develop following high-dose intravenous administration. The hearing loss is of the order of ca. 50 dB maximum and across all frequencies, although with somewhat greater effects on high frequencies (McGhan and Merchant, 2003). The symptoms disappear within a day or two of cessation of treatment. In patients, the onset of effects is reported to occur within two days of the start of treatment, but in experimental studies of animals given doses similar to those administered to patients, OAEs are affected within minutes (Uzun *et al.*, 2001). While changes in OAE and the level of maximal threshold shift indicate an effect on the cochlear amplifier, this is most likely due to effects on the stria vascularis. In animals, high intravenous doses of erythromycin cause a dose-dependent decline in EP within a few minutes, followed shortly after by decline in CM response (Kobayashi *et al.*, 1997), though the decrease in EP is not as great as that caused with loop diuretics. Experiments with isolated tissues maintained *in vitro* also show that the drug acts on the baso-lateral side of the marginal cells and of vestibular dark cells affecting ion transport by these cells (Liu, Marcus and Kobayashi, 1996), but the actual molecular target of action appears to be different from that of the loop diuretics. Consistent with inhibition of ion transport in the stria vascularis as the site of action in humans, sections of temporal bone from patients who have died during a course of erythromycin therapy have shown extensive oedema of the stria vascularis (McGhan and Merchant, 2003). This is apparent in all cochlear turns in correspondence with hearing losses at all tested frequencies. It has been recommended that patients receiving macrolide antibiotics be monitored for ototoxic side-effects, perhaps by use of OAEs, as these seem to be a sensitive measure to detect initial effects (Uzun *et al.*, 2001).

VANCOMYCIN

Vancomycin is a glycopeptide; despite the 'mycin' in the name it is not an aminoglycoside. There are various clinical reports of vancomycin producing transient hearing loss and/or tinnitus, but many of these derive from cases in which it has been used in combination with other potentially ototoxic drugs. From careful analyses of case reports it is not entirely clear whether vancomycin on its own has significant adverse effects on the cochlea (Brummett, 1993b). There are few experimental studies, but those that have been performed suggest that polypeptide antibiotics when administered systemically at even very high doses do not cause loss of hair cells or permanent hearing impairment. However, vancomycin when co-administered with an aminoglycoside appears to enhance the effects of aminoglycoside, producing much greater hair cell loss and hearing impairment than would have occurred with the aminoglycoside alone (Brummett *et al.*, 1990).

OTHER ANTIBIOTICS

Evidence for ototoxicity of the other antibiotics listed in Table 13.1 is relatively sparse. Viomycin has been reported to be vestibulotoxic rather than cochleotoxic, with ototoxic characteristics similar to streptomycin, following chronic treatment regimes (Daly and Cohen, 1965; Nakayama, Miura and Kamei, 1991), although in many cases viomycin was not the only potentially ototoxic drug that the patients received. Nevertheless, studies in animals have confirmed that viomycin causes hair cell death in the vestibular sensory organs, in a pattern similar to that seen with aminoglycosides, after repeated systemic injections of relatively high doses (Kanda and Igarashi, 1969). Chloramphenicol, which is used in some ear drop preparations usually in combination with other antibiotics, has been shown to cause irreversible hearing loss following infusion into the middle ear cavity in animals (Morizono and Johnstone, 1975). Presumably, it can gain access to the perilymph following uptake across the round window membrane. Interaction between chloramphenicol and noise that enhances development of permanent hearing loss has also been demonstrated in animal models (Henley *et al.*, 1984). However, clinical reports of hearing loss following use of chloramphenicol only are rare. Likewise polymyxin B, also a component of some ear drop preparations, may have ototoxic potential. In experimental studies in animals, perfusion of polymyxin B through the perilymphatic spaces caused an almost immediate decline in CM followed shortly after by a decline in EP, suggesting separate effects on both the organ of Corti and the stria vascularis (Komiya and Tachibana, 1990). However, the rarity of clinical reports in which an ototoxic effect can be attributed directly to polymyxin B suggests that the use of this antibiotic does not present a significant risk to the inner ear. The reports of ototoxicity following the use of other antibiotics listed in Table 13.1 are often anecdotal and there are no rigorous, well-controlled clinical studies or experimental studies in animal models to confirm and define their ototoxic effects.

DESFERRIOXAMINE

Desferrioxamine (deferoxamine mesylate, DFO) binds iron and is used in patients with β-thalassaemia to remove excess iron from the serum. In support of iron chelation as a means to ameliorate aminoglycoside toxicity, in cultured explants of inner ear sensory epithelia DFO attenuates aminoglycoside-induced hair cell loss (Forge and Li, 2000). However, repeated high-dose systemic administration of DFO to patients has been reported to cause high-frequency hearing loss in about 20 and 40% of those receiving long-term therapy (Olivieri *et al.*, 1986; Chiodo *et al.*, 1997; Karimi *et al.*, 2002). The total dose of drug given, the maximal plasma concentration, i.e. the clearance rate, and low serum ferritin levels have been suggested as risk factors (Porter *et al.*,

1989; Karimi *et al.*, 2002). In experimental studies in birds (which show oto-toxic responses similar to mammals) high-dose chronic treatment with DFO produced hair cell loss in the high-frequency region of the auditory organ in a pattern similar to that caused by gentamicin (Ryals, Westbrook and Schacht, 1997), suggesting that DFO may kill hair cells in a pattern similar to that caused by aminoglycosides. On the other hand, other clinical studies failed to identify a direct ototoxic effect of DFO (Masala *et al.*, 1988; Cohen *et al.*, 1990) and experimental studies with a mammalian model (chinchilla) could find no effects on cochlear physiology following long-term systemic treatment (Shirane and Harrison, 1987). The reasons for these apparent discrepancies have not been resolved. Differences between experimental models may derive from the differences in susceptibility between species, known to be the case for aminoglycosides (Forge and Schacht, 2000), and differing treatment regimes and/or patient groups may account for differences in clinical reports. Further work is clearly necessary, but it would seem that desferrioxamine may have ototoxic potential; however, the risks can be minimised by attention to dosing regimes and patient monitoring (Porter *et al.*, 1989; Karimi *et al.*, 2002).

Conclusions

Several different groups of therapeutic agents can have adverse effects in the inner ear. Other drugs listed in Table 13.1 but not discussed perhaps should also be used with caution, although evidence for their ototoxicity is limited. Drugs that normally do not have direct ototoxic effects may interact with others, resulting in damage in the inner ear that would not normally occur. Awareness of environmental and occupational factors that can have effects on the auditory system is also important. Some drugs may enhance suscep-tibility to noise-induced damage. Exposure to certain organic solvents (listed in Table 13.1) also can result in hair cell death. Interestingly, the pattern of damage with organic solvents is rather different from that of aminoglycosides or *cis*-platinum. Generally their initial effects are in the mid-frequency range, with corresponding damage in the lower-middle coil of the organ of Corti, with hearing impairment spreading to both lower and higher frequencies (Campo *et al.*, 1997; Morata, 1998; Lataye *et al.*, 2003). This pattern of damage may also confound drug-induced damage as well as interpretation of auditory assess-ments, so an attention to patient history is important.

To reduce the risk of ototoxic damage, ideally careful auditory monitoring of patients receiving any of the drugs listed is desirable to detect early indi-cations of adverse side-effects on the ear so treatment can be terminated. However, this may be difficult with sick patients and the need in many cases to use fairly sophisticated techniques such as high-frequency audiometry. Monitoring serum levels is also valuable to allow maintenance of drug concentrations below those that would cause ototoxic effects. The understanding of the underlying mechanisms by which damage to the inner ear is caused is leading to potential therapies to prevent or reduce the progression of ototoxic injury. Future progress in this area may allow the safe use of many otherwise highly effective therapeutic agents without compromising the functioning of the inner ear.

14 LABORATORY DIAGNOSIS, TREATMENT AND PREVENTION OF INFECTION LEADING TO HEARING LOSS

P.E. Klapper and P.J. Vallely

Introduction

The preceding chapters describe the numerous infectious organisms that may cause or contribute to hearing impairment in humans and what is known about the significance of each as a contributor to hearing impairment in studied populations. However, identification of an organism as the cause of the hearing loss in an individual patient is often problematic: the majority of intrauterine or perinatal infections are inapparent or symptoms are mild and nonspecific. Associated hearing loss may not be apparent for months or even years after the initial infection. Similarly, though less often, infections in the older child or adult may result in hearing loss as the only apparent manifestation and an infectious cause may not be suspected until well after the event has occurred. In such circumstances conventional diagnostic procedures designed to culture the pathogen or identify some component (e.g. antigen or nucleic acid) of the causative organism will fail. Often serological investigation will be the only viable route to establish a diagnosis and, because of the length of time elapsing between infection and observation of deafness or investigation of an infectious cause, such evidence may at best be circumstantial. That said, identifying a specific cause is often the key to optimal management of the patient and can help with parental understanding and acceptance of the problem. Thus it is important wherever possible to strive to identify the cause.

Infection and Hearing Impairment. Edited by V.E. Newton and P.J. Vallely
© 2006 John Wiley & Sons, Ltd

The purpose of this chapter is to present the opportunities that currently exist for diagnosing an infectious cause of hearing loss in the hope that an increased awareness of the causes will lead to improvement in the strategies for treating and preventing such infections and reduce the major contribution that they make to hearing impairment on a worldwide basis.

There are two potential situations that face the physician: firstly, the need to recognise and diagnose an infection where intervention may prevent hearing loss and, secondly, the need to determine a cause of hearing loss in an already deaf or hearing-impaired patient,

Recognising congenital and perinatal infections that may cause hearing loss

In the majority of cases of congenital infection maternal infection may be so mild and nonspecific that the infection is not recognised, reported or investigated during pregnancy. Similarly, at birth only the more severe cases in neonates with overt physical symptoms will be recognised and investigated. Hearing loss may not be apparent for months or years postnatally. Determination of a cause outside the immediate neonatal period may be problematic as postnatally acquired infections (unrelated to hearing loss) will be difficult to distinguish from congenitally acquired infection. Prevention of maternal infection remains the major method by which infectious causes of hearing impairment can be prevented. The success of childhood vaccination programmes using the combined measles, mumps and rubella (MMR) vaccine in developed countries has brought about a dramatic reduction in the incidence of rubella virus associated congenital deafness and indicates how public health preventative measures can make a real and effective difference (Figure 14.1).

An important development in the investigation of childhood hearing loss has been the introduction of universal neonatal hearing screening programmes. Audiological screening identifies those with existing audiological impairment and brings forth the possibility of intervention to prevent further progressive hearing loss via diagnosis and treatment of ongoing infection. It must be remembered of course that not all cases of audiological impairment arising from congenital or perinatal infection will be apparent upon first screening. Just as with the inherited causes of deafness, where many of the dominant genes for deafness are associated with late progressive hearing impairment, the effects of congenital or perinatal infection may not be immediately apparent. Nevertheless, universal audiological screening remains an extremely powerful tool and provides the impetus for investigation of the child and its mother in an appropriate time-frame.

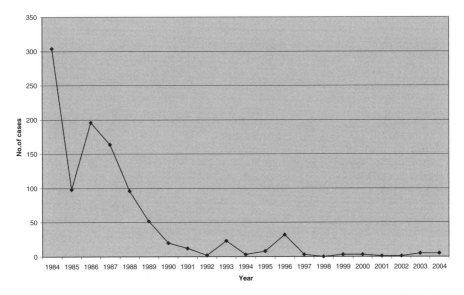

Figure 14.1. Reports to the Communicable Disease Surveillance Centre of the Health Protection Agency of rubella in pregnancy 1984–2004

Recognising an infectious cause in a deaf or hearing impaired child

Regrettably, for many congenitally or perinatally infected children access to universal audiological screening was not available at the time of their birth, and in many parts of the world universal audiological screening programmes are not yet in place or even in prospect. Those children acquiring hearing impairment by postnatal acquisition of an infection will also elude the screening programme. For these children and for children where there is late onset of hearing problems identification of a causal agent may be difficult. Furthermore, as the period of time elapsing between infection and the identification of an audiological problem may be long, the opportunity to intervene to prevent progressive loss may not be available.

The first and most important stage in diagnosis is to obtain a detailed clinical and family history (Table 14.1). A failure to develop speech or articulation difficulty is often the driver for postnatal investigation for hearing loss. The family history may lead to an indication of a genetic predisposition to hearing loss and direct investigation away from an infectious cause. Evidence of unsteadiness of gait or reports of recurrent meningitis may indicate deficits within the inner ear. Postnatal meningitis is known to be a major cause of acquired hearing loss (Chapter 11) and fibrosis and ossification of the cochlear

Table 14.1. Investigation of sensorineural hearing loss – general approaches

- Familial history: may indicate inherited disorders
- Past medical history: particularly concerning meningitis, recurrent meningitis or head trauma
- Travel history: may widen the search for a causal infective agent or exposure to ototoxic drugs
- Pregnancy
  - exposure to potential teratogens, use of drugs of abuse, prescription drugs
  - prematurity, infection during pregnancy
- Physical examination
- Neurological examination
- Ocular examination
- CT imaging

scalae occurs in 2–4% of cases (Fortnum, 1992). An account of head trauma, particularly to the temporal bone, may suggest a physical cause for hearing impairment. A history of recent foreign travel in the case of sudden onset hearing loss may raise suspicion of involvement of a particular organism or use of travel-related ototoxic drugs. Immunisation records for a child and details of known recent exposure to common infectious agents can all provide valuable clues to aid the search for an infective agent (Tables 14.1 and 14.2).

The history of the pregnancy should be reviewed. The gestational age and possible maternal exposure to teratogens or drugs of abuse may give clues as to the aetiology of hearing loss. Use of prescription medicines during pregnancy such as aminoglycosides, retinoids and diuretics should be reviewed. It is important to test the mother for serological evidence of possible exposure to infective agents such as human cytomegalovirus (HCMV) and particularly rubella virus during the first trimester of pregnancy (Table 14.3). Wherever possible any maternal blood samples collected during pregnancy, such as those obtained at an early antenatal care visit, should be recovered and tested together with the postnatal maternal blood specimen (Table 14.4). A detailed maternal sexual history will also be appropriate as this may raise an index of suspicion for sexually transmitted infections associated with neonatal hearing deficit such as syphilis or HIV.

In a general examination, the stature of the patient may provide evidence of a genetic cause; e.g. the Marfan or Stickler syndrome may be suggested if the child is very tall or alternatively, if small, their size may indicate Turner's syndrome or achondroplasia, all of which are associated with hearing loss. A 'small for dates' neonate may indicate prematurity or intrauterine growth retardation, both of which may be caused by unidentified congenital infection. Fused digits may indicate Aperts syndrome, broad distal phalanges may indicate otopalatodigital syndrome and brittle bones may indicate ostogenesis imperfecta, all of which are associated with hearing loss.

Table 14.2. Acquired infectious causes of auditory impairment

Perinatal and postnatally *acquired* infection	Risk of residual deafness
Bacterial meningitis	*Streptococcus pneumoniae*: 18–30% *Neisseria meningitidis*: 10% *Haemophilus influenzae*: 6% *Mycobacterium tuberculosis*: NK (probably rare) *Borrelia burgdorferi*: low frequency, hearing loss in 2% of cases
Chronic otitis media	NK (rare)
Fungal infection	NK (rare, but more common in immunocompromised)
Parasitic infection	*Treponema pallidum, Leishmania donovani, Fasciola hepaticum*: NK (rare)
Viral infection	Measles virus: 1 per 1000 cases of measles Mumps virus: 1 per 10 000 cases of mumps Rubella virus: NK (rare) Herpes simplex viruses: NK (rare) Varicella zoster virus: NK (rare, but 48% in cases of the Ramsay–Hunt syndrome) Human immunodeficiency virus: NK (rare, but HIV infection may increase risk of auditory morbidity from other infections)

NK = not known.

Table 14.3. Investigation of possible congenital infection – maternal serology

Blood samples taken	IgM	IgG	IgG avidity	Interpretation
First trimester	+	+	Low	Infection likely to have occurred in first trimester of pregnancy
Postnatal	−	+	High	
First trimester	−	−	–	Infection likely to have occurred in third trimester of pregnancy or perinatally
Postnatal	+	+	Low	
First trimester	−	+	High	Likely false positive IgM, or possible recurrence or reinfection during pregnancy
Postnatal	+/−	+	High	

The physical and audiological examination of the child should include neurological and ocular tests as these can often guide laboratory investigation. Pupillary response and a visual field tracking test require functional activity of the majority of the cranial nerves and can be tested in children as young as 6 weeks of age (Doyle, 2000). The corneal and gag reflex, presence of symmetrical facial movements and the midline tongue thrust are all indicators of cranial nerve function. Facial nerve function is a particularly valuable

Table 14.4. Investigation of possible congenital or
perinatal infection – appropriate serological
investigations of the mother

- Rubella virus
- Human cytomegalovirus
- *Treponema pallidum*
- *Toxoplasma gondii*
- Human immunodeficiency virus
- Herpes varicella zoster virus
- Herpes simplex virus

Where possible antenatal blood specimens should be examined in parallel
with the postnatal blood sample.

indicator of congenital, inherited, disorders such as the Goldenhar syndrome
and is reinforced by ocular examination, which in the Goldenhar syndrome
may reveal epibulbar dermoids. Careful external and internal examination
of the eye is a valued technique in pointing towards an infective cause; the
presence of cataracts may point towards a diagnosis of rubella, while the
presence of chorioretinitis may indicate a diagnosis of toxoplasmosis or of
congenital HCMV infection for example.

Detailed otolaryngeal examination of both the inner and the outer ear is an
essential part of assessment and is an important aid in the differentiation of
inherited and infective causes of impaired hearing. Routine X-ray, CT and possibly also MR imaging has been advocated in all children with sensorineural
hearing loss as 20–50% of children with a nonsyndromic sensorineural hearing
loss have abnormalities visible on CT scan (Doyle, 2000; Mafong, Shin and
Lalwani, 2002). This systematic evaluation of a child with sensorineural deafness will allow focusing of the search for a cause; relevant information should
then be communicated to the diagnostic microbiology and virology services to
enable appropriate laboratory investigations to be carried out.

The nonspecific application of laboratory tests is of little value in determining an aetiological diagnosis. The difficulties involved with retrospective
identification of a cause for hearing loss are illustrated in a study by Mafong,
Shin and Lalwani (2002). These authors conducted a retrospective analysis
of 114 children (<18 years of age) with sensorineural hearing loss in San
Francisco, US. They examined laboratory test results such as blood metabo-
lite, hormone and glucose levels and radiological imaging to try to establish a
syndromic aetiology for the hearing loss. They concluded that such laboratory
tests were unhelpful for establishing a diagnosis although radiological imaging
was helpful for identifying inner ear malformation. Interestingly, although
they excluded children for whom the hearing loss was attributed to maternal
infections such as rubella, toxoplasmosis or HCMV, they found that 22% of
the cases could still be attributed to environmental or nongenetic causes,
presumably including unidentified infectious causes.

Diagnosis of an infectious cause of hearing impairment

CONGENITAL AND PERINATAL INFECTION

The diagnosis of congenital infection *in utero* is not the subject of this chapter; interested readers are directed to comprehensive reviews of this topic which form the subject of several major textbooks and comprehensive reviews (Greenhough, Osbourne and Sutherland, 1991; Revello and Gerna, 2002; Banatvala and Brown, 2004; Saloojee *et al.*, 2004). During investigation of possible congenital infection in an infant, it is important to always consider the source of the infection. All too often the mother is not investigated in parallel with the infant, yet serological investigation of the mother is generally a much more rewarding endeavour than serological investigation of the infant. Congenital infection may delay or ablate the production of humoral immunity (antibody) directed against the causal agent, because infection has occurred prior to the maturation of the infant's immune system. The mother, however, as the source of infection, will have developed an immune response to the disease-causing agent. Serological investigation of the maternal blood post-delivery can thus provide valuable information to direct diagnostic investigation of the infant. If a blood specimen was taken during antenatal care this specimen can often be retrieved from the testing laboratory and examined in parallel with the postnatal sample. Immunoglobulin M (IgM) antibody is the first antibody to appear in systemic blood circulation following an infection. It is, however, a short-lived antibody that typically persists for only 3 to 6 months post-infection. Almost as soon as IgM antibody is detectable in peripheral blood, immunoglobulin G (IgG) antibody also appears. IgG antibody will persist for years after the acute infection. However, in the early stages of its production IgG antibody has lower avidity (effectively the strength of binding of the antibody to its antigen) than in the later stages of its production when high avidity antibody is produced. Typically this switch from low avidity to high avidity IgG antibody production occurs at about 16 weeks post-infection. The application of these three test procedures, appearance of IgM, appearance of IgG and IgG avidity, can help to identify and to pinpoint the timing of the maternal infection, as illustrated in Table 14.3.

While similar serological approaches can be applied to neonatal blood samples it is important to remember that because the immune system of a neonate is still maturing in the neonatal period, negative serological results do not rule out infection. Clinicians need to be made aware that the old procedure of taking a single sample of blood from a neonate and requesting 'TORCH' screening is not now considered an appropriate method for the investigation of possible congenital infection. Direct detection of a causal agent in appropriate body fluids and/or tissue samples is considered the method of choice for diagnosis. For example, congenital HCMV infection can be identified by detection of the virus in neonatal urine specimens via culture, antigen detection or virus-specific nucleic acid detection (Revello and Gerna, 2002).

For infection acquired perinatally an identical approach to that adopted for congenital infection is appropriate, provided that investigation commences within the neonatal period. However, as outlined below, investigation of possible congenital or perinatal infection outside the neonatal period brings additional difficulty. A range of specimens from the infant is needed if an infectious cause is to be properly delineated and, again, a maternal blood specimen is always of value in causal identification (Tables 14.3 and 14.4).

IDENTIFICATION IN THE IMMEDIATE POSTNATAL PERIOD

Identification of the causative agent is most easily achieved in the period immediately following birth. However, as many of the congenital infections that may result in later hearing loss are asymptomatic at birth, it is usually only the minority of cases exhibiting severe symptoms that will be investigated at this time. Culture of virus and detection of virus antigen in cells from the urine, or detection of virus by nucleic acid amplification techniques, such as the polymerase chain reaction (PCR), represent reliable methods for the detection of HCMV excretion (Revello and Gerna, 2002). It is probable that virus isolation from saliva is also a good marker of infection (Balcarek *et al.*, 1993). Symptomatic neonates with congenital HCMV infection shed virus in urine for periods of two or more years post-partum. The congenitally infected fetus appears to develop immunological 'tolerance' to the pathogen and an appropriate immunological response is delayed. Prolonged excretion of virus thus provides clear evidence of congenital infection, and failure to identify an immune response to the virus in the neonate does not preclude intrauterine infection.

In contrast to HCMV congenital infection, infections with rubella virus or *Treponema pallidum* usually result in production of specific IgM antibody in the neonate. In the case of syphilis, if papules or mucosal ulcers are available for examination *T. pallidum* may be observed in these samples using dark-ground microsocopy or by *T. pallidum* specific PCR. The diagnosis of congenital infection with herpes simplex virus (HSV) or varicella zoster viruses (VZV) may be achieved by virus culture, detection of viral DNA and by electron microscopic examination of vesicle fluids. Maternal serology will usually reveal the presence of virus-specific IgM in initial samples, followed by IgG in later sera. The neonate may initially be seronegative with the appearance of IgM antibody delayed for 6 months or more. Negative neonatal serology does not, therefore, preclude a diagnosis of HSV or VZV infection. Investigation of possible maternal infection is as important and urgent as investigation of the neonate. The maternal antenatal serological specimen should be retrieved wherever possible to allow comparative pre- and postnatal serology. Diagnosis of congenital infection is best established by comparison of the results obtained in the maternal and the neonatal specimens.

IDENTIFICATION AFTER THE NEONATAL PERIOD

While a universal audiological screening programme is available in some developed countries its availability is variable, and not all infants born with audiological problems will be identified and investigated within the neonatal period. Furthermore, a number of congenital and perinatal infections mediate late-onset hearing loss. Perhaps the best-known example of this is congenital HCMV infection: as outlined in Chapter 4 on HCMV by Britt and Boppana most babies born with congenital HCMV infection are asymptomatic at birth, but up to 15% of these may develop late-onset hearing loss. The challenge lies in identifying the infection as the cause in such cases.

During the first 6 to 9 months of life caution must be exercised in interpretation of serological test results since the detection of antibody may merely reflect passively transferred maternal antibody rather than infection. Serological investigation of a child that reveals *T. pallidum* infection (Table 14.5) after 6 to 9 months of age provides supportive evidence for congenital or early infection with this agent since syphilis would be an extremely rare infection of childhood. At 12 to 15 months of age detection of antibody to rubella may or may not reflect congenital infection since immunisation against rubella is given at this time. Similarly, the detection of HCMV, HSV or herpes VZV antibody cannot provide clear evidence of congenital infection since most primary infections with these viruses occur in childhood (Van Loon, Cleator and Klapper, 2003).

In the past, infants and children presenting for investigation of hearing loss were often examined at a time point remote from the time at which infection leading to hearing loss occurred. Investigation of a 4 year old child for possible congenital infection is not practicable; while serological evidence of infection may be found, it is not possible to determine whether this infection occurred congenitally, perinatally or at any time in the intervening postnatal period. Identification of maternal infection at a remote time point is also impractical since the vital antenatal blood specimens giving the mother's serological status at an early stage of pregnancy are unlikely to be retained more than 12 months after their collection. In these circumstances an alternative approach must be sought.

In developed countries it is usual to collect blood specimens from newborn infants on to so-called 'Guthrie' cards. These blood samples are utilised in tests for inborn error of metabolism among other markers. They are often stored for extended periods of time. If the Guthrie card prepared during the neonatal period can be located, nucleic acid amplification techniques can be applied in a search for viral nucleic acid within the dried blood spot (Fischler *et al.*, 1999; Caroppo *et al.*, 2001). However, some caution is warranted in the

Table 14.5. Tools for preventing and controlling maternal and congenital syphilis in different settings. (Reproduced by permission of the World Health Organization from Peeling and Ye, 2004, *Bulletin of the World Health Organization*)

	Tests for diagnosis of screening			Tests for surveillance	
	Local	Regional laboratory	Reference laboratory	Senitinel sites	Reference laboratory
Maternal syphilis					
Symptomatic	RPR or VDRL; rapid treponemal tests	Dark-field microscopy; DFA-TP; EIA-IgM; quantitative RPR or VDRL; rapid treponemal tests	Molecular tests; quantitative RPR or VDRL; TPHA-TPPA or FTA-ABS	Dark-field microscopy; DFA-TP-RPR or VDRL; rapid treponemal tests; EIA-IgM	Molecular tests; RPR or VDRL; EIA; TPHA-TPPA or FTA-ABS
Asymptomatic	RPR or VDRL; rapid treponemal tests	Quantitative RPR or VDRL; EIA-IgM; rapid treponemal tests	RPR or VDRL; EIA; TPHA-TPPA or FTA-ABS	RPR or VDRL; rapid treponemal tests	RPR or VDRL; EIA; TPHA-TPPA or FTA-ABS
Congenital syphilis[a]					
Symptomatic	None	Dark-field microscopy; DFA-TP; EIA-IgM; quantitative RPR or VDRL	Molecular tests; EIA-IgM; quantitative RPR or VDRL	Dark-field microscopy; DFA-TP-RPR or VDRL; rapid treponemal tests; EIA-IgM	Molecular tests; EIA-IgM; quantitative RPR or VDRL
Asymptomatic[b]	None	Quantitative RPR or VDRL	Quantitative RPR or VDRL	RPR or VDRL; rapid treponemal tests	Quantitative RPR or VDRL

RPR = rapid plasma reagin test; VDRL = Veneral Disease Research Laboratory test; DFA-TP = direct fluorescent antibody-*Treponema pallidum* testing; EIA = enzyme immunoassay; TPHA-TPPA = *T. pallidum* haemagglutination assay-*T. pallidum* particle agglutination test; FTA-ABS = fluorescent treponemal antibody absorption test.
[a] The lack of sensitive and specific tests for diagnosing congenital syphilis means that all infants born to mothers with syphilis should be treated regardless of test results.
[b] Serodiagnosis of an infant born to an infected mother who is reactive in treponemal tests is not recommended because of the passive transfer of IgG antibodies through the placenta; suspected congenital syphilis can be confirmed by an RPR titre in the infant ≥4 times that of the maternal titre. However, a negative result does not exclude syphilis in the infant. EIA-IgM is not recommended for asymptomatic infants due to low sensitivity.

interpretation of such results; the cards are often stored stacked together and a study of detection of herpes simplex virus DNA in such samples (Lewenson-Fuchs *et al.*, 2003) showed that the DNA from a positive sample could contaminate the card stacked above and beneath the positive sample card and produce false positive indication of infection in the patients represented by the adjacent cards. Where a positive result is obtained it is a sensible precaution to test adjacent stored cards to ensure that results are not compromised by such cross-contamination. The success of this approach is also determined by the sensitivity of the technique, the amount of DNA present within the original sample and the preservation of that DNA during storage.

Notwithstanding these caveats, dried blood spot testing appears to offer a valuable investigative procedure. Haginoya *et al.* (2002) describe two cases where asymptomatic congenital HCMV infection was diagnosed retrospectively as the cause of hearing loss. The first case was a 9 year old girl who had been delivered apparently normal and developed without any cause for concern until approximately 16 months of age, at which time it was noticed that she had difficulty hearing. A CT scan showed she had multiple areas of low density in the cerebral white matter, and 4 months later these had evolved to high-density lesions. Her auditory brainstem response was flat on both sides. Electroencephalogram (EEG) and ophthalmic examinations were normal. Examination of her cerebrospinal fluid (CSF) was normal and no oligoclonal IgG bands were identified to indicate central nervous system (CNS) infection. A hearing test showed she had severe bilateral sensorineural hearing loss (80–90 dB). Serum analysis showed she had high levels of HCMV antibody (IgG titre 1:2816) and was negative for antibodies against herpes simplex, measles and varicella zoster viruses. The child was followed for several years and, interestingly, the MRI high-intensity lesions faded over time and her mental development proceeded normally with the exception of language skills. When the child was 7 years of age a retrospective PCR assay was performed for HCMV using DNA extracted from her Guthrie card (taken at age 5 days). The test was positive for HCMV DNA sequences. Thus, a diagnosis of hearing loss resulting from asymptomatic congenital HCMV infection was made 7 years retrospective to the infection. The second case was of a 4 year old girl who was found to have no response to sound stimuli at 3 months of age. Again EEG and ophthalmic examination were normal. MRI at 9 months showed lesions in the subcortical white matter and these increased in number and intensity in later scans at 20 months and 3 years. The child showed developmental delay and deafness in one ear. Again HCMV DNA was amplified from the stored Guthrie card for this patient.

As mentioned above, it is recognised that congenital HCMV infection can be responsible for delayed-onset hearing loss. Suggestions that the virus may persist in the inner ear for long periods before causing damage led Sugiara and colleagues (Sugiura *et al.*, 2003, 2004) to sample perilymph from patients undergoing surgery for cochlear implantation. In their first study, real-time

PCR was used to test samples from five patients for the presence of HCMV DNA. Viral DNA was detected in the perilymph of one of these patients at a concentration of three copies per µL (Sugiura *et al.*, 2003). In the second study, samples from 15 patients were tested in the same way for the presence of HCMV, HSV-1 and HHV-6 viral genomes. Two perilymph samples were found to contain HCMV DNA and none of the other viral genomes were identified in any sample (Sugiura *et al.*, 2004). However, as all of these patients had symptomatic congenital HCMV infection the diagnostic value of routinely assaying the perilymph is questionable.

SUDDEN-ONSET HEARING LOSS

Nonspecific application of infection screening is of little value in the patient presenting with sudden hearing loss. Gagnebin and Maire (2002) applied systematic serological investigations in the search for an aetiological diagnosis in 182 patients presenting with either sudden (106 patients) or progressive hearing loss (76 patients). No aetiological diagnoses were achieved. A more appropriate route of investigation is to tailor investigation to those cases where systematic physical and neurological examination has confirmed the likelihood of an infectious aetiology (Table 14.6).

Cases of sudden deafness following bacterial meningitis are usually readily diagnosed since the meningitis is often a life-threatening event leading to hospital admission and comprehensive microbiological examination. Rarely, atypical presentations of bacterial meningitis, perhaps where the early application of antimicrobial therapy has masked the presence of pathogenic bacteria, will remain without a firm aetiology. In these cases testing for antibody to *Haemophilus influenzae*, *Neisseria meningitides* or *Streptococcus pneumoniae* may be worthwhile. Infection with *Mycobacterium tuberculosis* may be suggested when immunisation history is revealed and, in those without a firm history of vaccination, established by performance of a *Heaf* test. Enquiry

Table 14.6. Acquired infection: diagnostic specimens and appropriate tests

	PCR	Culture	Serology (IgG and IgM)[b]
Urine[a]	+	+	−
Blood	+	+	+

[a] Important specimen for detection of HCMV congenital infection. Virus excretion can occur for 2 or more years postnatally.
[b] Serological diagnosis is likely to be the mainstay of diagnosis in the asymptomatic child or in a child being investigated at a late stage. Serological investigation should include investigation of both the child and mother and, if appropriate, siblings or other immediate family members. Where possible, examine the mother's routine antenatal blood specimen in parallel with a postnatal blood specimen. Select appropriate laboratory tests in relation to maternal, family and geographical history.

concerning recent travel history and of possible tick bites may lead to investigation for *Borrellia burgdorferi* infection, which may be confirmed by application of specialist serological diagnosis.

One of the most common causes of hearing impairment in young children and, more rarely, in adults is the development of otitis media. Epidemiological studies clearly implicate upper respiratory tract virus infections as a cause of the condition by provoking Eustachian tube dysfunction and middle ear underpressure, which are considered to be the preconditions for otitis media pathogenesis (Doyle and Alper, 2003). Effusion recovered from symptomatic acute otitis media will often be positive for bacterial pathogens such as *Streptococcus pneumoniae*, *Haemophilius influenzae* or *Moraxella catarrhalis*, but bacterial infection is currently thought to be only a component of the pathogenesis of the condition. The range of upper respiratory virus infections suggested to precipitate the process include influenza viruses, parainfluenza, adenovirus, rhinoviruses and Coxsackie viruses, as outlined by Doyle and Alper (2003). The range of sensitivity of the diagnostic procedures employed in the detection of infection and the seasonal variation in the relative importance of one respiratory virus infection over another means that it is not possible to define any particular type of respiratory virus as a causal agent; indeed, it seems likely that almost any respiratory virus can precipitate the process. Diagnosis of an infection prior to the development of otitis media and subsequent hearing loss is not possible in the majority of children who present for investigation of hearing loss since the initial viral infection will have been cleared by the immune response and replaced by subsequent bacterial colonisation. Circumstantial evidence for a particular upper respiratory infection can be obtained by serological testing; however, interpretation of results may be difficult because of the frequency of respiratory virus infections encountered in childhood. Nevertheless, given the strong association of viral upper respiratory tract infection as a prequel to acute otitis media, interventions to prevent or reduce the frequency of upper respiratory tract infections in childhood infection are being actively considered (see below).

Acute mumps virus infection is usually clinically apparent but may occasionally be confused with acute cytomegalovirus or Epstein–Barr virus infections. In the acute stages of infection virus may be excreted in saliva or urine. While mumps virus culture is recognised as being an insensitive test procedure, the giant cell (synctia) formation on culture of mumps virus in a diverse range of cell types (including monkey kidney, Vero or human embryo lung fibroblast cells) is characteristic. However, detection of the virus via nucleic acid amplification (i.e. polymerase chain reaction detection) is recognised as a more reliable and sensitive diagnostic procedure. Infection can be further confirmed by the detection of mumps virus specific IgM antibody and/or the detection of a significant rise in mumps virus specific antibody in specimens of blood drawn 10–14 days apart (i.e. during acute infection and in convalescence).

The typical rash symptoms of measles virus infection are usually readily apparent on the skin of Caucasian children but may be more difficult to discern in nonwhite children. As with mumps virus infection, the isolation of measles virus in cell culture is recognised as being an insensitive method for the diagnosis of infection. Polymerase chain reaction detection of viral nucleic acid in salivary specimens and/or the detection of measles virus specific IgM antibody in a blood sample collected during the acute infection provide a more reliable means of diagnosis. In very young children a general reluctance among clinicians to draw blood samples has led to the development of methods of detecting IgM antibody in crevicular fluid (i.e. the fluid surrounding teeth cavities, often mistakenly described as salivary fluid). It is important to appreciate that the amount of antibody present in such fluid is low; thus it is important to use specialist oral fluid collection devices to obtain the specimens and to ensure that immunoassays used to detect the antibody are specifically optimised for use in such fluids (Judd *et al.*, 2003)

Chronic infection may occasionally result in sudden hearing loss. Undiagnosed congenital syphilitic infection may be revealed by serological investigation. Serodiagnosis during the first 12 to 18 months of life is often confounded by the passive placental transfer of maternal immunoglobulin G antibody. Infants born to mothers with untreated syphilis should be treated regardless of their serological test results. An RPR (rapid plasma region) titre in the infant four times higher than that found in the mother strongly suggests congenital syphilis. However, only about 30% of congenitally infected infants will show such high titres (Peeling and Ye, 2004). Immunoglobulin M can be detected in 80% of symptomatic infants but data on sensitivity are lacking in asymptomatic infants. Immunoblot procedures are recommended in infants as these yield higher sensitivity for detection of IgM antibody than the FTA antibody IgM test or IgM specific ELISAs. As IgM responses may be delayed in infancy a negative IgM result does not rule out congenital syphilis (Table 14.5).

Late-onset hearing loss as a consequence of congenital HCMV infection may, for the reasons outlined above, present a more difficult diagnostic challenge. Serological evidence of past infection may be found, but to define such infection as being due to unrecognised congenital HCMV infection would require an attempt to obtain samples collected around the time of birth, such as investigation of postnatal Guthrie card blood spot samples to define the infection. Human immunodeficiency virus infection will in the late stages of infection (i.e. AIDS) result in abnormal audiometry in up to 33% of cases and abnormal brainstem auditory evoked potentials in up to 56% of cases leading to subjective hearing loss (Mata Castro *et al.*, 2000). Careful analysis to determine risk factors for HIV infection including obtaining, where appropriate, a full sexual history may lead to serological investigation of infection. Current serological tests for HIV infection are both highly sensitive and highly specific, although it is important to emphasise that no diagnosis of HIV infection should ever be made on the basis of a single serological test or indeed on the basis of a single sample of blood (Parry *et al.*, 2003).

Prevention of infections that can cause hearing loss

As outlined in the preceding sections diagnosis of infection in association with hearing loss can sometimes be made through a careful and systematic approach and, where this is possible, pinpointing a cause of hearing loss is important. Obtaining a definite diagnosis for the cause of hearing loss is helpful to the patient and, in the case of an infant or child, to the parents. It often aids acceptance of the condition, may provide a prognosis, help the parents to establish any risk for future pregnancies, or inform patient management strategies to prevent progression of hearing loss. However, it is a sad fact that in many cases such diagnosis is not possible, or is unhelpful in altering or managing the condition. Control of infections that result in hearing loss must thus be a major aim of modern medicine and, as will be outlined, planned intervention designed to interrupt transmission of infection has had, at least in the developed world, a major impact in reduction of hearing loss acquired through infection.

IMMUNISATION

Immunisation provides the major tool for control of infections that result in hearing loss.

Measles, mumps and rubella

Perhaps the best exemplar of this, and the most successful immunisation strategy yet applied, is that associated with rubella. As outlined in Chapter 5, infection during the first 11 weeks of pregnancy carries a 90% risk of the fetus developing the congenital rubella syndrome (Miller, Cradock-Watson and Pollock, 1982). Following the introduction of rubella immunisation in the United Kingdom in the 1970s for prepubertal girls and nonimmune women of child-bearing age, the number of cases of the syndrome decreased dramatically although there were still as many as 70 cases of congenital rubella syndrome and perhaps as many as 700 elective terminations of pregnancy occurring during rubella epidemic years. In 1988, a universal childhood immunisation programme was introduced using a combined measles, mumps and rubella (MMR) vaccine. The effective deployment of this vaccine rapidly led to the arrest of epidemics of rubella and by the year 2000 the number of cases of the congenital rubella syndrome had dropped to less than 5 per year, with almost all cases occurring in nonimmunised women who acquired the infection abroad. A similar success story is the reduction in the number of cases of sporadic sudden hearing loss associated with mumps virus infection and of cases of hearing loss associated with measles infection. In the UK, the intro-duction of universal childhood immunisation with the MMR vaccine very rapidly led to the stopping of the epidemic circulation of these viruses and consequent prevention of cases of infection-associated hearing loss.

Haemophilus influenzae type b

Similarly, introduction of a programme for *Haemophilus influenzae* type b immunisation has led to control of a serious infection and cause of audiologi-cal morbidity. In the United Kingdom *Haemophilus influenzae* type b was the most common cause of bacterial meningitis in children. Following the devel-opment of an effective vaccine consisting of the purified capsular polysaccha-rides of *Haemophilus influenzae* type b, conjugated with tetanus toxoid or diphtheria based carrier proteins, the vaccines were deployed within a uni-versal childhood vaccination programme. Prior to the introduction of the vaccine in 1992 there were 30 deaths each year due to *Haemophilus influenzae* type b infection and about 80 children per year were left with hearing loss and/or permanent brain damage. With the vaccine the number of cases of infection and meningitis have declined dramatically, not only in the young chil-dren targeted by the campaign but also in older children and in adults because of their reduced likelihood of exposure to the organism as the number of chil-dren carrying the bacteria and, therefore, capable of transmitting infection has fallen.

Neisseria meningitidis

Immunisation to prevent meningococcal meningitis has had a similar effect. However, to date the meningococcal campaign must be considered less suc-cessful than the *Haemophilus influenzae* type b campaign, because vaccines to combat all serogroups of *Neisseria meningitiditis* are not yet available. The major serogroups circulating in the UK are serogroups B and C. Polysaccha-ride meningococcal vaccines (prepared using highly purified polysaccharides derived from the capsule of *N. mengitiditis*) have been available to protect adults and older children from meningococcus since the early 1970s, but these vaccines do not provide protection for young children. This is because immu-nity developed to the capsule does not involve direct interaction with T cells; instead, immunity is developed via a T cell independent mechanism, and this pathway is lacking in children below the age of 2 years. A purified capsular polysaccharide vaccine for meningococcus type C, capable of inducing T cell dependent immunity by conjugating the polysaccharides to tetanus toxoid or diphtheria carrier proteins, was produced and deployed in 1999 in the UK for children under 18 years of age. Since the deployment of the vaccine a steady and sustained decline in cases of meningococcal type C infection has been achieved, from approximately 100 deaths in 1998 to 19 by 2003.

Streptococcus pneumoniae

The problems of failure to stimulate cell-mediated immunity, with consequent poor protection, in young children observed with conventional meningococcal vaccines have also been seen with vaccines developed against pneumococcal infections. Now, as for meningococcus type C, a new conjugated vaccine (polysaccharide conjugated with carrier protein) has been developed and is being administered to young children and others who have a high risk of developing severe pneumococcal disease (e.g. those with severe kidney disease) in an attempt to reduce the 203 cases of pneumococcal meningitis reported in the UK in 2003 and the numerous numbers of children who present each year with pneumococcal-associated otitis media.

Respiratory viruses

The use of influenza vaccine in the prevention of acute otitis media has provided direct evidence for the role of respiratory viruses in causation of this condition. In a trial of the use of influenza vaccine in a child day-care centre half of 374 children received a trivalent influenza vaccine and half did not. During a subsequent influenza outbreak the incidence of acute-onset otitis media was reduced by 83% in the vaccinated group (Heikken et al., 1991). These findings were later corroborated in several alternate studies (Heikkinenin and Chonmaitree, 2003). While influenza vaccine can protect against infection and subsequent induction of acute otitis media, vaccines to protect against other respiratory virus infections are presently not available. Passive immunisation using either RSV antibody enriched immune globulin or a recombinant humanised monoclonal antibody (Palivizumab) has been attempted in order to prevent acute otitis media following respiratory syncytial virus infection. However, these studies do not as yet provide conclusive evidence of benefit in prevention of the condition (Heikken and Chonmaitree, 2003).

ALTERNATIVE STRATEGIES

While the introduction of universal childhood immunisation against these major causes of hearing impairment has had a dramatic effect in reducing the incidence in both children and adults on a worldwide basis, much work remains to be done to sustain and maintain progress (Meissner, Strebel and Orenstein, 2004). The World Health Organization's targeted vaccination programme to reduce infant mortality (and *inter alia* audiological morbidity), ably aided by the efforts of governmental philanthropic donations and numerous charitable efforts of organisations such as the Bill and Melinda Gates Foundation, have led international efforts to control these infections and must ultimately aim to eradicate them.

As mentioned earlier, one option for control of a severe congenital infection such as that caused by rubella virus has been via a programme of elective termination when maternal infection is proven during the first 11 weeks of pregnancy. However, such a strategy was never straightforward and is particularly problematic as an option for control of the other major viral cause of severe congenital disease: HCMV. In contrast to rubella virus, it is known that infection with HCMV at any stage of pregnancy can result in congenital infection and residual morbidity. Furthermore, the virus can also cause congenital infection through reactivation of a latent maternal infection and probably also through reinfection. In addition, congenital infection in the majority of cases (95%) does not result in overt morbidity. Thus any programme of elective termination of pregnancy following a proven maternal infection would probably result in both unnecessary termination of a high proportion of healthy infants as well as missing those rare cases where a clinically significant congenital infection was caused by reactivation of maternal infection or reinfection. In the absence of any effective method of preventing mother-to-fetus transmission of virus and in the absence of an effective vaccine to protect the seronegative mother from infection, the introduction of screening for congenital infection during pregnancy or of *in utero* diagnosis remains controversial (Peckham *et al.*, 2001; Revello and Gerna, 2002; Collinet *et al.*, 2004).

Rubella virus infection was, until it was effectively controlled via preventative immunisation programmes, considered to be the major cause of hearing impairment due to congenital infection. Following its control, attention rapidly shifted with the realisation of the scale of hearing impairment associated with congenital HCMV infection. While there is evidence showing that reactivation of latent HCMV or reinfection occurring during pregnancy in mothers shown to be seropositive for HCMV antibody pre-pregnancy can result in fetal damage, the major cause of fetal damage occurs when a mother suffers primary infection with the virus during pregnancy. Prevention of primary infection might be achieved through the application of a vaccine to seronegative females pre-conception and, as reviewed by Revello and Gerna (2002), has led to more than 30 years of effort towards development of an HCMV vaccine designed to prevent the occurrence of primary HCMV infection during pregnancy. Vaccine development has encompassed a number of candidate live attenuated vaccines, recombinant virus vaccines, subunit vaccines, peptide vaccines and most recently DNA vaccines. These efforts have as yet failed to realise an effective vaccine although several candidate vaccines are undergoing clinical trial.

An alternative to active or passive immunisation is the prophylactic use of antiviral agents. A trial of administration of the anti-influenza drug oseltamavir within 48 hours of the commencement of acute respiratory symptoms during an influenza outbreak suggested that its administration resulted in a 44% reduction in the development of acute otitis media (Whitley *et al.*, 2001). As with both passive and active immunisation, the availability of antiviral agents to combat respiratory virus infections is at present very limited. Thus the prospect of prevention of respiratory infection leading on to acute otitis media is presently very limited.

ANTIMICROBIAL THERAPY

Otitis media and bacterial meningitis

Effusion recovered from acute otitis media that is culture positive for bacterial pathogens is usually treated with appropriate antibiotics because of the risk of development of meningitis or mastoiditis, both of which may threaten life. Eradication of bacterial pathogens leads to reduced duration of pain, but it is not certain whether such treatment is able to prevent sensorineural hearing loss (Doyle and Alper, 2003). Where the symptoms of meningitis and/or mastoiditis are apparent, rapid identification of the causal agent and prompt and aggressive application of appropriate antibiotic therapy are required together with full supportive neurological care in order to save the life of the victim. In certain circumstances the additional application of anti-inflammatory therapy may be appropriate to minimise the risk of the development of subsequent audiological damage.

Lyme disease

About 15% of people with *Borrelia burgdorferi* infection develop so-called neuroborrelia, which can be manifest in a range of symptoms, the most severe of which is meningoencephalitis, appearing between one and five weeks after the tick bite. Hospitalisation is urgent and intravenous administration of ceftriaxone or oral administration of doxycycline is important.

Syphilis

Prenatal screening for syphilis is commonplace in developed countries (Table 14.5). Because of the serious morbidity and risk of fetal mortality associated with the infection all pregnant women identified with syphilis require treatment. The WHO recommendation is that asymptomatic neonates born to RPR-positive women should receive 50 000 units/kg of benzathine penicillin G in a single intramuscular dose. Symptomatic infants should receive intramuscular or intravenous aqueous crystalline penicillin G administered at a dose of 50 000 units/kg every 12 hours for the first 7 days of life and then every 8 hours for 3 days or intramuscular procaine penicillin G at a dose of 50 000 IU/kg as a single dose daily for 10 days (Saloojee *et al.*, 2004). In the presence of HIV infection caution is warranted; the alteration of B cell function in HIV patients can result in both false positive and false negative testing for syphilis and women identified with HIV infection therefore require special attention.

HIV

Evidence of HIV infection is sought through prenatal screening programmes in developed countries. Guidelines on treatment of infection identified in pregnancy are continuously updated in response to an ever-evolving range of anti-retroviral treatment, their potential efficacy and toxicity during pregnancy and in the neonatal period. Interested readers are thus directed to consult up to date recommendations, which are freely available on the internet (e.g. in the UK http://www.bhiva.org, in the US http://www.aidsinfo.nih.gov or internationally accessed via http://hivinsite.ucsf.edu).

Once audiological damage is apparent the role of anti-infectives is usually of limited value. There is, however, one possible exception to this general rule and that is in the possible application of antiviral agents in the child with proven congenital HCMV infection. However, if preconception or *in utero* prevention of congenital HCMV infection is presently problematic, postnatal treatment of a child identified with congenital HCMV infection is only slightly less controversial.

Cytomegalovirus

As outlined by Revello and Gerna (2002), prenatal treatment or postnatal treatment of congenital HCMV infection could be contemplated. Hyperimmune HCMV immune globulin therapy, Foscarnet, a competitive inhibitor of pyrophosphate, and ganciclovir, a competitive inhibitor of guanosine in viral DNA synthesis, have all been utilised for *in utero* treatment of congenital HCMV. While suppression of intra-amniotic viral load can be achieved, a clear benefit of therapy has not been achieved in that treated infants were either stillborn or exhibited severe symptoms of congenital damage at birth. Postnatal antiviral treatment of infants with symptomatic disease has shown more promise. A limited trial of the effect of 6 weeks of intravenous therapy in patients with symptomatic congenital HCMV infection (Kimberlin *et al.*, 2003) showed that this therapy prevented hearing deterioration or further hearing deterioration at 6 months post-therapy and possibly also at 1 year. The use of intravenous therapy with ganciclovir does present major logistic difficulties and is associated with toxicity. Almost two-thirds of the infants enrolled in the study had significant neutropenia during the period of therapy. In a study of nine children with symptomatic congenital HCMV infection, extended intravenous ganciclovir therapy (median 1 year) was followed by oral ganciclovir therapy (median 0.83 year), but none of the enrolled children showed progressive hearing loss (Michaels *et al.*, 2003). Numerous complications of intravenous therapy were, however, noted. These studies provide some encouragement that treatment of congenital HCMV may prevent progression of hearing loss. However, the current high level of toxicity associated with antiviral treatment precludes their general use, especially in those infants with asymptomatic congenital HCMV infection. While the development of an orally administered pro-drug of ganciclovir – valganciclovir – eases some of the logistical problems associated with prolonged intravenous administration significant toxicity is still associated with its use. Drug or drug–immunoglobulin combinations of lower toxicity will be needed to allow more extensive evaluation of the possibility of treatment to arrest hearing deterioration in infants born with congenital HCMV infection.

Prospects for the future

The success of universal childhood vaccination programmes in reducing the number of infants, children and adults who suffer hearing impairment resulting from an infectious cause clearly illustrates the importance of prevention of infection in controlling acquired hearing impairment. To this end, the promotion of immunisation strategies in developing countries and sustaining these programmes in the developed world is of vital importance. Existing vaccines are being improved to allow their more widespread application and the development of new vaccines is being facilitated by novel molecular methods. Development of a wider range of vaccines for respiratory virus infections and new antiviral agents used in prophylaxis against respiratory infections will allow their wider use in the prevention of acute otitis media.

There is real scope for improvement in detection and prevention of HCMV-induced hearing loss. As discussed above and in detail in an earlier chapter, diagnosis of a symptomatic, severely affected infant with cytomegalic inclusion disease is relatively straightforward. However, the majority of congenitally infected infants are asymptomatic, and unless a primary infection is suspected in the mother, investigation is unlikely and the infection will be unnoticed. In most instances this will have no further consequence, but in an estimated 15% of infants late-onset hearing impairment will follow. Indeed, it is possible that this may be an underestimate because of the difficulties already described with assigning a congenital diagnosis to a late-onset hearing loss. Implementation of studies to systematically screen newborns for HCMV excretion would provide a good indication of current rates of congenital HCMV infection. A few such studies have been completed in the past (Revello and Gerna, 2002), but the age of HCMV acquisition and level of seropositivity in the population increases with economic and social development and determination of congenitally acquired HCMV infection rates around the world would be timely.

The relevance of this for identification of hearing-affected children is shown by an earlier study by Peckham *et al.* (1987) in the UK. Urine specimens from 1644 children (6 months to 4 years) attending the Nuffield Hearing and Speech

Centre were tested for HCMV. It was found that the prevalence of HCMV in urine from patients with SNHL but no immediate family history of deafness was 13%, compared with 7% in other children (including those with family history and normal children), suggesting that HCMV screening of urine could be useful for identifying asymptomatic children at risk for development of hearing impairment. Infected infants identified in this way may benefit from long-term audiological follow-up to identify any hearing loss at the earliest possible stage and intervene to prevent associated developmental delay. The development of new anti-HCMV chemotherapeutic agents of lower toxicity will be important to allow treatment to prevent progressive audiological damage. Advances in the science of pharmacogenetics, following on from the elucidation of the human genome, promise to provide an important future aid to this endeavour. Much remains to be done but there is hope that the identification of infective causes of hearing loss will not, in the future, be merely an academic driver and stimulus for the development and application of preventive strategies but will also stimulate a drive to intervene to prevent progressive hearing loss from infection.

Summary

Infection remains a major cause of congenital and acquired hearing loss and, as the success of childhood vaccination programmes for rubella, measles, meningococcus, *H. influenzae* and others illustrate, can result in a major reduction in infection-associated hearing impairment. Diagnosis can represent a challenge, but through an appreciation of the route by which infection occurs, awareness of the importance of testing at the right time and the provision of correct specimens, progress can be made. Most importantly, there is a need for greater awareness and cooperation between audiologists, virologists, microbiologists and infectious disease physicians in the investigation of audiological problems.

15 THE EXPERIENCE OF DEAFNESS – PSYCHOSOCIAL EFFECTS

A. Young

Introduction

The poet David Wright in his book *Deafness: A Personal Account* (1969) points out that while at University his difficulties did not lie in 'not hearing' but rather in not being able to 'overhear'. For it is through overhearing that hearing people pick up the incidental communication through which is built a sense of the characteristics of others, the culture of organisations, the trends and fashions of social groups, and simply a vast amount of information that enables one to fit in. His disability did not lie in his deafness, but in his restricted access to this texture of life.

This distinction is important in considering what we may mean by the psychosocial effects of deafness. The effect David Wright describes was not *because* of his deafness in any simple or direct sense, but rather a result of the interaction between the condition of not hearing and the characteristics of a social context in which he found himself. Changing the social condition can change the experience of deafness. Compare the relative ease with which some deaf people communicate on a one-to-one basis, with the observation that for lipreaders in a group context the edge of a conversation is a lonely place to be (Ladd, 2003).

Of course, the experience of deafness is not simply explicable by the characteristics of the circumstances in which individuals interact. In an audiological sense there are many varieties of not hearing and variables such as age of onset, aetiology, degree of deafness and additional needs do have distinguishing effects on the range of consequences and challenges experienced by deaf children and adults. The progressive hearing loss of old age is not easily com-

Infection and Hearing Impairment. Edited by V.E. Newton and P.J. Vallely
© 2006 John Wiley & Sons, Ltd

parable with profound deafness at birth. However, in thinking about the psychosocial effects of deafness the problem comes in deciding how much explanatory authority to give to such medical/audiological variables in tracing typical effects, if such things exist, of different kinds of deafness. This is not just a question of understanding that audiological variables interact with variations in social and developmental circumstances resulting in a range of potential outcomes. Rather the medical paradigm that constructs deafness as an impairment and a condition to be treated is itself open to challenge (Lane, 1993).

For Deaf[1] people who use signed languages such as the British Sign Language (BSL) or the American Sign Language (ASL), Deafness is a marker of cultural and linguistic identity, not a medical condition arising from the loss of something that is normal (to hear) (Padden and Humphries, 1988; Ladd, 2003). Through this lens, the psychosocial effects of deafness are largely regarded as being engendered by the medical paradigm rather than by deafness itself. For example, the personal and social consequences of constructing deaf children as defective and in need of habilitation to enable them to speak is contrasted with the psychological and social implications of recognising them as developmentally normal proto members of the signing Deaf community (Ladd, 2003).

In other words, in considering the psychosocial effects of deafness we are faced with not only the complexity of the individual experience of deafness but also of the complex interaction between social, medical and cultural–linguistic understandings of what it is to be Deaf (Gregory, 2003). In the limited space available, we will consider the psychosocial effects of deafness in only two domains: early childhood deafness and acquired hearing loss in adults. In each section close attention will be paid to the challenges posed by competing perspectives on Deafness to our understanding of the source and scope of the effects discussed.

Early childhood deafness

For many deaf children and their families, the greatest challenge of deafness at birth/early infancy lies in the acquisition of language and with it the development of complex and satisfying communication within both the immediate developmental environment and the wider social world (Robinson, 1987;

---

[1] Following Woodward (1972), it has become common to distinguish between upper case 'Deaf' and lower case 'deaf'. The latter refers to the condition of not being able to hear and is usually used in conjunction with deaf people who do not sign. Upper case 'D' distinguishes Deafness as a cultural identity much as we would use capitalisation for other ethnic identities such as Asian or Polish. It is intended to demonstrate affiliation with the Deaf community and culture and distance from the medical condition of not hearing.

Marschark, 1997). For Deaf children from Deaf families who share a common (signed) language that is not dependent on auditory function, we know that the language-acquisition process progresses much as that of spoken language for hearing children in hearing families (Volterra, 1981; Caselli, 1983; Woll and Kyle, 1989). Deafness of itself does not automatically cause problems of language acquisition. Synchronous, reciprocal communication is easily established from the earliest age.

However, for deaf children in hearing families or more particularly those with severe/profound losses, significant difficulties, delays and in some cases deficiencies in language acquisition are well documented (Marschark, 1993). Indeed, one of the most crucial supporting arguments for the implementation of universal newborn hearing screening lies in its role in offsetting such usual problems of language development and their consequential difficulties for the child and family (Davis *et al.*, 1997; Yoshinaga-Itano, 2003). Therefore, if we are faced by these two conditions that in one case (Deaf children in Deaf families) difficulties in the development of language are not usual and in the other (deaf children, usually with severe/profound losses in the context of hearing families) language development problems are very highly likely, what does this tell us about the psychosocial effects of early childhood deafness?

The first thing it does is point us to the issue of 'fit' and the developmental environment. For Deaf children developing language in a signing family environment the situation is relatively straightforward. The family is not required to adapt their communication other than the natural 'childese' – documented in signed languages as it is in spoken languages (Woll and Kyle, 1989; Harris, 1992). Also the child is not required to do anything particularly difficult or special because the visual linguistic environment is suited to the acquisition of a visual language. Child developmental needs and developmental environment resources generally fit. For these children, the greater challenge is likely to lie in the learning of a spoken/written language as their second language (Mayer and Wells, 1996; Mayer and Akamatsu, 1999) and with it extensive academic and social knowledge.

The situation is very different, however, for hearing families. Whether they choose to bring up their deaf child with spoken language or signed language, child and developmental environment do not easily fit. In terms of a spoken language developmental trajectory, the child's strengths and weaknesses have to be adapted (e.g. through hearing aids, cochlear implants, speech therapy, etc.) and the skills and resources of the parents require adaptation also (through deliberately learning communicative strategies and therapies with the child). Ensuring communication is accessible and the child develops spoken language to their full potential requires a great deal of effort on both parts. For hearing parents who choose signed language for their child, they are faced with the challenges involved in a situation when your child's mother tongue is not your mother's tongue (Maitland, 1994). The task is one of not only learning a new language and using it in common everyday situations within the family (Sutherland, Griggs and Young, 2003). It is also about developing understanding of Deaf culture and their child's Deaf identity (Young, 1999) as well as in drawing on the support and resources of the Deaf community (Canavan, 1999). Thus, whether in the case of spoken or signed language, there is, be it for different reasons, likely to be a lack of fit between child language and developmental environment.

Much of our understanding, therefore, of the psychosocial effects of deafness in early childhood is bound up with the consequences and variability in how such an issue of fit is tackled. As such the psychosocial effects of deafness are not the deaf child's but rather the whole family's (Henderson and Hendershot, 1991; Young, 2003). Much early intervention is firmly focused on assisting parents to develop the knowledge, understanding, resources and behaviours needed to maximise communicative fit (Marschark, 1997). As such the core issue is not how deafness might impede the accessibility and availability of language, but rather how it might interfere with the development of effective, meaningful and elaborated *reciprocal* communication (Marschark, 1993; Calderon and Greenberg, 2000).

In such a style of communication, the child experiences active participation, builds linguistic knowledge, social knowledge and social competence, cognitive and problem solving strategies, information about the self and others, and a sense of being a meaningful part of the familial and social world (Marschark, 2000). In turn all of these gains are vital for the development of positive self-esteem (Bat-Chava, 1993), reflective cognitive styles and an internal locus of control (Marschark, 1993). We know that deaf children who experience poor communication (both quantitatively and qualitatively) within the family and also the wider social world tend to have fewer and less flexible coping resources, an impoverished sense of self-worth, less trust in their ability to control their own lives, deficits in their ability to understand the social world and are more at risk of behaviour problems (Calderon and Greenberg, 2000).

In linking in this way the early issues of communicative fit and adaptation in the family environment with later developmental difficulties deaf children may experience, the intention is not to suggest any simple causality. Deaf children like all children experience a vast range of developmental influences and we do not yet fully understand the complex interactions between them (Marschark, 1993). Certainly the deaf child's individual characteristics (Calderon and Greenberg, 2000), the preexisting coping styles and resources of different families (Calderon and Greenberg, 1993), the experiential diversity of the child's developmental environment (Marschark, 2000), the nature of parental adjustment to childhood deafness (Luterman, 1999), the experience of education (Marschark, 1997), the culture, values and beliefs of the family (Bailey, 1987) and peer relationships (Hindley, 2000) all exert major effects. Nonetheless, the most profound effect of early childhood deafness is on the development of communication, which in turn has long-term consequences for deaf children's academic (Powers, Gregory and Thoutenhoofd,

1998) and socioemotional development (Hindley, 2000). Therefore, in think-ing about the psychosocial effects of early childhood deafness one always has to return to the psychosocial effects for the family of having a deaf child and how they tackle the most significant challenge of building a communicative and developmental fit that works for all (Knight and Swanick, 1999; Young, 2002).

Acquired hearing loss in adulthood

If the central challenge in early childhood deafness is how to ensure optimal language development in the first place, then a central challenge for those with an acquired hearing loss in adulthood is in many ways the opposite – how to cope with the disruption to previously established patterns of communication. Such a transition and its consequences are only very inadequately understood by thinking in terms of not hearing, or missed information. Rather, as Morgan Jones (2001) points out, acquired hearing loss disrupts the very fabric of per-sonal, familial and social relationships. Its effects are felt in self-image, employ-ment, mental health, future aspiration and life chances (Jones, Kyle and Wood, 1987). In other words, while changed or disrupted communication may be the nexus for the psychosocial effects of acquired hearing impairment, it is not descriptively or explanatorily adequate for those effects. Furthermore, while research and personal accounts (e.g. Ashley, 1973) have provided us with a detailed understanding of the range of experiences associated with hearing loss in adult life, what remains less clear is exactly what the relationship might be between those experiences and the fact of losing one's hearing. For example, we know that loneliness and isolation are very common and often extreme experiences both for those with traumatic and those with progressive losses (Thomas and Herbst, 1980; Thomas, 1984). However, what are the path-ways that might take one individual with a hearing loss into extreme social isolation but which leaves another, with a comparable hearing loss, relatively untouched by such effects? In what follows, commonly cited psychosocial effects of losing one's hearing will be discussed alongside a consideration of the range of dynamic relationships that will influence and underpin such outcomes.

Challenges to self-identity, self-confidence and self-esteem are fundamental experiences of those with acquired hearing loss (Jones, Kyle and Wood, 1987). As Hogan (2001) states: 'The onset of deafness ... challenges one's very notion of who you are, how you fit into the world and how you will live out the rest of your life. The onset of deafness signals not just the loss of hearing but also the loss of a sense of self ...' (page 12). Indeed, he goes on to suggest that the central task of rehabilitation will be to support the individual in how they 'remake' that identity and return to a state of satisfaction with who they are, what they do and the aspirations they seek for their future. Hearing loss underpins such disruption in the sense of self because it renders the communicative exchanges by which we both know others and we are known by them problematic and unpredictable. Professional, personal or social situations that previously would have been handled with ease become instead potential sources of embarrassment, stress or anxiety because it is not possible to predict whether one will be able to understand or be understood (Morgan Jones, 2001). If we are known by what we do, what we say and the roles we take then such a problematical social world directly threatens and distorts those sources of identity. Hogan (2001) goes so far as to suggest that the primary emotion underlying the challenges to identity experienced is one of fear. Fear of seeming stupid, fear of being 'caught out' (if others are unaware of your hearing loss), fear of loss of control and independence (Jones, Kyle and Wood, 1987), fear you will not be able to manage the situation in which you are required to act, fear you are no longer the person you always thought you were.

However, such fundamental challenges to self and identity are not simply a result of the interaction between the self, one's particular social world and one's particular variety of not hearing. There are also macro considerations that operate outside but affect the psychosocial circumstances of any given individual or context. Society is not benign about deafness. Certainly within Western European society dominant perceptions reinforce the spurious connections between deafness, stupidity, stubbornness and suspicion. How many times in the popular media or from your own tongue have you heard the exasperated expression 'Are you deaf or something?' As Jones and colleagues (1987) point out, it is ironic that many of the response behaviours to acquired hearing loss only serve to reinforce such stereotypes. For example, people who feel forced to withdraw from friends and society, do not participate in discussion or feel that they have little to offer become unconfident and unassertive. In coming to terms with deafness one is also coming to terms with society's perceptions, expectations, discriminations and prejudices (Corker, 1998). These in turn also assault one's sense of self.

A second oft-cited psychosocial effect of acquired deafness has already been implied in the previous discussion, namely that of impaired social interaction. In this respect, Thomas and Herbst (1980) make a distinction between social isolation and emotional isolation. The former refers to a restricted ability to initiate and maintain relationships outside the home, the latter to feeling less involved and supported by immediate family, and a loss of intimacy (Morgan Jones, 2001). Thomas and Herbst (1980) go on to suggest that the overriding social effect of acquired deafness is 'loneliness' and interestingly that this is the case regardless of the degree of hearing loss. They account for this finding by pointing out that *any* perceived breakdown in communication will be sufficient to engender feelings of loneliness; it is not dependent on the severity of the breakdown. While later work has pointed to more complex models for understanding the relationship between communicative breakdown and feelings of personal and social isolation (e.g. Jones, Kyle and Wood, 1987), the connection between acquired hearing loss and loneliness remains.

Once again, however, it is important to put the resultant effect (social isolation) into a dynamic context rather than simply see it as caused by hearing loss. The difficulties in understanding experienced by the deafened person must be set alongside factors such as others' failure to adjust to changed communication patterns, particularly within home and family (Morgan Jones, 2001), society's orientation towards and privileging of auditory/spoken communication (Corker, 1998) and variations in the extent to which individuals are able to tolerate changes in access to communication and styles of interaction (Jones, Kyle and Wood, 1987). In other words, both the phonocentrism (Corker, 1998) of modern society and one's psychosocial predisposition (Hogan, 2001) also play their part.

Finally, stress has been extensively investigated in relation to those with acquired hearing loss and the connection between the two has been found to be strong (Jones, Kyle and Wood, 1987). In many respects stress is a response to a range of circumstances we have already discussed – the unpredictability of communicative and social circumstances, perceived loss of control and independence, changes in self-identity, the sheer hard work involved in finding one's way through an 'uncommunicating' world (Wright, 1969). Also medical/audiological factors that might accompany hearing loss such as vertigo or tinnitus are further potential sources of stress (Thomas and Herbst, 1980). Specific stress factors have also been investigated within the context of family and social relationships. In this respect, Morgan Jones (2001) interestingly focused on the stress involved in the communication tactics used within relationships and in particular those associated with lipreading. She identified five major stress factors (Morgan Jones, 2001, page 234):

1. The stress caused through encountering strangers
2. Stress with unlipreadable children
3. Stress for men who feel threatened or provoked by the intimacy required in the act of 'looking' in order to lipread
4. Stress in being forced to change long-established marital communication patterns
5. Stress due to the forced 'looking' required when marital intimacy was experienced as frightening because of past failed relationships

As with any discussion on stress in any context, the extent to which an individual will experience a circumstance as stressful is governed by a whole web of other intervening variables such as social support, preexistent coping resources and strategies, life stage, other personal and familial events and variations in one's psychological ability to admit and respond to change. Consequently, as Hogan (2001) suggests, when an individual with an acquired hearing loss seeks help/rehabilitation he or she is not simply seeking assistance with hearing and communication but rather assistance with managing such complex background variables in interaction with that hearing loss.

Conclusions

Seeking to explore the psychosocial effects of deafness as a general topic is rather like trying to capture a shape that is in constant motion. Rarely is it possible to be definitive or predictive because resultant effects are exactly that – resultant – from complex interactions of psychological and sociological variables that are themselves open to multiple definition. So are there any bottom lines? In the case of early childhood deafness the psychosocial effects for the child will always come back to two factors: the challenges involved in establishing reciprocal, synchronous, quality communication and the impact on the family of having a deaf child. In the case of acquired hearing loss in adults, if there is one central message it has to be that attention must be paid not only to individual coping but to the contribution that others make to that process in both creating some of the problems and in mediating some of the solutions.

Although the remit of this chapter has been to provide a general introduction to the psychosocial effects of deafness and not a specific focus on deafness and infectious diseases, within the context of this book a final word perhaps should be offered on that particular context. Particularly, for hearing families with deaf children the key challenges we have identified concerning reciprocal quality communication and the impact on the family are themselves mediated by a range of issues associated with the psychosocial challenge of coming to terms with having a deaf child (Luterman, 1999). Within that process, 'why is my child deaf?' is a common and understandable question for many families and for the majority it is still the case that the answer will be that cause is unknown. However, for some an answer will be possible and among aetiologies that can be defined is that of some infections such as meningitis. However, once again there is not an easy relationship to be established between the fact of knowing why one's child is deaf and subsequent responses and reactions. For some parents the knowledge is comforting because uncertainty causes greater anxiety. There is closure in the knowledge. For some it will be profoundly disturbing raising questions of guilt and responsibility and whether something could have been done to prevent it. There is no easy connection to be established between the identification of a cause of deafness, the response of parents and how subsequently the challenges of language and family adaptation are pursued. Once again the psychosocial effects of deafness, in this aspect, will be multifactorial, complex and messy to understand, as indeed are most of our own familial, social and emotional lives.

REFERENCES

Adler, S.P. (1985) The molecular epidemiology of cytomegalovirus transmission among children attending a day care center. *Journal of Infectious Diseases*, **152**, 760–8.

Adler, S.P. (1988) Cytomegalovirus transmission among children in day care, their mothers and caretakers. *Pediatric Infectious Diseases Journal*, **7**, 279–85.

Adler, S.P. (1989) Cytomegalovirus and child day care. Evidence for an increased infection rate among day-care workers. *New England Journal of Medicine*, **321**, 1290–6.

Adler, S.P., Starr, S.E., Plotkin, S.A., Hempfling, S.H., Bus, J., Manning, M.L. and Best, A.M. (1995) Immunity induced by primary human cytomegalovirus infection protects against secondary infection among women of childbearing age. *Journal of Infectious Diseases*, **171**, 26–32.

Adler, S.P., Plotkin, S.A., Gonzol, E., Cadoz, M., Meric, C., Wang, J.B., Dellamonica, P., Best, A.M., Zahradnik, J., Pinuis, S., Berenci, K., Cox, W.I. and Gyulai, Z. (1999) A canarypox vector expressing cytomegalovirus (CMV) glycoprotein B primes for antibody responses to a live attenuated CMV vaccine (Towne). *Journal of Infectious Diseases*, **180**, 843–6.

Afzal, M.A., Yates, P.J. and Minor, P.D. (1988) Nucleotide sequence at position 1081 of the haemagglutinin-neuraminidase gene in the mumps Urabe vaccine strain. *Journal of Infectious Diseases*, **177**, 265–6.

Ahlfors, K. and Ivarsson, S.A. (1985) Cytomegalovirus in breast milk of Swedish milk donors. *Scandinavian Journal of Infectious Diseases*, **17**, 11–3.

Ahlfors, K., Ivarsson, S.A. and Harris, S. (1999) Report on a long-term study of maternal and congenital cytomegalovirus infection in Sweden. Review of prospective studies available in the literature. *Scandinavian Journal of Infectious Diseases*, **31**, 443–57.

Ahlfors, K., Ivarsson, S.A. and Harris, S. (2001) Secondary maternal cytomegalovirus infection: a significant cause of congenital disease. *Pediatrics*, **107**, 1227–8.

Ahlfors, K., Ivarsson, S.A., Harris, S., Svanberg, L., Holmquist, R., Lemmark, B. and Theander, G. (1984) Congenital cytomegalovirus infection and disease in Sweden and the relative importance of primary and secondary maternal infections. *Scandinavian Journal of Infectious Diseases*, **16**, 129–37.

Ahmad, I. and Lee, W.C. (1999) Otosyphilis masquerading as neurofibromatosis type II. *Otorhinolaryngology*, **61**, 37–40.

Alberola, J., Tamarit, A., Igual, R. and Navarro, D. (2000) Early neutralizing and glycoprotein B (gB)-specific antibody responses to human cytomegalovirus (HCMV) in immunocompetent individuals with distinct clinical presentations of primary HCMV infection. *Journal of Clinical Virology*, **16**, 113–22.

Infection and Hearing Impairment. Edited by V.E. Newton and P.J. Vallely
© 2006 John Wiley & Sons, Ltd

Alford, C.A., Hayes, K. and Britt, W. (1988) Primary cytomegalovirus infection in pregnancy: comparison of antibody responses to virus encoded proteins between women with and without intrauterine infection. *Journal of Infectious Diseases*, **158**, 917–24.

Alford, C.A. and Pass, R.F. (1981) Epidemiology of chronic congenital and perinatal infections of man. *Clinics in Perinatology*, **8**, 397–414.

Alford, C.A., Stagno, S. and Pass, R.F. (1980) Natural history of perinatal cytomegalovirus infection, in *Perinatal Infections*, Excerpta Medica, Amsterdam, pp. 125–47.

Alford, C.A., Stagno, S., Pass, R.F. and Huang, E.S. (1981) Epidemiology of cytomegalovirus, in *The Human Herpesviruses: An Interdisciplinary Perspective* (eds A. Nahmais, W. Dowdle and R. Schinazi), Elsevier, New York, pp. 159–71.

Alicata, J.E. (1991) The discovery of *Angiostrongylus cantonensis* as a cause of human eosinophilic meningitis. *Parasitology Today*, **7**, 151–3.

Al-Khabori, M., Mohammed, A.J., Khandekar, R. and Prakesh, N. (1996) National survey for causes of deafness and common ear disorders in Oman. Oman Ear Study (OES '96) survey report. Sultanate of Oman Ministry of Health, World Health Organization.

Al-Muhaimeed, H. (1996) Hearing impairment among 'at risk' children. *International Journal of Pediatric Otorhinolaryngology*, **34**, 75–85.

Al-Sous, M.W., Bohlega, S., Al-Kawi, M.Z., Alwatban, J. and McLean, D.R. (2004) Neurobrucellosis: clinical and neuroimaging correlation. *American Journal of Neuroradiology*, **25**, 395–401.

Alvan, G., Karlsson, K.K., Hellgren, U. and Villen, T. (1991) Hearing impairment related to plasma quinine concentration in healthy volunteers. *British Journal of Clinical Pharmacology*, **31**, 409–12.

Ames, M.D., Plotkin, S.A., Winchester, R.A. and Atkins, T.E. (1970) Central auditory imperception: a significant factor in congenital rubella deafness. *Journal of the American Medical Association*, **213**, 419–21.

Ammerman, K., Schessel, D.A., Simon, G.L. and Parenti, D.M. (2000) Acute deafness due to syphilitic meningitis in a patient with HIV. *Infectious Diseases in Clinical Practice*, **9**, 131–3.

Andersen, J., Christensen, R. and Hertel, J. (2004) Clinical features and epidemiology of septicaemia and meningitis in neonates due to *Streptococcus agalactiae* in Copenhagen County, Denmark: a 10 year survey from 1992 to 2001. *Acta Paediatrica*, **93**, 1334–9.

Anderson, R.M. and May, R.M. (1991) *Infectious Diseases Inhumana: Dynamics and Control*, Open University Press, Oxford.

Angeli, S. (2003) Value of vestibular testing in young children with sensorineural hearing loss. *Archives of Otolaryngology – Head and Neck Surgery*, **129**, 478–82.

Anon (1996a) Replacement Chapter 25: Pneumococcal. September 2004, in *Immunisation against Infectious Disease 1996* (eds D. Salisbury and N. Begg) On-line publication at http://www.dh.gov.uk/PolicyAndGuidance/HealthAndSocialCareTopics/GreenBook/GreenBookGeneralInformation/GreenBookGeneralArticle/fs/en?CONTENT_ID=4097254&chk=isTfGX.

Anon (1996b) Replacement Chapter 16: *Haemophilus influenzae* b (Hib). August 2004, in *Immunisation against Infectious Disease 1996* (eds D. Salisbury and N. Begg). On-line publication at http://www.dh.gov.uk/PolicyAndGuidance/HealthAndSocial

CareTopics/GreenBook/GreenBookGeneralInformation/GreenBookGeneral Article/fs/en?CONTENT_ID=4097254&chk=isTfGX.

Anon (1996c) Replacement Chapter 23: Meningococcal. April 2004, in *Immunisation against Infectious Disease 1996* (eds D. Salisbury and N. Begg). On-line publication at http://www.dh.gov.uk/PolicyAndGuidance/HealthAndSocialCareTopics/Green Book/GreenBookGeneralInformation/GreenBookGeneralArticle/fs/en?CONTEN T_ID=4097254&chk=isTfGX.

Anon (2002) Prevention of perinatal group B streptococcal disease. Revised guidelines from CDC. *Morbidity and Mortality Weekly Report*, **51**, 1–23.

Anon (2003) Pneumococcal vaccination for cochlear implant candidates and recipients: Updated Recommendations of the Advisory Committee on Immunization Practices. *Morbidity and Mortality Weekly Report*, **52**, 739–40.

Anton, E., Otegui, A. and Alonso, A. (2000) Meningoencephalitis and *Chlamydia pneumoniae* infection. *European Journal of Neurology*, **7**, 586.

Arends, J.P. and Zanen, H.C. (1988) Meningitis caused by *Streptococcus suis* in humans. *Reviews in Infectious Diseases*, **10**, 131–7.

Arguedas, A., Dagan, R., Soley, C., Loaiza, C., Knudsen, K., Porat, N., Perez, A., Brilla, E. and Herrera, M.L. (2003) Microbiology of otitis media in Costa Rican children, 1999 through 2001. *Paediatric Infectious Disease Journal*, **22**, 1063–8.

Arita, M., Ueno, Y. and Masuyama, Y. (1981) Complete heart block in mumps myocarditis. *British Heart Journal*, **46**, 342–4.

Arnold, W. and Friedmann, I. (1988) Otosclerosis – an inflammatory disease of the otic capsule of viral aetiology? *The Journal of Laryngology and Otology*, **102**, 865–71.

Arnold, W., Nadol, J.B. and Weidauer, H. (1981) Temporal bone histopathology in human ototoxicity due to loop diuretics. *Scandinavian Audiology Supplement*, **14**, 201–13.

Arnold, W., Niedermeier, H.P., Lehn, N., Neubert, W. and Hoeffler, H. (1996) Measles virus in otosclerosis and the specific immune response of the inner ear. *Acta Otolaryngologica*, **116**, 705–9.

Arola, M., Ruuskanen, O., Ziegler, T., Mertsola, K., Nanto-Salonen, K., Putto-Laurila, A., Viljanen, M.K. and Halonen, P. (1990) Clinical role of respiratory virus infections in acute otitis media. *Pediatrics*, **86**, 848–55.

Aron, J.L. and May, R.M. (1982) The population dynamics of malaria, in *Population Dynamics of Infectious Diseases* (ed. R.M. Anderson), Chapman and Hall, London, pp. 139–79.

Asanuma, H., Numazaki, K., Nagata, N., Hotsubo, T., Horino, K. and Chiba, S. (1996) Role of milk whey in the transmission of human cytomegalovirus infection by breast milk. *Microbiology and Immunology*, **40**, 201–4.

Ashley, J. (1973) *Journey into Silence*, Bodley Head, London.

Atkinson, P., Taylor, H., Sharland, M. and Maguire, H. (2002) Resurgence of paediatric tuberculosis in London. *Archives of Disease in Childhood*, **86**, 264–5.

Aust, G. (2001) Vestibulotoxicity and ototoxicity of gentamicin in newborns at risk. *International Tinnitus Journal*, **7**, 27–9.

Autran, B., Carcelain, G., Li, T.S., Blanc, C., Mathez, D., Tubiana, R., Katlama, C., Debre, P. and Leibowitch, J. (1997) Positive effects of combined antiretroviral therapy on CD4+ T cell homeostasis and function in advanced HIV disease. *Science*, **277**, 112–6.

Axon, P.R., Temple, R.H., Saeed, S.R. and Ramsden, R.T. (1998) Cochlear ossification after meningitis. *American Journal of Otology*, **19**, 724–9.

Azimi, P.H., Cramlett, H.G. and Haynes, R.E. (1969) Mumps meningoencephalitis in children. *Journal of the American Medical Association*, **207**, 509–12.

Bachor, E. and Karmody, C.S. (2001) Neural hearing loss in a child with poliomyelitis: a histopathological study. *Journal of Laryngology and Otology*, **115**, 243–6.

Badiaga, S., Levy, P.Y., Brouqui, P., Delmont, J. and Bourgeade, A. (1993) Méningite á éosinophiles. Revue de la littérature a propos d'un nouveau cas en provenance de la Réunion (Eosinophilic meningitis. Review of the literature and a new case originating from Reunion Island). *Bulletin de la Societe de Pathologie Exotique*, **86**, 277–81.

Bailey, D.P. (1987) Collaborative goal setting with families: resolving differences in values and priorities for services. *Topics in Early Childhood Special Education*, **7**, 59–71.

Baker, R.C., Kummer, A.W., Schultz, J.R., Ho, M. and Gonzalez del Rey, J. (1996) Neurodevelopmental outcome of infants with viral meningitis in the first three months of life. *Clinical Pediatrics*, **35**, 295–301.

Bakshi, S.S. and Cooper, L.Z. (1990) Rubella and mumps vaccines. *Pediatric Clinics of North America*, **37**(3), 651–68.

Balcarek, K.B., Warren, W., Smith, R.J., Lyon, M.D. and Pass, R.F. (1993) Neonatal screening for congenital cytomegalovirus infection by detection of virus in saliva. *Journal of Infectious Disease*, **167**, 1433–6.

Bale Jr, J.F., Petheram, S.J., Souza, I.E. and Murph, J.R. (1996) Cytomegalovirus reinfection in young children. *Journal of Pediatrics*, **128**, 347–52.

Balkany, T.J. and Dans, P.E. (1978) Reversible sudden deafness in early acquired syphilis. *Archives of Otolaryngology*, **104**, 66–8.

Balls, M.J., Bødker, R., Thomas, C.J., Kisinza, W., Msangeni, H.A. and Lindsay, S.W. (2004) Effect of topography on the risk of malaria infection. *Transactions of the Royal Society of Tropical Medicine & Hygiene*, **98**, 400–8.

Balmer, P., Borrow, R. and Miller, E. (2002) Impact of meningococcal C conjugate vaccine in the UK. *Journal of Medical Microbiology*, **51**, 717–22.

Balthesen, M., Messerle, M. and Reddehase, M.J. (1993) Lungs are a major organ site of cytomegalovirus latency and recurrence. *Journal of Virology*, **67**, 5360–6.

Banatvala, J.E. and Best, J.M. (1998) Rubella, in *Topley and Wilson's Microbiology and Microbial Infections: Virology* (eds B.W.J. Mahy and L. Collier), 9th edn, Arnold, London, pp. 551–77.

Banatvala, J.E. and Brown, D.W. (2004) Rubella. *Lancet*, **363**, 1127–37.

Bang, H.O. and Bang, J. (1943) Involvement of the central nervous system in mumps. *Acta Medica Scandinavica*, **13**, 487–505.

Bankaitis, A.E. and Schountz, T. (1998) HIV related ototoxicity. *Seminars in Hearing*, **19**, 155–61.

Barenfanger, J., Lawhorn, J. and Drake, C. (2004) Nonvalue of culturing cerebrospinal fluid for fungi. *Journal of Clinical Microbiology*, **42**, 236–8.

Barry, B., Delattre, J., Vie, F., Bedos, J.-P. and Gehano, P. (1999) Otogenic intracranial infections in adults. *Laryngoscope*, **109**, 483–7.

Basavaraj, S., Najaraj, S., Shanks, M., Wardrop, P. and Allen, A.A. (2004) Short-term versus long-term antibiotic prophylaxis in cochlear implant surgery. *Otology and Neurotology*, **25**, 720–2.

Bastos, I., Reimer, A. and Lundegren, K. (1993) Chronic otitis media and hearing loss in urban schoolchildren in Angola – a prevalence study. *Journal of Audiological Medicine*, **2**, 129–40.

Bastos, I., Mallya, J., Bastos Ingvarsson, L., Reimer, A. and Andreasson, L. (1995) Middle ear disease and hearing impairment in northern Tanzania. A prevalence study of schoolchildren in the Moshi and Monduli districts. *International Journal of Pediatric Otorhinolaryngology*, **32**, 1–12.

Batayneh, N. and Bdour, S. (2002) Mumps: immune status of adults and epidemiology as a necessary background for choice of vaccination strategy in Jordan. *Acta Pathologica, Microbiologica et Immunologica Scandinavica*, **110**, 528–34.

Bat-Chava, Y. (1993) Antecedents of self esteem in deaf people: a meta-analytic review. *Rehabilitation Psychology*, **38**, 221–34.

Bausch, D.G., Demby, A.H., Coulibaly, M., Kanu, J., Goba, A., Bah, A., Conde, N., Wurtzel, H.L., Cavallaro, K.F., Lloyd, E., Baldet, F.B., Cisse, S.D., Fofona, D., Savane, I.K., Tolno, R.T., Mahy, B., Wagoner, K.D., Ksiazek, T.G., Peters, C.J. and Rollin, P.E. (2001) Lassa fever in Guinea: I. Epidemiology of human disease and clinical observations. *Vector Borne and Zoonotic Diseases*, **1**, 269–81.

Beal, D.D., Davey, P.R. and Lindsay, J.R. (1967) Inner ear pathology of congenital deafness. *Archives of Otolaryngology*, **85**, 134–42.

Beckman, J.S. and Koppenol, W.H. (1996) Nitric oxide, superoxide, and peroxynitrite: the good, the bad, and the ugly. *American Journal of Physiology* (*Cell Physiology*), **271**, C1424–37.

Becroft, D.M.O. (1981) Prenatal cytomegalovirus infection: epidemiology, pathology, and pathogenesis, in *Perspective in Pediatric Pathology* (eds H.S. Rosenberg and J. Bernstein), Vol. 6, Masson Press, New York, pp. 203–41.

Begg, N., Cartwright, K.A., Cohen, J., Kaczmarski, E.B., Innes, J.A., Leen CL Nathwani, D., Singer, M., Southgate, L., Todd, W.T., Welsby, P.D. and Wood, M.J. (1999) Consensus statement on diagnosis, investigation, treatment and prevention of acute bacterial meningitis in immunocompetent adults. British Infection Society Working Party. *Journal of Infection*, **39**, 1–15.

Benirschke, K. (1974) Syphilis – the placenta and the fetus. *American Journal of Diseases in Childhood*, **128**, 142–3.

Berencsi, K., Endresz, V., Klurfeld, D., Kari, L., Kritchevsky, D. and Gonczol, E. (1998) Early atherosclerotic plaques in the aorta following cytomegalovirus infection of mice. *Cell Adhesion and Communication*, **5**, 39–47.

Berenguer, J., Moreno, S., Laguna, F., Vicente, T., Adrados, M., Ortega, A., Gonzalez-LaHoz, J. and Bouza, E. (1992) Tuberculous meningitis in patients infected with the human immunodeficiency virus. *New England Journal of Medicine*, **326**, 668–72.

Bergman, I., Painter, M.J., Wald, E.R., Chiponis, D., Holland, A.L. and Taylor, I. (1987) Outcome in children with enteroviral meningitis during the first year of life. *Journal of Pediatrics*, **110**, 705–9.

Bergström, T., Vahlne, A., Alestig, K., Jeansson, S., Forsgren, M. and Lycke, E. (1990) Primary and recurrent herpes simplex virus type 2-induced meningitis. *Journal of Infectious Diseases*, **162**, 322–30.

Beria, J. (2003) Prevalence of deafness and hearing impairment: preliminary results of a population-based study in southern Brazil, in *Informal Consultation on Epidemiology of Deafness and Hearing Impairment in Developing Countries and Update of the WHO Protocol*, World Health Organization, Geneva.

Beria, J.U., Warth Raymann, B.C., Gigante, L.P., Figueiredo, A., Jotz, G., Roithmann, R., Selaimen da Costa, S., Garcez, V., Scherer, C. and Smith, A. (2005) Hearing impairment and socio-economic factors: a population-based survey in Southern Brazil (unpublished paper).

Bernit, E., de Lamballerie, X., Zandotti, C., Berger, P., Veit, V., Schleinitz, N., de Micco, P., Harle, J.R. and Charrel, R.N. (2004) Prospective investigations of a large outbreak of meningitis due to echovirus 30 during summer 2000 in Marseilles, France. *Medicine*, **83**, 245–53.

Bernstein, J.M. (2002) Immunologic aspects of otitis media. *Current Allergy and Asthma Reports*, **2**, 309–15.

Bernstein, D.I. and Bourne, N. (1999) Animal models for cytomegalovirus infection: guinea-pig CMV, in *Handbook of Animal Models of Infection* (ed. M.S.O. Zak), Academic Press, London, pp. 935–41.

Bess, F.H. and Tharpe, A.M. (1984) Unilateral hearing impairment in children. *Pediatrics*, **74**, 206–16.

Best, J.M., O'Shea, S., Tipples, G., Davies, N., Al-Khusaiby, S.M., Krause, A., Hesketh, L.M., Jin, L. and Enders, G. (2002) Interpretation of rubella serology in pregnancy – pitfalls and problems. *British Medical Journal*, **325**, 147–8.

Bhatia, K., Gibbin, K.P., Nikolopoulos, T.P. and O'Donoghue, G.M. (2004) Surgical complications and their management in a series of 300 consecutive pediatric cochlear implantations. *Otology and Neurotology*, **25**, 730–9.

Bhatt, S., Halpin, C. and Hsu, W. (1991) Hearing loss and pneumococcal meningitis: an animal model. *Laryngoscope*, **101**, 1285–92.

Bhatt, S.M., Lauretano, A., Cabellos, C., Halpin, C., Levine, R.A., Xu, W.Z., Nadol Jr, J.B. and Tuomanen, E. (1993) Progression of hearing loss in experimental pneumococcal meningitis: correlation with cerebrospinal cytochemistry. *Journal of Infectious Diseases*, **167**, 675–83.

Bia, F.J., Griffith, B.P., Tarsio, M. and Hsiung, G.D. (1980) Vaccination for the prevention of maternal and fetal infection with guinea pig cytomegalovirus. *Journal of Infectious Diseases*, **142**, 732–8.

Bia, F.J., Griffith, B.P., Fong, C.K. and Hsiung, G.D. (1983) Cytomegalovirus infections in the guinea pig: experimental models for human disease. *Review of Infectious Diseases*, **5**, 177–95.

Bia, F.J., Miller, S.A., Lucia, H.L., Griffith, B.P., Tarsio, M. and Hsiung, G.D. (1984) Vaccination against transplacental cytomegalovirus transmission: vaccine reactivation and efficacy in guinea pigs. *Journal of Infectious Diseases*, **149**, 355–62.

Bibas, A., Liang, J., Michaels, L. and Wright, A. (2000) The development of the stria vascularis in the human foetus. *Clinical Otolaryngology*, **25**, 126–9.

Biedenbach, D.J., Stephen, J.M. and Jones, R.N. (2003) Antimicrobial susceptibility profile among beta-haemolytic *Streptococcus* spp. collected in the SENTRY Antimicrobial Surveillance Program – North America, 2001. *Diagnostic Microbiology and Infectious Disease*, **46**, 291–4.

Bifrare, Y.D., Kummer, J., Joss, P., Tauber, M.G. and Leib, S.L. (2005) Brain-derived neurotrophic factor protects against multiple forms of brain injury in bacterial meningitis. *Journal of Infectious Diseases*, **191**, 40–5.

Billings, K.R. and Kenna, M.A. (1999) Causes of pediatric sensorineural hearing loss: yesterday and today. *Archives of Otolaryngology – Head and Neck Surgery*, **125**, 517–21.

Birchall, M.A., Wight, R.G., French, P.D., Cockbain, Z. and Smith, S.J. (1992) Auditory function in patients infected with the human immunodeficiency virus. *Clinical Otolaryngology*, **17**, 117–21.

Biron, C.A. and Brossay, L. (2001) NK cells and NKT cells in innate defense against viral infections. *Current Opinion in Immunology*, **13**, 458–64.

Biron, C.A., Byron, K.S. and Sullivan, J.L. (1989) Severe herpesvirus infections in an adolescent without natural killer cells (comment). *New England Journal of Medicine*, **320**, 1731–5.

Bissinger, A.L., Sinzger, C., Kaiserling, E. and Jahn, G. (2002) Human cytomegalovirus as a direct pathogen: correlation of multiorgan involvement and cell distribution with clinical and pathological findings in a case of congenital inclusion disease. *Journal of Medical Virology*, **67**, 200–6.

Bistrian, K.B., Phillips, C.A. and Kaye, I.C. (1972) Fatal mumps meningeoencephalitis: isolation of virus premortem and postmortem. *Journal of the American Medical Association*, **222**, 478–9.

Bitnum, S., Rakover, Y. and Rosen, G. (1986) Acute bilateral total deafness complicating mumps. *The Journal of Laryngology and Otology*, **100**, 943–5.

Bitnun, A., Ford-Jones, E.L., Petric, M., MacGregor, D., Heurter, H., Nelson, S., Johnson, G. and Richardson, S. (2001) Acute childhood encephalitis and *Mycoplasma pneumoniae*. *Clinical Infectious Diseases*, **32**, 1674–84.

Black, F.O., Pesznecker, S. and Stallings, V. (2004) Permanent gentamicin vestibulotoxicity. *Otology and Neurotology*, **25**, 559–69.

Block, S.L. (1999) Strategies for dealing with amoxicillin failure in acute otitis media. *Archives of Family Medicine*, **8**, 68–78.

Bluestone, C.D., Stephenson, J.S. and Martin, L.M. (1992) Ten year review of otitis media pathogens. *Paediatric Infectious Disease Journal*, 11 (Suppl.), S7–11.

Bodur, H., Erbay, A., Akinci, E., Colpan, A., Cevik, M.A. and Balaban, N. (2003) Neurobrucellosis in an endemic area of brucellosis. *Scandinavian Journal of Infectious Diseases*, **35**, 94–7.

Boeckh, M., Leisenring, W., Riddell, S.R., Bowden, R.A., Huang, M.L., Myerson, O., Stevens-Ayers, T., Flowers, M.E., Cunningham, T. and Corey, L. (2003) Late cytomegalovirus disease and mortality in recipients of allogeneic hematopoietic stem cell transplants: importance of viral load and T-cell immunity. *Blood*, **101**, 407–14.

Boettcher, F.A., Bancroft, B.R. and Salvi, R.J. (1990) Concentration of salicylate in serum and perilymph of the chinchilla. *Archives of Otolaryngology*, **116**, 681–4.

Bogaert, D., van Belkum, A., Sluijter, M., Luijendijk, A., de Groot, R., Rumke, H.C., Verbrugh, H.A. and Hermans, P.W.M. (2004) Colonisation by *Streptococcus pneumoniae* and *Staphylococcus aureus* in healthy children. *The Lancet*, **363**, 1871–2.

Boongird, P., Phuapradit, P., Siridej, N., Chirachariyavej, T., Chuahirun, S. and Vejjajiva, A. (1977) Neurological manifestations of gnathostomiasis. *Journal of the Neurological Sciences*, **31**, 279–91.

Boppana, S.B. and Britt, W.J. (1995) Antiviral antibody responses and intrauterine transmission after primary maternal cytomegalovirus infection. *Journal of Infectious Diseases*, **171**, 1115–21.

Boppana, S.B., Fowler, K.B. *et al.* (1992a) Newborn findings and outcome in children with symptomatic congenital CMV infection. *Pediatric Research*, **31**, 158A.

Boppana, S.B., Pass, R.F., Britt, W.J., Stagno, S. and Alford, C.A. (1992b) Symptomatic congenital cytomegalovirus infection: neonatal morbidity and mortality. *Pediatric Infectious Diseases Journal*, **11**, 93–9.

Boppana, S.B., Polis, M.A., Kramer, A.A., Britt, W.J. and Koenigs, S. (1995) Virus specific antibody responses to human cytomegalovirus (HCMV) in human immunodeficiency virus type 1-infected individuals with HCMV retinitis. *Journal of Infectious Diseases*, **171**, 182–5.

Boppana, S.B., Fowler, K.B., Vaid, Y., Hedlund, G., Stagno, S., Britt, W.J. and Pass, R.F. (1997) Neuroradiographic findings in the newborn period and long-term outcome in children with symptomatic congenital cytomegalovirus infection. *Pediatrics*, **99**, 409–14.

Boppana, S.B., Fowler, K.B., Britt, W.J., Stagno, S. and Pass, R.F. (1999) Symptomatic congenital cytomegalovirus infection in infants born to mothers with pre-existing immunity to cytomegalovirus. *Pediatrics*, **104**, 55–60.

Boppana, S.B., Rivera, L.B., Fowler, K.B., Mach, M. and Britt, W.J. (2001) Intrauterine transmission of cytomegalovirus to infants of women with preconceptional immunity. *New England Journal of Medicine*, **344**, 1366–71.

Bordley, J.E., Brookhouser, P.E. and Worthington, E.L. (1972) Viral infections and hearing: a critical review of the literature, 1969–1970. *The Laryngoscope*, **82**, 557–77.

Bordley, J.E. and Kapur, Y.P. (1977) Histopathologic changes in the temporal bone resulting from measles infection. *Archives of Otolaryngologica*, **103**, 162–8.

Borisch, B., Jahn, G., Scholl, B.C., Filger-Brillinger, J., Heymer, B., Fleckengstein, B. and Muller-Hermelink, H.K. (1988) Detection of human cytomegalovirus DNA and viral antigens in tissues of different manifestations of CMV infections. *Virchow's Archive B Cell Pathology including Molecular Pathology*, **55**, 93–9.

Borisenko, K.K., Tichonova, L.I. and Renton, A.M. (1999) Syphilis and other sexually transmitted infections in the Russian Federation. *International Journal of Sexually Transmitted Diseases and AIDS*, **10**, 665–8.

Böttcher, T., Gerber, J., Wellmer, A., Smirnov, A.V., Fakhrjanali, F., Mix, E., Pilz, J., Zettl, U.K. and Nau, N. (2000) Rifampin reduces production of reactive oxygen species of cerebrospinal fluid phagocytes and hippocampal neuronal apoptosis in experimental *Streptococcus pneumoniae* meningitis. *Journal of Infectious Diseases*, **181**, 2095–8.

Bourne, N., Rosteck, R., Fox, D., Schleiss, M.R. and Bernstein, D.I. (1996) Immunization with a cytomegalovirus (CMV) glycoprotein vaccine improves pregnancy outcome in an animal model of congenital CMV infection (abstract). *Program and Abstracts*, 36th International CAAC, p. 179.

Bourne, N., Schleiss, M., Bravo, F.J. and Bernstein, D.I. (2001) Preconception immunization with a cytomegalovirus (CMV) glycoprotein vaccine improves pregnancy outcome in a guinea pig model of congenital CMV infection. *Journal of Infectious Diseases*, **183**, 59–64.

Bowden, R.A. (1995) Transfusion-transmitted cytomegalovirus infection. *Hematology–Oncology Clinics of North America*, **9**, 155–66.

Bowden, R.A., Sayers, A.M., Flournoy, N., Newton, B., Banaji, M., Thomas, E.D. and Meyers, J.D. (1986) Cytomegalovirus immune globulin and seronegative blood products to prevent primary cytomegalovirus infection after marrow transplantation. *New England Journal of Medicine*, **314**, 1006–10.

Brewis, C. and McFerran, D.J. (1997) Farmer's ear: sudden sensorineural hearing loss due to *Chlamydia psittaci* infection. *Journal of Laryngology and Otology*, **111**, 855–7.

British National Formulary (2004) **48**, 267.

Brook, I. (1995) Role of anaerobic bacteria in chronic otitis media and cholesteatoma. *International Journal of Otorhinolaryngology*, **31**, 153–7.

Brook, I., Yocum, P., Shah, K., Feldman, B. and Epstein, S. (1983) Aerobic and anaerobic bacteriologic features of serious otitis media in children. *American Journal of Otology*, **4**, 389–92.

Brookhouser, P.E. and Auslander, M.C. (1989) Aided auditory thresholds in children with postmeningitic deafness. *Laryngoscope*, **99**, 800–8.

Brown, M.R., Allison, D.G. and Gilbert, P. (1988) Resistance of bacterial biofilms to antibiotics: a growth-related effect? *Journal of Antimicrobial Chemotherapy*, **22**, 777–83.

Brown, E.G., Dimock, K. and Wright, K.E. (1996) The Urabe AM9 mumps vaccine is a mixture of viruses differing at amino acid 335 of the hemagglutinin-neuraminidase gene with one form associated with disease. *Journal of Infectious Diseases*, **174**, 619–22.

Brown, N.J. and Richmond, S.J. (1980) Fatal mumps myocarditis in an 8-month-old child. *British Medical Journal*, **281**, 356–7.

Brown, E.G. and Wright, K.E. (1998) Genetic studies on a mumps vaccine strain associated with meningitis. *Reviews in Medical Virology*, **47**, 128–33.

Brown, T.J., Yen-Moore, A. and Tyring, S.K. (1999) An overview of sexually transmitted diseases. Part I. *Journal of the American Academy of Dermatology*, **41**, 511–32.

Browne, E.P., Wing, B., Coleman, D. and Shenk, T. (2001a) Altered cellular mRNA levels in human cytomegalovirus-infected fibroblasts: viral block to the accumulation of antiviral mRNAs. *Journal of Virology*, **75**, 12319–30.

Browne, G., Whitworth, C., Bellamy, C. and Ogilvie, M.M. (2001b) Acute allograft glomerulopathy associated with CMV viraemia. *Nephrology Dialysis Transplantation*, **16**, 861–2.

Bruce-Chwatt, L.J. (1988) History of malaria from prehistory to eradication, Chapter 1 in *Malaria; Principles and Practice of Malariology* (eds W.H. Wernsdorfer and I.A. McGregor), Vol. 1, Churchill Livingstone, Edinburgh, pp. 1–59.

Brummett, R.E. (1981) Effects of antibiotic-diuretic interactions in the guinea pig model of ototoxicity. *Review of Infectious Diseases*, **3**(Suppl.), 216–23.

Brummett, R.E. (1993a) Ototoxic liability of erythromycin and analogues. *Otolaryngological Clinics of North America*, **26**, 811–9.

Brummett, R.E. (1993b) Ototoxicity of vancomycin and analogues. *Otolaryngological Clinics of North America*, **26**, 821–8.

Brummett, R.E., Fox, K.E., Jacobs, F., Kempton, J.B., Stokes, Z. and Richmond, A.B. (1990) Augmented gentamicin ototoxicity induced by vancomycin in guinea pigs. *Archives of Otolaryngology – Head and Neck Surgery*, **116**, 61–4.

Brunello, F., Favari, F. and Fontana, R. (1999) Comparison of the MB/BacT and BACTEC 460 TB systems for recovery of mycobacteria from various clinical specimens. *Journal of Clinical Microbiology*, **37**, 1206–9.

Bruning, J.H., Persoons M, Lemstrom, K., Stals, F.S., De Clercq, E. and Bruggeman, C.A. (1994). Enhancement of transplantation-associated atherosclerosis by CMV, which can be prevented by antiviral therapy in the form of HPMPC. *Transplant International*, **7**(Suppl. 1), S365–70.

Bu, X. (2002) Report of the pilot study on WHO Ear and Hearing Disorders Survey Protocol, Jiangsu Province, China, Nanjing Medical University.

Bu, X. (2002) The Report of Results from the Pilot Study on WHO Ear and Hearing Disorders Survey Protocol, Jiangsu Province, China, in *Informal Consultation on Epidemiology of Deafness and Hearing Impairment in Developing Countries and Update of the WHO Protocol*, World Health Organization, Geneva.

Bunnag, T., Comer, D.S. and Punyagupta, S. (1970) Eosinophilic myeloencephalitis caused by *Gnathostoma spinigerum*. Neuropathology of nine cases. *Journal of the Neurological Sciences*, **10**, 419–34.

Buruelt, C.H. (1877) *Treatise on the Ear*. Philadelphia: Lea and Sons, at p. 269.

Byl, F.M. and Adour, K.K. (1976) Auditory symptoms associated with herpes zoster or idiopathic facial paralysis. *Laryngoscope*, **86**, 372–9.

Bylander, A. (1984) Function and dysfunction of the Eustachian tube in children. *Acta Otolaryngologica (Belgium)*, **38**, 238–45.

Calderon, L. and Greenberg, M. (1993) Considerations in the adaption of families with school-aged deaf children, in *Psychological Perspectives on Deafness* (eds M. Marschark and M.D. Clark), Lawrence Erlbaum Associates, Hillsdale, New Jersey.

Calderon, R. and Greenberg, M. (2000) Challenges to parents and professionals in promoting socioemotional development in deaf children, in *The Deaf Child in the Family and at School: Essays in Honour of Kathryn P. Meadow-Orlans* (eds P.E. Spencer, C. Erting and M. Marschark), Lawrence Erlbaum Associates, Hillsdale, New Jersey, pp. 167–85.

Campo, P., Latayer, R., Cossesc, B. and Placidi, V. (1997) Toluene-induced hearing loss: a mid-frequency location of the cochlear lesions. *Neurotoxicology and Teratology*, **19**, 129–40.

Canavan, F. (1999) A parent's response to Alys Young's article. *Journal of Social Work Practice*, **13**, 172–3.

Carbone, K.M. and Wolinsky, J.S. (2001) Mumps virus, in *Fields Virology* (eds D.M. Knipe and P.M. Howley), 4th edn, Lippincott-Raven Publishers Philadelphia, pp. 1381–400.

Caroppo, B.S., Dido, P., Primache, V., Guidotti, P., Sergi, P., Pastorino, G. and Barbi, M. (2001) Cytomegalovirus DNA detection on Guthrie cards: a useful method to identify hearing loss cases due to congenital infection. *International Pediatrics*, **16**, 1–3.

Carroll, K.J. and Carroll, C.A. (1994) Prospective investigation of the longterm auditory-neurological sequelae associated with bacterial meningitis: a study from Vanuatu. *Journal of Tropical Medicine and Hygiene*, **97**, 145–50.

Carroll, E.D., Clark, J.E. and Cant, A.J. (2001) Non-pulmonary tuberculosis. *Paediatric Respiratory Reviews*, **2**, 113–9.

Caselli, M.C. (1983) Communication to language: deaf children's and hearing children's development compared. *Sign Language Studies*, **39**, 113–24.

Casey, J.R. and Pichichero, M.E. (2004) Changes in frequency and pathogens causing otitis media in 1995–2003. *Paediatric Infectious Disease Journal*, **23**, 824–8.

Casselbrant, M.L., Mandel, E.M., Kurs-Lasky, M., Rockette, H.E. and Bluestone, C.D. (1995) Otitis media in a population of black American and white American infants, 0–2 years of age. *International Journal of Pediatric Otorhinolaryngology*, **33**, 1–16.

Casteels, A., Naessens, A., Gordts, F., De Catte, L., Bougatef, A. and Foulon, W. (1999) Neonatal screening for congenital cytomegalovirus infections. *Journal of Perinatal Medicine*, **27**, 116–21.

Castillo-Solorzano, C., Carrasco, P., Tambini, G., Reef, S., Brana, M. and de Quadros, C.A. (2003) New horizons in the control of rubella and prevention of congenital rubella syndrome in the Americas. *Journal of Infectious Diseases*, **187**(Suppl. 1), S146–52.

CDSC (Communicable Diseases Surveillance Centre) (2000) *Antimicrobial Resistance in 2000. England and Wales*, Public Health Laboratory Service, pp. 16–7.

Centers for Disease Control and Prevention (2002) Sexually transmitted diseases treatment guidelines 2002. *Morbidity and Mortality Weekly Report*, **51**(RR-6).

Chan, Y.C., Ho, K.H., Chuah, Y.S., Lau, C.C., Thomas, A. and Tambyah, P.A. (2004) Eosinophilic meningitis secondary to allergic *Aspergillus sinusitis*. *Journal of Allergy and Clinical Immunology*, **114**, 194–5.

Chandler, S.H., Handsfield, H.H. and McDougall, J.K. (1987) Isolation of multiple strains of cytomegalovirus from women attending a clinic for sexually transmitted disease. *Journal of Infectious Diseases*, **155**, 655–60.

Chang, Y.C., Huang, C.C. and Liu, C.C. (1996) Frequency of linear hyperechogenicity over the basal ganglia in young infants with congenital rubella syndrome. *Clinical Infectious Diseases*, **22**, 569–71.

Chappuis, F., Farinelli, T. and Loutan, L. (2001) Ivermectin treatment of a traveler who returned from Peru with cutaneous gnathostomiasis. *Clinical Infectious Diseases*, **33**, E17–9.

Chatterjee, A., Harrison, C.J., Britt, W.J. and Bewtra, C. (2001) Modification of maternal and congenital cytomegalovirus infection by anti-glycoprotein b antibody transfer in guinea pigs. *Journal of Infectious Diseases*, **183**, 1547–53.

Chaudhuri, A. (2004) Adjunctive dexamethasone treatment in acute bacterial meningitis. *Lancet Neurology*, **3**, 54–62.

Chee, M.S., Bankier, A.T., Beck, S., Bohni, R., Brown, C.M., Cerny, R., Hasnell, T., Hutchinson, C.A., Kouzarides, T., Martignetti, J.A. *et al.* (1990) Analysis of the protein-coding content of the sequence of human cytomegalovirus strain AD169. *Current Topics in Microbiology and Immunology*, **154**, 125–70.

Chen, M.C., Harris, J.P. and Keithley, E.M. (1998) Immunohistochemical analysis of proliferating cells in a sterile labyrinthitis animal model. *Laryngoscope*, **108**, 651–6.

Cherukupally, S.R. and Eavey, R. (2004) Vaccine-preventable pediatric postmeningitic sensorineural hearing loss in southern India. *Otolaryngology – Head and Neck Surgery*, **130**, 339–43.

Chiba, Y., Dzierba, J.L., Morag, A. and Ogra, P.L. (1976) Cell-mediated immune response to mumps virus infection in man. *Journal of Immunology*, **116**, 12–5.

Child, S.J., Jarrahian, S., Harper, V.M. and Geballe, A.P. (2002) Complementation of vaccinia virus lacking the double-stranded RNA-binding protein gene E3L by human cytomegalovirus. *Journal of Virology*, **76**, 4912–8.

Chiodo, A.A., Alberti, P.W., Sher, G.D., Francombe, W.H. and Tyler, B. (1997) Desferrioxamine ototoxicity in an adult transfusion-dependent population. *Journal of Otolaryngology*, **26**, 116–22.

Chitanondh, H. (1963) Gnathostomiasis, in *Tropical Neurology* (eds L. van Bogaert, J.P. Käfer and G.F. Poch), Lopez Libreros Editores, Buenos Aires.

Chomarat, M., Fredenucci, I., Barbe, G., Boucaud-Maitre, Y., Boyer, M., Carricajo, A., Celard, M., Clergeau, P., Croize, J., Delubac, F., Fevre, D., Fuhrmann, C., Gilles, Y., Gravagna, B., Helfre, M., Letouzey, M.N., Lelievre, H., Mandjee, A., Marchal, M.F., Marthelet, P., Meley, R., Perrier-Gros-Claude, J.D., Bercion, R., Reverdy, M.E., Ros,

A., Roure, C., Sabot, O., Smati, S., Thierry, J., Tixier, A., Tous, J., Verger, P. and Zaoui, E. (2002) Observatoire Rhône-Alpes du pneumocoque en 1999: 35 cas de meningitis. *Pathologie Biologie*, **50**, 595–8.

Chonmaitree, T., Owen, M.J., Patel, J.A., Hedgpeth, D., Horlick, D. and Howie, V.M. (1992a) Presence of cytomegalovirus and herpes simplex virus in middle ear fluids from children with acute otitis media. *Clinical Infectious Diseases*, **15**, 650–3.

Chonmaitree, T., Owen, M.J., Patel, J.A., Hedgpeth, D., Horlick, D. and Howie, V.M. (1992b) Effect of viral respiratory tract infection on outcome of acute otitis media. *Journal of Paediatrics*, **120**, 856–62.

Chotmongkol, V., Yimtae, K. and Intapan, P.M. (2004) Angiostrongylus eosinophilic meningitis associated with sensorineural hearing loss. *Journal of Laryngology and Otology*, **118**, 57–8.

Christensen, L.A., Morehouse, C.R., Powell, T.W., Alchediak, T. and Silio, M. (1998) Antiviral therapy in a child with pediatric human immunodeficiency virus (HIV): case study of audiologic findings. *Journal of American Audiology*, **9**, 292–8.

Christenson, B. and Bottiger, M. (1994) Long-term follow-up study of rubella antibodies in naturally immune and vaccinated young adults. *Vaccine*, **12**, 41–5.

Chukuezi, A. (1995) Hearing loss: a possible consequence of malaria. *African Health*, **17**, 18–9.

Ciana, G., Parmar, N., Antonio, C., Pivetta, S., Tamburlini, G. and Cuttani, M. (1995) Effectiveness of adjuvant treatment with steroids in reducing short term mortality in a high risk population of children with bacterial meningitis. *Journal of Tropical Pediatrics*, **41**, 164–7.

Çiftçi, E., Erden, İ. and Akyar, S. (1998) Brucellosis of the pituitary region: MRI. *Neuroradiology*, **40**, 383–4.

Clark, G. (2003) Cochlear implants in children: safety as well as speech and language. *International Journal of Pediatric Otorhinolaryngology*, **67**(Suppl. 1), S7–20.

Clarke, C.E., Ray, P.S. and Abdelhadi, H.A. (1999) An adolescent Pakistani girl with chronic meningitis. *Postgraduate Medical Journal*, **75**, 47–9.

Clarkson, M.G. and Clifton, R.K. (1985) Infant pitch perception: evidence for responding to pitch categories and the missing fundamental. *Journal of the Acoustic Society of America*, **77**, 1521–8.

Cobbs, C.S., Harkins, L., Samanta, M., Gillespie, G.Y., Bharara, S., King, P.H., Nabors, L.B., Cobbs, C.G. and Britt, W.J. (2002) Human cytomegalovirus infection and expression in human malignant glioma. *Cancer Research*, **62**, 3347–50.

Cohen, J. (2003) Management of bacterial meningitis in adults. *British Medical Journal*, **326**, 996–7.

Cohen, A., Martin, M., Mizanin, J., Konkle, D.F. and Schwartz, E. (1990) Vision and hearing during deferoxamine therapy. *Journal of Pediatrics*, **117**, 326–30.

Collier, A.C., Handsfield, H.H., Ashley, R., Roberts, P.L., De Rouen, T., Meyers, J.D. and Corey, L. (1995) Cervical but not urinary excretion of cytomegalovirus is related to sexual activity and contraceptive practices in sexually active women. *Journal of Infectious Diseases*, **171**, 33–8.

Collinet, P., Subtil, D., Houfflin-Debarge, V., Kacet, N., Dewilde, A. and Puech, F. (2004) Routine CMV screening during pregnancy. *European Journal of Obstetrics and Gynecology Reproductive Biology*, **114**, 3–11.

Comacchio, F., D'Eredità, R. and Marchiori, C. (1996) MRI evidence of labyrinthine and eighth nerve bundle involvement in mumps virus sudden deafness and vertigo. *Otorhinolaryngology*, **58**, 295–7.

Compton, T., Kurt-Jones, E.A., Boehme, K.W., Belko, J., Latz, E., Golenbock, D.T. and Finberg, R.W. (2003) Human cytomegalovirus activates inflammatory cytokine responses via CD14 and Toll-like receptor 2. *Journal of Virology*, **77**, 4588–96.

Cooper, L.Z., Preblud, S.R. and Alford, C.A. (1995) Rubella, in *Infectious Diseases of the Fetus and Newborn Infant* (eds J.S. Remington and J.O. Klein), 4th edn, W.B. Saunders Company, Philadelphia, pp. 268–311.

Cooper, C.B., Gransden, W.R., Webster, M., King, M., O'Mahony, M., Young, S. and Banatvala, J.E. (1982) A case of Lassa fever: experience at St Thomas's Hospital. *British Medical Journal*, **285**, 1003–5.

Cope, A.V., Sabin, C., Burroughs, A., Rolles, K.,Griffiths, P.D. and Emery, V.C. (1997a) Interrelationships among quantity of human cytomegalovirus (HCMV) DNA in blood, donor-recipient serostatus, and administration of methylprednisolone as risk factors for HCMV disease following liver transplantation. *Journal of Infectious Diseases*, **176**, 1484–90.

Cope, A.V., Sweny, P., Rees, L., Griffiths, P.D. and Emery, V.C. (1997b) Quantity of cytomegalovirus viruria is a major risk factor for cytomegalovirus disease after renal transplantation. *Journal of Medical Virology*, **52**, 200–5.

Corbacella, E., Lanzoni, I., Ding, D., Previati, M. and Salvi, R. (2004) Minocycline attenuates gentamicin induced hair cell loss in neonatal cochlear cultures. *Hearing Research*, **197**, 11–8.

Corker, M. (1998) *Deaf and Disabled or Deafness Disabled*, Open University Press, Buckingham.

Corless, C.E., Guiver, M., Borrow, R., Edwards-Jones, V., Fox, A.J. and Kaczmarski, E.B. (2001) Simultaneous detection of *Neisseria meningitidis*, *Haemophilus influenzae*, and *Streptococcus pneumoniae* in suspected cases of meningitis and septicemia using real-time PCR. *Journal of Clinical Microbiology*, **39**, 1553–8.

Cotanche, D.A. (1999) Structural recovery from sound and aminoglycoside damage in the avian cochlea. *Audiology and Neurootology*, **4**, 271–85.

Cox, F.E.G. (ed.) (1996) *The Wellcome Trust Illustrated History of Tropical Diseases*, Wellcome Trust, London.

Cox, D.L., Chang, P., McDowall, A. and Radolf, J.D. (1992) The outer membrane, not a coat of host proteins, limits the antigenicity of virulent *Treponema pallidum*. *Infection and Immunity*, **60**, 1076–83.

Creagh, E.M. and Martin, S.J. (2001) Caspases: cellular demolition experts. *Biochemical Society Transactions*, **29**, 696–701.

Cripps, A.W., Otczyk, D.C. and Kyd, J.M. (2005) Bacterial otitis media: a vaccine preventable disease? *Vaccine*, **23**, 2304–10.

Crowley, B. and Afzal, M.A. (2002) Mumps virus reinfection – clinical findings and serological vagaries. *Communicable Diseases and Public Health*, **5**, 311–3.

Cruickshanks, K., Klein, R., Klein, B., Wiley, T., Nondahl, D. and Tweed, T. (1998a) Cigarette smoking and hearing loss: The Epidemiology of Hearing Loss Study. *Journal of the American Medical Association*, **279**, 1715–9.

Cruickshanks, K., Klein, R., Klein, B., Wiley, T., Nondahl, D., Tweed, T., Mares-Perlman, J.A. and Nondahl, D.M. (1998b) Prevalence of hearing loss in older adults in Beaver,

Dam, Wisconsin: The Epidemiology of Hearing Loss Study. *American Journal of Epidemiology*, **148**, 879–86.

Cummins, D., McCormick, J.B., Bennett, D., Samba, J.A., Farrar, B., Machin, S.J. and Fisher-Hoch, S.P. (1990) Acute sensorineural deafness in Lassa fever. *Journal of the American Medical Association*, **264**, 2093–6.

Dacou-Voutetakis, C., Constantiniidis, M., Moschos, A., Viachou, C. and Matsaniotis, N. (1974) Diabetes mellitus following mumps; insulin reserve. *American Journal of Diseases of Childhood*, **127**, 890–1.

Daengsvang, S. (1968) Further observations on the experimental transmission of *Gnathostoma spinigerum*. *Annals of Tropical Medicine and Parasitology*, **62**, 88–94.

Dagan, R. (2004) The potential effect of widespread use of pneumococcal conjugate vaccines on the practice of pediatric otolaryngology: the case of acute otitis media. *Current Opinion in Otolaryngology and Head and Neck Surgery*, **12**, 488–94.

Dahle, A.J., McCollister, F.P., Stagno, S., Reynolds, D.W. and Hoffman, H.E. (1979) Progressive hearing impairment in children with congenital cytomegalovirus infection. *Journal of Speech and Hearing Disorders*, **44**, 220–9.

Dahle, A.F., Fowler, K.B., Wright, J.D., Boppana, S.B., Britt, W.J. and Pass, R.F. (2000) Longitudinal investigation of hearing disorders in children with congenital cytomegalovirus. *Journal of the American Academy of Audiology*, **11**, 283–90.

Dallos, P. and Fakler, B. (2002) Prestin, a new type of motor protein. *Nature Reviews. Molecular Cell Biology*, **3**, 104–11.

Dalton, D., Cruickshanks, K., Klein, R., Klein, B. and Wiley, T. (1998) Association of NIDDM and hearing loss. *Diabetes Care*, **21**, 1540–4.

Daly, J.F. and Cohen, N.L. (1965) Viomycin ototoxicity in man: a cupulometric study. *Annals of Otology, Rhinology and Laryngology*, **74**, 521–34.

Danielssen, D.C. and Boeck, C.W. (1847) Om Spedalskhed. Udginet efter Foraustaltning af den Kongelige Norske Regjenings Department fer det Indre. C. Gröndaw, Christiania (now called Bergen).

Darmstadt, G.L. and Harris, J.P. (1989) Luetic hearing loss: clinic presentation, diagnosis and treatment. *American Journal of Otolaryngology*, **10**, 410–21.

Darrow, D.H., Dash, N. and Derkay, C.S. (2003) Otitis media: concepts and controversies. *Current Opinion in Otolaryngology and Head and Neck Surgery*, **11**, 416–23.

Das, V.K. (1996) Aetiology of bilateral sensorineural hearing impairment in children: a 10 year study. *Archives of Disease in Childhood*, **74**, 8–12.

Davey, P.G., Jabeen, F.J., Harpur, E.S., Shenoi, P.M. and Geddes, A.M. (1983) A controlled study of the reliability of pure tone audiometry for the detection of gentamicin auditory toxicity. *Journal of Laryngology and Otology*, **97**, 27–36.

Davidson, J., Hyde, M.L. and Alberti, P.W. (1988) Epidemiology of hearing impairment in childhood. *Scandinavian Audiology Supplementum*, **30**, 13–20.

Davidson, J., Hyde, M.L. and Alberti, P.W. (1989) Epidemiologic patterns in childhood hearing loss: a review. *International Journal of Pediatric Otorhinolaryngology*, **17**, 239–66.

Davis, A.C. (1989) The prevalence of hearing impairment and reported hearing disability among adults in Great Britain. *International Journal of Epidemiology*, **18**, 911–7.

Davis, L.E. (1990) Comparative experimental viral labyrinthitis. *American Journal of Otolaryngology*, **11**, 382–8.

Davis, A. (1994) Hearing in adults. The prevalence and distribution of hearing impairment and reported hearing disability, in *The MRC Institute of Hearing Research's National Study of Hearing*, London.

Davis, L.E. and Greenlee, J.E. (2003) Pneumococcal meningitis: antibiotics essential but insufficient. *Brain*, **126**, 1013–4.

Davis, G.L. and Hawrisiak, M.M. (1977) Experimental cytomegalovirus infection and the developing mouse inner ear: *in vivo* and *in vitro* studies. *Laboratory Investigation*, **37**, 20–9.

Davis, L.E. and Johnson, R.T. (1976) Experimental viral infections of the inner ear: I. Acute infections of the newborn hamster labyrinth. *Laboratory Investigation*, **34**, 349–56.

Davis, L.E. and Johnsson, L.G. (1983) Viral infections of the inner ear: clinical, virologic and pathologic studies in humans and animals. *American Journal of Otolaryngology*, **4**, 347–62.

Davis, L.E., Shurin, S. and Johnson, R.T. (1975) Experimental viral labyrinthitis. *Nature*, **254**, 329–31.

Davis, G.L., Spector, G.J., Strauss, M. and Middlekamp, J.N. (1977) Cytomegalovirus endolabyrinthitis. *Archives of Pathology and Laboratory Medicine*, **101**, 118–21.

Davis, L.E., Rarey, K.E., Stewart, J.A. and McLaren, L.C. (1987) Recovery and probable persistence of cytomegalovirus in human inner ear fluid without cochlear damage. *Annals of Otology, Rhinology and Laryngology*, **96**, 380–3.

Davis, A., Bamford, J., Wilson, I., Ramkalawan, T., Forshaw, M. and Wright, S. (1997) A critical review of the role of neonatal hearing screening in the detection of congenital hearing impairment. *Health Technology Assessment*, **1**, 1–76.

Davison, S.P. and Marion, M.S. (1998) Sensorineural hearing loss caused by NSAID-induced aseptic meningitis. *Ear, Nose and Throat Journal*, **77**, 824–6.

Dawson, K.G., Emerson, J.C. and Burns, J.L. (1999) Fifteen years of experience with bacterial meningitis. *Pediatric Infectious Disease Journal*, **18**, 816–22.

de Azavedo, J.C.S., McGavin, M., Duncan, C., Low, D.E. and McGeer, A. (2001) Prevalence and mechanisms of macrolide resistance in invasive and noninvasive group B streptococcus isolates from Ontario, Canada. *Antimicrobial Agents and Chemotherapy*, **45**, 3504–8.

Deben, K., Janssens de Varebeke, S., Cox, T. and Van de Heyning, P. (2003) Epidemiology of hearing impairment at three Flemish institutes for deaf and speech defective children. *International Journal of Pediatric Otorhinolaryngology*, **67**, 969–75.

de Gans, J. and van de Beek, D. (2002) Dexamethasone in adults with bacterial meningitis. *New England Journal of Medicine*, **347**, 1549–56.

de Godoy, C.V.F., de Brito, T., Tiriba, A.C. and de Campos, C.M. (1969) Fatal mumps meningoencephalitis: isolation of virus from human brain. *Reviews of the Institute of Tropical Medicine, Sao Paulo*, **11**, 436–41.

del Castillo, F., Garcia-Perea, A. and Baquero-Artigao, F. (1996) Bacteriology of acute otitis media in Spain: a prospective study based on tympanocentesis. *Paediatric Infectious Disease Journal*, **15**, 541–3.

de Mouy, D., Cavallo, J.-D., Leclercq, R., Fabre, R. and The Aforcopi-Bio Network (2001) Antibiotic susceptibility and mechanisms of erythromycin resistance in clinical isolates of *Streptococcus agalactiae*: French multicenter study. *Antimicrobial Agents and Chemotherapy*, **45**, 2400–2.

Deng, G.-M., Liu, Z.-Q. and Tarkowski, A. (2001) Intracisternally localized bacterial DNA containing CpG motifs induces meningitis. *Journal of Immunology*, **167**, 4616–26.

Department of Health (1996) *Immunisation against Infectious Diseases*, HMSO, London.

Dereköy, F.S. (2000) Etiology of deafness in Afyon school for the deaf in Turkey. *International Journal of Paediatric Otorhinolaryngology*, **55**, 125–31.

DeStefano, F. and Thompson, W.W. (2004) MMR vaccine and autism: an update of the scientific evidence. *Expert Review of Vaccines*, **3**, 19–22.

de Vries, P.J., Kerst, J.M. and Kortbeek, L.M. (2001) Migrerende zwellingen uit Azie: gnathostomiasis (Migrating swellings from Asia: gnathostomiasis). *Nederlands Tijdschrift voor Geneeskunde*, **145**, 322–5.

Dias, J.A., Cordeiro, M., Afzal, M.A., Freitas, M.G., Morgado, M.R., Silva, J.L., Nunes, L.M., Lima, M.G. and Avilez, F. (1996) Mumps epidemic in Portugal despite high vaccine coverage – preliminary report. *European Surveillance*, **1**, 25–8.

Dickson, G.R., Shirodaria, P.V., Kanis, J.A., Bnmeton, M.N., Carr, K.E. and Mollan, R.A. (1991) Familial expansile osteolysis; a morphological, histomorphometric and serological study. *Bone* **12**, 331–8.

Dobbins, J.G., Adler, S.P., Pass, R.F., Bale Jr, JF., Grillner, L. and Stewart, J.A. (1993) The risks and benefits of cytomegalovirus transmission in child day care. *American Journal of Public Health*, **94**, 1016–8.

Dodds, A., Tyszkiewicz, E. and Ramsden, R. (1997) Cochlear implantation after bacterial meningitis: the dangers of delay. *Archives of Disease in Childhood*, **76**, 139–40.

Dodge, P.R., Davis, H., Feigin, R.D., Holmes, S.J., Kaplan, S.L., Jubelirer, D.P., Stechenberg, B.W. and Hirsh, S.K. (1984) Prospective evaluation of hearing impairment as a sequela of acute bacterial meningitis. *New England Journal of Medicine*, **311**, 869–74.

Donald, P.R. and Schoeman, J.F. (2004) Tuberculous meningitis. *New England Journal of Medicine*, **351**, 1719–20.

Donley, D.K. (1993) TORCH infections in the newborn. *Seminars in Neurology*, **13**, 106–15.

Donsakul, K., Dejthevaporn, C. and Witoonpanich, R. (2003) *Streptococcus suis* infection: clinical features and diagnostic pitfalls. *Southeast Asian Journal of Tropical Medicine and Public Health*, **34**, 154–8.

Doyle, K.J. (2000) Otologic diagnosis and treatment after newborn hearing screening. *Seminars in Hearing*, **21**, 389–97.

Doyle, W.J. and Alpers, C.M. (2003) Prevalence of otitis media caused by viral upper respiratory tract infection vaccines, antivirals and other approaches. *Current Allergy and Asthma Reports*, **3**(4), 326–34.

Drew, W.L. and Mintz, L. (1984) Cytomegalovirus infection in healthy and immune-deficient homosexual men, in *The Acquired Immune Deficiency Syndrome and Infections of Homosexual Men* (eds P. Ma and D. Armstrong), Yorke Medical Books, New York, pp. 117–23.

Drew, W.L., Sweet, E.S., Minor, R.C. and Mocarski, E.S. (1984) Multiple infections by cytomegalovirus in patients with acquired immune deficiency syndrome: documentation by Southern blot hybridization. *Journal of Infectious Diseases*, **150**, 952–3.

Drummond, A. (1968) Deafness in Malawi: case finding survey. Unpublished Report to the Commonwealth Foundation and the Commonwealth Society for the Deaf.

D'Souza, R.M. and D'Souza, R. (2002) Vitamin A for treating measles in children. *Cochrane Database Systematic Reviews*, **22**, CD001479.

Dudgeon, J.A., Peckham, C.S., Marshall, W.C. and Smithells, R.W. (1973) National Congenital Rubella Surveillance Programme. *Health Trends*, **5**, 75–9.

Dummer, J.S. (1990) Cytomegalovirus infection after liver transplantation: clinical manifestations and strategies for prevention. *Reviews of Infectious Diseases*, **12**(S), 767–75.

Dung, T.T. (2003) The Preliminary Results of Survey 'Ear and Hearing Disorders in Vietnam', Informal Consultation on Epidemiology of Deafness and Hearing Impairment in Developing Countries and Update of the WHO Protocol, World Health Organization, Geneva, March 2003.

Dung, T.T., Cio, P.T. and Thuy, N.B. (2003) Nguyen bich thuy. Preliminary result of survey 'Ear and Hearing Disorder' in Vietnam, in *Informal Consultation on Epidemiology of Deafness and Hearing Impairment in Developing Countries and Update of the WHO Protocol*, World Health Organization, Geneva, March 2003.

Dunn, D., Wallon, M., Peyron, F., Pedersen, E., Peckham, C. and Gilbert, R. (1999) Mother to child transmission of toxoplasmosis: risk estimates for clinical counselling. *Lancet*, **353**, 1829–33.

Dunne, A.A., Wiegand, A., Prinz, H., Slenczka, W. and Werner, J.A. (2004) *Chlamydia pneumoniae* IgA seropositivity and sudden sensorineural hearing loss. *Otolaryngologia Polska*, **58**, 427–8.

Durand, M.L., Calderwood, S.B., Weber, D.J., Miller, S.I., Southwick, F.S., Caviness Jr, V.S. and Swartz, M.N. (1993) Bacterial meningitis in adults – a review of 493 episodes. *New England Journal of Medicine*, **328**, 21–8.

Dussaix, E., Lebon, P., Ponsot, G., Huault, G. and Tardieu, M. (1985) Intrathecal synthesis of different alpha-interferons in patients with various neurological diseases. *Acta Neurologica Scandinavica*, **71**, 504–9.

Dwivedi, G.S. and Mehra, Y.N. (1978) Ototoxicity of chloroquine phosphate. A case report. *Journal of Laryngology and Otology*, **92**, 701–3.

Dworsky, M., Yow, M., Stagno, S., Pass, R.F. and Alford, C. (1983) Cytomegalovirus infection of breast milk and transmission in infancy. *Pediatrics*, **72**, 295–9.

Dylewski, J.S. and Bekhor, S. (2004) Mollaret's meningitis caused by herpes simplex virus type 2: case report and literature review. *European Journal of Clinical Microbiology and Infectious Diseases*, **23**, 560–2.

Eckel, H.E., Richling, F., Streppel, M., Roth, B., Walger, M. and Zorowka, P. (1998) Ätiologie mittel- und hochgradiger Schwerhörig-keiten im Kindersalter. *Phonatrie und Pädaudiologie*, **46**, 252–63.

Edwards, M.S. and Baker, C.J. (2002) Bacterial infections in the neonate, in *Principles and Practice of Pediatric Infectious Diseases* (eds S.S. Long, L.K. Pickering and C.G. Prober), 2nd edn, Churchill Livingstone, Edinburgh.

Eichenwald, H.F. (1960) A study of congenital toxoplasmosis with particular emphasis on clinical manifestations and sequelae and therapy, in *Human Toxoplasmosis* (ed. J.C. Siim), Munksgaard, Copenhagen, pp. 41–58.

Eisenhut, M., Meehan, T. and Batchelor, L. (2003) Cerebrospinal fluid glucose levels and sensorineural hearing loss in bacterial meningitis. *Infection*, **31**, 247–50.

El-Hakim, H., Levasseur, J., Papsin, B.C., Mount, R.J., Stevens, D. and Harrison, R.V. (2001a) Assessment of vocabulary development in children after cochlear implantation. *Archives of Otolaryngology – Head and Neck Surgery*, **127**, 1053–9.

El-Hakim, H., Papsin, B., Mount, R.J., Levasseur, J., Panesar, J., Stevens, D. and Harrison, R.V. (2001b) Vocabulary acquisition rate after pediatric cochlear implantation and the impact of age at implantation. *International Journal of Paediatric Otorhinolaryngology*, **59**, 187–94.

Elliman, D.A. and Bedford, H.E. (2001) MMR vaccine: worries are not justified. *Archives of Disease in Childhood*, **85**, 271–4.

Ellis, R.W. and Sobanski, M.A. (2000) Diagnostic particle agglutination using ultrasound: a new technology to rejuvenate old microbiological methods. *Journal of Medical Microbiology*, **49**, 853–9.

Emery, V.C. (1999) Viral dynamics during active cytomegalovirus infection and pathology. *Intervirology*, **42**, 405–11.

Emery, V.C., Sabin, C.A., Cope, A.V., Gor, D., Hassan-Walker, A.F. and Griffiths, P.D. (2000) Application of viral-load kinetics to identify patients who develop cytomegalovirus disease after transplantation (comment). *Lancet*, **355**, 2032–6.

Emond, R.T.D., Bannister, B., Lloyd, G., Southee, T.J. and Bowen, E.T.D. (1982) A case of Lassa fever: clinical and virological findings. *British Medical Journal*, **285**, 1001–2.

Enders, G., Miller, E., Nickerl-Pacher, U. and Cradock-Watson, J.E. (1988) Outcome of confirmed periconceptional maternal rubella. *Lancet*, **1**(i), 1445–7.

Epstein, S.E., Zhou, Y.F. and Zhu, J. (1999) Infection and atherosclerosis: emerging mechanistic paradigms. *Circulation*, **100**, e20–8.

Epstein, S.E., Speir, E., Zhou, Y.F., Guetta, E., Leon, M. and Finkel, T. (1996). The role of infection in restenosis and atherosclerosis: focus on cytomegalovirus. *Lancet*, **348**(Suppl. 1), s13–17.

Escajadillo, J.R., Alatorre, G. and Zarate, A. (1982) Typhoid fever and cochleovestibular lesions. *Annals of Otology, Rhinology and Laryngology*, **91**, 220–4.

Eshragi, A.A., Telischi, F.F., Hodges, A.V., Odabasi, O. and Balkany, T.J. (2004) Changes in programming over time in postmeningitis cochlear implant users. *Otolaryngology – Head and Neck Surgery*, **131**, 885–9.

Eskola, J., Kilpi, T., Palmu, A., Jokinen, J., Haapakoski, J., Herva, E., Takala, A., Kayhty, H., Karma, P., Kohberger, R., Siber, G., Makela, H., for the Finnish Otitis Media Study Group (2001) Efficacy of a pneumococcal conjugate vaccine against acute otitis media. *New England Journal of Medicine*, **344**, 403–9.

Esterly, J.R. and Oppenheimer, E.H. (1969) Pathological lesions due to congenital rubella. *Archives of Pathology*, **87**, 380–8.

Evans, H.E. and Frenkel, L.D. (1994) Congenital syphilis. *Clinics in Perinatology*, **21**, 149–62.

Evans, P.C., Coleman, N., Wreggitt, T.G., Wight, D.J.G. and Alexander, G.J. (1999) Cytomegalovirus infection of bile duct epithelial cells, hepatic artery and portal venous endothelium in relation to chronic rejection of liver grafts. *Journal of Hepatology*, **31**, 913–20.

Everberg, G. (1957) Deafness following mumps. *Acta Otolaryngologica (Stockholm)*, **48**, 397–403.

Everberg, G. (1960) Etiology of unilateral total deafness. *Annals of Otology Rhinology and Laryngology*, **69**, 711–30.

Everett, J.P., Hershberger, R.E., Norman, D.J., Chou, S., Ratkovec, R.M., Cobanoglu, A., Oh, G.T. and Hosenpud, J.D. (1992) Prolonged cytomegalovirus infection with viremia is associated with development of cardiac allograft vasculopathy. *Journal of Heart and Lung Transplantation*, **11**, 5133–7.

Fabiyi, A. (1976) Lassa fever (arenaviruses) as a public health problem. *Bulletin of the Pan American Health Organization*, **10**, 335–7.

Falser, N. (1981) Experimental infection of the guinea pig inner ear with *Toxoplasma gondii. Archives of Otorhinolaryngology*, **233**, 219–25.

Fausti, S.A., Rappaport, B.Z., Schechter, M.A., Frey, R.H., War, T.T. and Brummett, R.E. (1984) Detection of aminoglycoside ototoxicity by high frequency auditory evaluation: selected case studies. *American Journal of Otolaryngology*, **5**, 177–82.

FDA (2003) Public Health Web Notification: risk of bacterial meningitis in children with cochlear implants (Updated: 25 September 2003), published online www.fda.gov/cdrh/safety/cochlear.pdf.

Feinmesser, R., Weissel, M.J., Levi, H. and Weiss, S. (1980) Bullous myringitis: its relation to sensorineural hearing loss. *Journal of Laryngology and Otology*, **94**, 643–7.

Feldstein, J.D., Johnson, F.R., Kallick, C.A. and Doola, A. (1974) Acute hemorrhagic pancreatitis and pseudocyst due to mumps. *Annals of Surgery*, **180**, 85–8.

Fenoll, A., Jado, I., Vicioso, D., Perez, A. and Casal, J. (1998) Evolution of *Streptococcus pneumoniae* serotypes and antibiotic resistance in Spain: update (1990 to 1996). *Journal of Clinical Microbiology*, **36**, 3447–54.

Fergie, N., Bayston, R., Pearson, J.P. and Birchall, J.P. (2004) Is otitis media with effusion a biofilm infection? *Clinics in Otolaryngology*, **29**, 38–46.

Fernando, R.L., Fernando, S.S.E. and Leong, A.S.-Y. (2001) *Tropical Infectious Diseases: Epidemiology, Investigation, Diagnosis and Management*, Greenwich Medical Media, London.

Finlay, F.O., Witherow, H. and Rudd, P.T. (1995) Latex agglutination testing in bacterial meningitis. *Archives of Disease in Childhood*, **73**, 160–1.

Fireman, B., Black, S.B., Shinefield, H.R., Lee, J., Lewis, E. and Ray, P. (2003) Impact of the pneumococcal conjugate vaccine on otitis media. *Paediatric Infectious Disease Journal*, **22**, 10–6.

Fischler, B., Rodensjo, P., Nemeth, A., Forsgren, M. and Lewensohn-Fuchs, I. (1999) Cytomegalovirus DNA detection on Guthrie cards in patients with neonatal cholestasis. *Archives of Diseases of Childhood: Fetal and Neonatal Edition*, **80**, F130–4.

Fish, K.N., Britt, W. and Nelson, J.A. (1996) A novel mechanism for persistence of human cytomegalovirus in macrophages. *Journal of Virology*, **70**, 1855–62.

Fish, K.N., Stenglein, S.G., Ibanez, C. and Nelson, J.A. (1995) Cytomegalovirus persistence in macrophages and endothelial cells. *Scandinavian Journal of Infectious Diseases* (Suppl. 99), 34–40.

Fish, K.N., Soderberg-Naucler, C., Mills, L.K., Stenglein, S. and Nelson, A. (1998) Human cytomegalovirus persistently infects aortic endothelial cells. *Journal of Virology*, **72**, 5661–8.

Fisher-Hoch, S.P., Tomori, O., Nasidi, A., Perez-Oronoz, G.I., Fakile, Y., Hutwagner, L. and McCormick, J.B. (1995) Review of cases of nosocomial Lassa fever in Nigeria: the high price of poor medical practice. *British Medical Journal*, **311**, 857–9.

Fisher-Hoch, S.P., Hutwagner, L., Brown, B. and McCormick, J.B. (2000) Effective vaccine for lassa fever. *Journal of Virology*, **74**, 677–83.

Fiumara, N.J. and Lessell, S. (1970) Manifestations of late congenital syphilis. Analysis of 271 patients. *Archives Dermatology*, **102**, 78–83.

Fleischer, B. and Kreth, H.W. (1982) Mumps virus replication in human lymphoid cell lines and in peripheral blood lymphocytes: preference for T cells. *Infection and Immunity*, **35**, 25–31.

Fluegge, K., Supper, S., Siedler, A. and Berner, R. (2004) Antibiotic susceptibility in neonatal invasive isolates of *Streptococcus agalactiae* in a 2-year nationwide surveillance study in Germany. *Antimicrobial Agents and Chemotherapy*, **48**, 4444–6.

Forge, A. (1981) Ultrastructure in the stria vascularis of the guinea pig following intraperitoneal injection of ethacrynic acid. *Acta Otolaryngologica*, **92**, 439–57.

Forge, A. and Brown, A.M. (1982) Ultrastructural and electrophysiological studies of acute ototoxic effects of furosemide. *British Journal of Audiology*, **16**, 109–16.

Forge, A. and Harpur, E.S. (2002) Ototoxicity, in *General and Applied Toxicology* (eds B. Ballantyne, T.C. Marrs and T. Syversen), 2nd edn, Macmillan Reference Ltd, Basingstoke, pp. 775–801.

Forge, A. and Li, L. (2000) Apoptotic death of hair cells in mammalian vestibular sensory epithelia. *Hearing Research*, **139**, 97–115.

Forge, A., Li, L. and Nevill, G. (1988) Hair cell recovery in the vestibular sensory epithelia of mature guinea pigs. *Journal of Comparative Neurology*, **397**, 69–88.

Forge, A. and Schacht, J. (2000) Aminoglycoside antibiotics. *Audiology and Neurootology*, **5**, 3–22.

Forge, A., Wright, A. and Davies, S.J. (1987) Analysis of structural changes in the stria vascularis following chronic gentamicin treatment. *Hearing Research*, **31**, 253–66.

Forge, A., Li, L., Corwin, J.T. and Nevill, G. (1993) Ultrastructural evidence for hair cell regeneration in the mammalian inner ear. *Science*, **259**, 1616–9.

Forrest, J.M., Turnbull, F.M., Sholler, G.F., Hawker, R.E., Martin, F.J., Doran, T.T. and Burgess, M.A. (2002) Gregg's congenital rubella patients 60 years later. *Medical Journal of Australia*, **177**, 664–7.

Fortnum, H.M. (1992) Hearing impairment after bacterial meningitis: a review. *Archives of Diseases of Childhood*, **67**, 1128–53.

Fortnum, H. and Davis, A. (1997) Epidemiology of permanent childhood hearing impairment in Trent Region, 1985–1993. *British Journal of Audiology*, **31**, 409–46.

Fortnum, H., Farnsworth, A. and Davis, A. (1993) The feasibility of evoked otoacoustic emissions as an in-patient hearing check after meningitis. *British Journal of Audiology*, **27**, 227–31.

Foulon, W., Villena, I., Stray-Pedersen, B., Decoster, A., Lappalainen, M., Pinon, M., Jenum, P.A., Hedman, K. and Naessens, A. (1999) Treatment of toxoplasmosis during pregnancy: a multicenter study of impact on fetal transmission and children's sequelae at one year of age. *American Journal of Obstetrics and Gynecology*, **180**, 410–5.

Fowler, K.B., Stagno, S. and Pass, R.F. (1993) Maternal age and congenital cytomegalovirus infection: screening of two diverse newborn populations, 1980–1990. *Journal of Infectious Diseases*, **168**, 552–6.

Fowler, K.B., Stagno, S. *et al.* (1991) Rates of congenital cytomegalovirus infection based on newborn screening in two populations over an eleven year interval. *Pediatric Research*, **29**, 90A.

Fowler, K.B., Stagno, S., Pass, R.F., Britt, W.J., Bole, T.J. and Alford, C.A. (1992) The outcome of congenital cytomegalovirus infection in relation to maternal antibody status. *New England Journal of Medicine*, **326**, 663–7.

Fowler, K.B., Stagno, S. *et al.* (1996) Maternal cytomegalovirus immunity and risk of congenital cytomegalovirus infection in future pregnancies (abstract). *Pediatric Research*, **39**, 171A.

Fowler, K.B., McCollister, F.P., Dahle, A.J., Boppana, S., Britt, W.J. and Pass, R.F. (1997) Progressive and fluctuating sensorineural hearing loss in children with asymptomatic congenital cytomegalovirus infection. *Journal of Pediatrics*, **130**, 624–30.

Fowler, K.B., Dahle, A.J., Boppana, S.B. and Pass, R.F. (1999) Newborn hearing screening: will children with hearing loss caused by congenital cytomegalovirus infection be missed? *Journal of Pediatrics*, **135**, 60–4.

Fowler, M.I., Weller, R.O., Heckels, J.E. and Christodoulides, M. (2004) Different meningitis-causing bacteria induce distinct inflammatory responses on interaction with cells of the human meninges. *Cellular Microbiology*, **6**, 555–67.

Fox, J.C., Kidd, I.M., Griffiths, P.D., Sweny, P. and Emery, V.C. (1995) Longitudinal analysis of cytomegalovirus load in renal transplant recipients using a quantitative polymerase chain reaction: correlation with disease. *Journal of General Virology*, **76**, 309–19.

Fraser, C.M., Norris, S.J., Weinstock, G.M., White, O., Sutton, G.G., Dodson, R., Gwinn, M., Hickey, E.K., Clayton, R., Ketchum, K.A., Sodergren, E., Hardham, J.M., McLeod, M.P., Salzberg, S., Peterson, J., Khalak, H., Richardson, D., Howell, J.K., Chidambaram, M., Utterback, T., McDonald, L., Artiach, P., Bowman, C., Cotton, M.D., Fujii, C., Garland, S., Hatch, B., Horst, K., Roberts, K., Sandusky, M., Weidman, J., Smith, H.O. and Venter, J.C. (1998) Complete genome sequence of *Treponema pallidum*, the syphilis spirochete. *Science*, **281**, 375–88.

Friedmann, I. (1974) *Pathology of the Ear*, Blackwell Scientific Publications, Oxford, pp. 1–607.

Friedmann, I. and Wright, M.I. (1966) Histopathologic changes in the fetal and infantile inner ear caused by rubella. *British Medical Journal*, **504**, 20–3.

Fritsch, M.H. and Sommer, A. (1991) Embryology of the ear, in *Handbook of Congenital and Early Onset Hearing Loss*, Igaku-Shoin, New York, pp. 3–7.

Fritzsch, B., Barald, K.F. and Lomax, M.I. (1998) Ototoxity: of mice and men, in *Early Embryology of the Vertebrate Ear* (eds E.W. Rubel, A.N. Popper and R.R. Fay), Springer-Verlag, New York, pp. 80–145.

Fukuda, S., Keithley, E.M. and Harris, J.P. (1988) Experimental cytomegalovirus infection: viremic spread to the inner ear. *American Journal of Otolaryngology*, **9**, 135–41.

Fukuda, S., Chida, E., Kuroda, T., Kashiwamura, M. and Inuyama, Y. (2001) An anti-mumps IgM antibody level in the serum of idiopathic sudden sensorineural hearing loss. *Auris Nasus Larynx*, **28**(Suppl.), S3–5.

Furuta, S., Ogura, M., Higano, S., Takahashi, S. and Kawase, T. (2000) Reduced size of the cochlear branch of the vestibulocochlear nerve in a child with sensorineural hearing loss. *American Journal of Neuroradiology*, **21**, 328–30.

Fuse, T., Inamura, H., Nakamura, T., Suzuki, T. and Aoyagi, M. (1996) Bilateral hearing loss due to viral infection. *Otorhinolaryngology*, **58**, 175–7.

Gabutti, G., Rota, M.C., Salmaso, S., Bruzzone, B.M., Bella, A. and Crovari, P. (2002) Epidemiology of measles, mumps and rubella in Italy. *Epidemiology and Infection*, **129**, 543–50.

Gagnebin, J. and Maire, R. (2002) Infection screening in sudden and progressive idiopathic sensorineural hearing loss: a retrospective study of 182 cases. *Otolaryngology Neurotology*, **23**, 160–2.

Gallant, J.E., Moore, R.D., Richman, D.D., Keruly, J. and Chaisson, R.C. (1992) Incidence and natural history of cytomegalovirus disease in patients with advanced human immunodeficiency virus disease treated with zidovudine. The Zidovudine Epidemiology Study Group. *Journal of Infectious Diseases*, **166**, 1223–7.

Garcia d'Orta (1563) *Coloquios dos simples, e drogas he cousas medicinais da India*, Joannes, Goa (cited by Norman, 1993).

Garetz, S.L., Altschuler, R.A. and Schacht, J. (1994) Attenuation of gentamicin ototoxicity by glutathione in the guinea pig *in vivo*. *Hearing Research*, **77**, 81–7.

Garetz, S.L. and Schacht, J. (1996) Ototoxicity: of mice and men, in *Handbook of Auditory Research; Clinical Aspects of Hearing* (eds T.R. van de Water, R.R. Fay and A.N. Popper), Vol. VII, Springer, Berlin, pp. 116–54.

Garty, B.Z., Danon, Y.L. and Nitzan, M. (1985) Hearing loss due to mumps. *Archives of Diseases of Childhood*, **63**, 105–6.

Gates, G. and Miyamato, R.T. (2003) Cochlear implants. *New England Journal of Medicine*, **349**, 421–3.

Gehrz, R.C., Marker, S.C., Knorr, S.O., Kalis, J.M., Balfour Jr, H.H. (1977) Specific cell-mediated immune defect in active cytomegalovirus infection of young children and their mothers. *Lancet*, **2**, 844–7.

Gehrz, R.C., Christianson, W.R., Linner, K.M., Conroy, M.M., McCue, S.A. and Balfour Jr, H.H. (1981) Cytomegalovirus-specific humoral and cellular immune responses in human pregnancy. *Journal of Infectious Diseases*, **143**, 391–5.

Gerber, J., Lotz, M., Ebert, S., Kiel, S., Kuhnt, U. and Nau, R. (2005) Melatonin is neuroprotective in experimental *Streptococcus pneumoniae* meningitis. *Journal of Infectious Diseases*, **191**, 783–90.

Gerhardt, K.J. and Abrams, R.M. (2000) Fetal exposures to sound and vibroacoustic stimulation. *Journal of Perinatology*, **20**, S21–30.

Germann, R., Schachtele, M., Nessler, G., Seitz, U. and Kniehl, E. (2003) Cerebral gnathostomiasis as a cause of an extended intracranial bleeding. *Klinische Padiatrie*, **215**, 223–5.

Gerna, G., Zavattoni, M., Baldanti, F., Furione, M., Chezzi, L. and Revello, M.G. (1998) Circulating cytomegalic endothelial cells are associated with high human cytomegalovirus (HCMV) load in AIDS patients with late-stage disseminated HCMV disease. *Journal of Medical Virology*, **55**, 64–74.

Gerna, G., Percivalle, E., Baldanti, F., Sozzani, S., Lanzarini, P., Genini, E., Lilleri, D. and Revello, M.G. (2000) Human cytomegalovirus replicates abortively in polymorphonuclear leukocytes after transfer from infected endothelial cells via transient microfusion events. *Journal of Virology*, **74**, 5629–38.

Gerna, G., Percivalle, E., Sarasini, A. and Revello, M.G. (2002) Human cytomegalovirus and human umbilical vein endothelial cells: restriction of primary isolation to blood samples and susceptibilities of clinical isolates from other sources to adaptation. *Journal of Clinical Microbiology*, **40**, 233–8.

Gilles, H.M. and Kent, J.C. (1976) Lassa fever: retrospective diagnosis of two patients seen in Great Britain in 1971. *British Medical Journal*, **2**, 1173.

Gnann Jr, J.W., Ahlmen, J., Svlander, C., Olding, L., Oldstone, M.B. and Nelson, J.A. (1988) Inflammatory cells in transplantation kidneys are infected by human cytomegalovirus. *American Journal of Pathology*, **132**, 239–48.

Gonczol, E. and Plotkin, S. (1990) Progress in vaccine development for prevention of human cytomegalovirus infection. *Current Topics in Microbiology and Immunology*, **154**, 255–74.

Goodrich, J.M., Boeckh, M. and Bowden, R. (1994) Strategies for the prevention of cytomegalovirus disease after marrow transplantation. *Clinical Infectious Diseases: An Official Publication of the Infectious Diseases Society of America*, **19**, 287–98.

Gor, D., Sabin, C., Prentice, H.G., Vyas, N., Man, S., Griffiths, P.D. and Emery, V.C. (1998) Longitudinal fluctuations in cytomegalovirus load in bone marrow transplant patients: relationship between peak virus load, donor/recipient serostatus, acute GVHD and CMV disease. *Bone Marrow Transplant*, **21**, 597–605.

Government Statistical Service (2004) *NHS Immunisation Statistics, England: 2002–03*, Department of Health.

Gow, J.A., Ostler, H.B. and Schachter, J. (1974) Inclusion conjunctivitis with hearing loss. *Journal of the American Medical Association*, **229**, 519–20.

Gower, D. and McGuirt, W.F. (1983) Intracranial complications of acute and chronic infectious ear disease: a problem still with us. *Laryngoscope*, **93**, 1028–33.

Goycoolea, M.V. (1995) Oval and round window membrane changes in otitis media in the human. *Acta Otolaryngologica (Stockholm)*, **115**, 282–3.

Graber, D., Hebert, J.C., Jaffar-Bandjee, M.C., Alessandri, J.L. and Combes, J.C. (1999) Formes graves de méningites á éosinophiles chez le nourrisson a Mayotte. A propos de 3 observations. (Severe forms of eosinophilic meningitis in infants of Mayotte. Apropos of 3 cases). *Bulletin de la Société de Pathologie Exotique*, **92**, 164–6.

Graham, D.Y., Brown, C.H., Benrey, J. and Butel, J.S. (1974) Thrombocytopenia: a complication of mumps. *Journal of the American Medical Association*, **227**, 1162–4.

Grattan, M.T., Moreno-Cabral, C.E., Starnes, V.A., Oyer, P.E., Stinson, E.B. and Shumway, N.E. (1989) Cytomegalovirus infection is associated with cardiac allograft rejection and atherosclerosis. *Journal of the American Medical Association*, **261**, 3561–6.

Gray, J.A., Moffat, M.A.J. and Sangster, D. (1969) Viral meningitis: a 10 year study. *Scottish Medical Journal*, **14**, 234–42.

Gray, S.J., Sobanski, M.A., Kaczmarski, E.B., Guiver, M., Marsh, W.J., Borrow, R., Barnes, R.A. and Coakley, W.T. (1999) Ultrasound-enhanced latex immunoagglutination and PCR as complementary methods for non-culture-based confirmation of meningococcal disease. *Journal of Clinical Microbiology*, **37**, 1797–801.

Grayeli, A.B., Palmer, P., Tran, B.H.P., Soudant, J., Sterkers, O., Lebon, P. and Ferrary, E. (2000) No evidence of measles virus in stapes samples from patients with otosclerosis. *Journal of Clinical Microbiology*, **38**, 2655–60.

Grazia Revello, M., Baldanti, F., Percivalle, E., Sagrasini, A., De Giuli, L., Genini, E., Lilleri, D., Labo, N. and Gerna, G. (2001) *In vitro* selection of human cytomegalovirus variants unable to transfer virus and virus products from infected cells to polymorphonuclear leukocytes and to grow in endothelial cells. *Journal of General Virology*, **82**, 1429–38.

Greenhough, A., Osbourne, J. and Sutherland, S. (eds) (1991) *Congenital, Perinatal and Neonatal Infections*, Churchill Livingstone, London.

Gregg, N.M. (1941) Congenital cataract following german measles in the mother. *Transactions of the Ophthalmological Society Australia*, **3**, 35–46.

Green, K.M.J., Bhatt, Y.M., Saeed, S.R. and Ramsden, R.T. (2004) Complications following adult cochlear implantation: experience in Manchester. *Journal of Laryngology and Otology*, **118**, 417–20.

Greenwood, B. (1999) Manson Lecture. Meningococcal meningitis in Africa. *Transactions of the Royal Society of Tropical Medicine and Hygiene*, **93**, 341–53.

Gregory, S. (2003) Models of deafness and the implications for families of deaf children; www.deafnessatbirth.org.uk.

Gremillion, D.H. and Crawford, G.E. (1981) Measles pneumonia in young adults. An analysis of 106 cases. *American Journal of Medicine*, **71**, 539–42.

Grenfell, B.T., Bjornstad, O.N. and Kappey, J. (2001) Travelling waves and spatial hierarchies in measles epidemics. *Nature*, **414**, 716–23.

Griffin, D.E. (2001) Measles virus, in *Fields Virology* (eds B.N. Fields, D.M. Knipe and P.M. Howley), Lippincott-Raven Publishers, Philadelphia, pp. 1401–42.

Griffith, B.P., Lucia, H.L. and Hsiung, G.D. (1982) Brain and visceral involvement during congenital cytomegalovirus infection of guinea pigs. *Pediatric Research*, **16**, 455–9.

Griffith, B.P., Lucia, H.L., Bia, F.J. and Hsiung, G.D. (1981) Cytomegalovirus-induced mononucleosis in guinea pigs. *Infection and Immunity*, **32**, 857–63.

Griffith, B.P., McCormick, S.R., Booss, J. and Hsiung, G. (1986) Inbred guinea pig model of intrauterine infection with cytomegalovirus. *American Journal of Pathology*, **122**, 112–9.

Griffiths, P.D. and Baboonian, C. (1984) A prospective study of primary cytomegalovirus infection during pregnancy: final report. *British Journal of Obstetrics and Gynaecology*, **91**, 307–15.

Griffiths, P.D., Stagno, S., Pass, R.F., Smith, R.J. and Alford Jr, C.A. (1982) Infection with cytomegalovirus during pregnancy: specific IgM antibodies as a marker of recent primary infection. *Journal of Infectious Diseases*, **145**, 647–53.

Grimaldi, L.M.E., Luzi, L., Martino, G.V., Furlan, R., Nemni, R., Antonelli, A., Canal, N. and Pozza, G. (1993) Bilateral eighth cranial nerve neuropathy in human immunodeficiency virus infection. *Journal of Neurology*, **240**, 363–6.

Gross, U. and Pelloux, H. (2000) Diagnosis in pregnant woman, in *Congenital Toxoplasmosis* (eds P. Ambroise-Thomas and E. Petersen), Springer-Verlag, France, pp. 121–30.

Gruber J. (1870) *Lehrbuch der Ohlenheilkunde,* Leipzig: Carl Gerold's Sohn, at p. 319. Translated by E. Law and C. Jewell into the English, *A Textbook of Diseases of the Ear.* London: H.K. Lewis, 1893.

Grzimek, N.K., Dreis, D., Schmalz, S. and Reddehase, M.J. (2001) Random, asynchronous, and asymmetric transcriptional activity of enhancer-flanking major immediate–early genes ie1/3 and ie2 during murine cytomegalovirus latency in the lungs. *Journal of Virology*, **75**, 2692–705.

Guerra, B., Lazzorotto, T., Quarta, S., Lanari, M., Bovicelli, L., Nicolosi, A. and Landini, M.P. (2000) Prenatal diagnosis of symptomatic congenital cytomegalovirus infection. *American Journal of Obstetrics and Gynaecology*, **183**, 476–82.

Guiscafre, H., Benitez-Diaz, L., Martinez, M.C. and Munoz, O. (1984) Reversible hearing loss after meningitis. Prospective assessment using auditory evoked responses. *Annals of Otology, Rhinology and Laryngology*, **93**, 229–32.

Gunther, S., Weisner, B., Roth, A., Grewing, T., Asper, M., Drosten, C., Emmerich, P., Petersen, J., Wilczek, M. and Schmitz, H. (2001) Lassa fever encephalopathy: Lassa virus in cerebrospinal fluid but not in serum. *Journal of Infectious Diseases*, **184**, 345–9.

Gut, J.-P., Lablache, C., Behr, S. and Kirn, A. (1995) Symptomatic mumps virus reinfections. *Journal of Medical Virology*, **45**, 17–23.

Guthrie, D. (1945) *A History of Medicine*, Nelson, London.

Hackett, S.J., Carrol, E.D., Guiver, M., Marsh, J., Sills, J.A., Thomson, A.P., Kaczmarski, E.B. and Hart, C.A. (2002a) Improved case confirmation in meningococcal disease with whole blood Taqman PCR. *Archives of Disease in Childhood*, **86**, 449–52.

Hackett, S.J., Guiver, M., Marsh, J., Sills, J.A., Thomson, A.P., Kaczmarski, E.B. and Hart, C.A. (2002b) Meningococcal bacterial DNA load at presentation correlates with disease severity. *Archives of Disease in Childhood*, **86**, 44–6.

Hadi, U., Nuwayhid, N. and Hasbini, A.S. (1996) Chloroquine ototoxicity: an idiosyncratic phenomenon? *Otolaryngology – Head and Neck Surgery*, **114**, 491–3.

Haginoya, K., Osura, T., Kon, K., Yagi, T., Sawaishi, Y., Ishii, K.K., Funato, T., Higano, S., Takahashi, S. and Iinuma, K. (2002) Abnormal white matter lesions with sensorineural hearing loss caused by congenital cytomegalovirus infection: retrospective diagnosis by PCR using Guthrie cards. *Brain and Development*, **24**, 710–4.

Hale, D.C., Blumberg, L. and Frean, J. (2003) Case report: gnathostomiasis in two travelers to Zambia. *American Journal of Tropical Medicine and Hygiene*, **68**, 707–9.

Hall III, J.W. and Penn, T. (2002) Neurodiagnostic paediatric audiology, in *Paediatric Audiological Medicine* (ed. V.E. Newton), Whurr Publishers, London.

Hall, R. and Richard, H. (1987) Hearing loss due to mumps. *Archives of Diseases in Childhood*, **62**, 189–91.

Halsey, N.A. and Smith, M.H.D. (1984) Diphtheria, Chapter 84 in *Tropical and Geographical Medicine* (eds K.S. Warren and A.A.F. Mahmoud), McGraw-Hill, New York.

Halwachs-Baumann, G., Wilders-Truschnig, M., Desoye, G., Hahn, T., Kiesel, L., Klingel, K., Rieger, P., Jahn, G. and Sinzger, C. (1998) Human trophoblast cells are permissive to the complete replicative cycle of human cytomegalovirus. *Journal of Virology*, **72**, 7598–602.

Hamprecht, K., Maschmann, J., Vochem, M., Dietz, K., Speer, C.P. and Jahn, G. (2001) Epidemiology of transmission of cytomegalovirus from mother to preterm infant by breastfeeding. *Lancet*, **357**, 513–8.

Hanshaw, J.B., Scheiner, A.P., Moxley, A.W., Gaev, L., Abel, V. and Scheiner, B. (1976) School failure and deafness after 'silent' congenital cytomegalovirus infection. *New England Journal of Medicine*, **295**, 468–70.

Harada, T., Sando, I. and Myers, E.N. (1979) Temporal bone histopathology in deafness due to cryptococcal meningitis. *Annals of Otology, Rhinology and Laryngology*, **88**, 630–6.

Harada, T., Semba, T., Suzuki, M., Kikuchi, S. and Murofushi, T. (1988) Audiological characteristic of hearing loss following meningitis. *Acta Otolaryngologia*, **456**(Suppl.), 61–7.

Hariri, M. (1990) Sensorineural hearing loss in bullous myringitis. A prospective study of eighteen patients. *Clinical Otolaryngology and Allied Sciences*, **15**, 351–3.

Harkins, L., Volk, A.L., Samanta, M., Mikolaenko, I., Britt, W.J., Bland, K.I. and Cobbs, C.S. (2002) Specific localisation of human cytomegalovirus nucleic acids and proteins in human colorectal cancer. *Lancet*, **360**, 1557–63.

Harris, M. (1992) Early language development in deaf children, in *Language Experience and Early Language Development from Input to Uptake*, Lawrence Erlbaum Associates, Hove.

Harris, J.P., Fan, J.T. and Keithley, E.M. (1990) Immunologic responses in experimental cytomegalovirus labyrinthitis. *American Journal of Otolaryngology*, **11**, 304–8.

Harris, J.P. and Keithley, E.M. (1993) Inner ear inflammation and round window otosclerosis. *American Journal of Otology*, **14**, 109–12.

Harris, J.P. and Ryan, A.F. (1995) Fundamental immune mechanisms of the brain and inner ear. *Otolaryngology – Head and Neck Surgery*, **112**, 639–53.

Harris, S., Ahlfors, K., Ivarsson, S., Lemmark, B. and Svanberg, L. (1984) Congenital cytomegalovirus infection and sensorineural hearing loss. *Ear and Hearing*, **5**, 352–5.

Harris, J.P., Heydt, J., Keithley, E.M. and Chen, M.C. (1997) Immunopathology of the inner ear: an update. *Annals of the New York Academy of Sciences*, **830**, 166–78.

Harrison, R.V., Gordon, K.A. and Mount, R.J. (2005) Is there a critical period for cochlear implantation in congenitally deaf children? Analyses of hearing and speech perception performance after implantation. *Developmental Psychobiology*, **46**, 252–61.

Harrison, C.J., Marks, M.I. and Welch, D.F. (1985) Microbiology of recently treated acute otitis media compared with previously untreated acute otitis media. *Paediatric Infectious Disease Journal*, **20**, 641–6.

Harrison, R.V., Nagasawa, A., Smith, D.W., Stanton, S. and Mount, R.J. (1991) Reorganisation of auditory cortex after neonatal high frequency cochlear hearing loss. *Hearing Research*, **54**, 11–9.

Harrison, C.J., Britt, W.J., Chapman, N.M., Mullican, J. and Tracy, S. (1995) Reduced congenital cytomegalovirus (CMV) infection after maternal immunization with a guinea pig CMV glycoprotein before gestational primary CMV infection in the guinea pig model. *Journal of Infectious Diseases*, **172**, 1212–20.

Harter, C.A. and Benirschke, K. (1976) Fetal syphilis in the first trimester. *American Journal of Obstetrics and Gynaecology*, **124**, 705–11.

Hartmann *Zeitschrift für Ohrenheilkunde*, **8**, 209.

Hartmann, R., Shepherd, R., Heid, S. and Klinke, R. (1997) Response of the primary auditory cortex to electrical stimulation of the auditory nerve in the congenitally deaf white cat. *Hearing Research*, **112**, 115–33.

Hartnick, C.J., Kim, H.Y., Chute, P.M. and Parisier, S.C. (2001) Preventing labyrinthitis ossificans. The role of steroids. *Archives of Otolaryngology – Head and Neck Surgery*, **127**, 180–3.

Hassan-Walker, A.F., Kidd, I.M., Sabin, C., Sweny, P., Griffiths, P.D. and Emery, V.C. (1999) Quantity of human cytomegalovirus (CMV) DNAemia as a risk factor for CMV disease in renal allograft recipients: relationship with donor/recipient CMV serostatus, receipt of augmented methylprednisolone and antithymocyte globulin (ATG). *Journal of Medical Virology*, **58**, 182–7.

Hatcher, J., Smith, A., Mackenzie, I., Thompson, S., Bal, I., Macharia, I., Mugwe, P., Okoto-Olende, C., Oburra, H. and Wanjohi, Z. (1995) A prevalence study of ear problems in school children in Kiambu district, Kenya, May 1992. *International Journal of Pediatric Otorhinolaryngology*, **33**, 197–205.

Haviland, A. (1879) The geographical distribution of disease. *The Sanitary Record*, **10**, 88–9.

Hawkins, R.D. and Lovett, M. (2004) The developmental genetics of auditory hair cells. *Human Molecular Genetics*, **13**(Special Note 2), R289–96.

Health Protection Agency (2004a) Enhanced tuberculosis surveillance: 2002 final and 2003 preliminary results. *Communicable Disease Report Weekly*, **14** (52), published online www.hpa.org.uk/cdr/PDFfiles/2004/cdr5204.pdf.

Health Protection Agency (2004b) HIV and AIDS in the UK quarterly update: data to the end of December 2004. *Communicable Disease Report Weekly*, **14**, 8.

Heath, P.T., Nik Yusoff, N.K. and Baker, C.J. (2003) Neonatal meningitis. *Archives of Disease in Childhood Fetal and Neonatal Edition*, **88**, F173–8.

Heaton, D.C. and Gutteridge, B.H. (1980) Angiostrongyliasis in Australia. *Australian and New Zealand Journal of Medicine*, **10**, 255–6.

Heikkinen, T. and Chonmaitree, T. (2003) Importance of respiratory viruses in acute otitis media. *Clinical Microbiology Reviews*, **16**, 230–41.

Heikkinen, T., Thint, M. and Chonmaitree, T. (1999) Prevalence of various respiratory viruses in the middle ear during acute otitis media. *The New England Journal of Medicine*, **340**, 260–4.

Heikkinen, T., Ruuskanen, O., Waris, M., Ziegler, T., Arola, M. and Halonen, P. (1991) Influenza vaccination in the prevention of acute otitis media in children. *American Journal of Diseases of Childhood*, **145**, 445–8.

Henderson, D. and Hendershot, A. (1991) ASL and the family system. *American Annals of the Deaf*, **136**, 325–9.

Henderson, D., Hu, B., McFadden, S. and Zheng, X. (1999) Evidence of a common pathway in noise-induced hearing loss and carboplatin ototoxicity. *Noise and Health*, **2**, 53–70.

Hengge, U.R., Tannapfel, A., Tyring, S.K., Erbel, R., Arendt, G. and Ruzicka, T. (2003) Lyme borreliosis. *Lancet Infectious Diseases*, **3**, 489–500.

Henley, C.M., Brown, R.D., Penny, J.E., Kupetz, S.A., Hodges, K.B. and Jobe, P.C. (1984) Impairment in cochlear function produced by chloramphenicol and noise. *Neuropharmacology*, **23**, 197–202.

Hennebert, D. (1959) Ototoxicity of quinine in experimental animals. *Archives of Otolaryngology*, **70**, 312–23.

Herndon, R.M., Johnson, R.T., Davis, L.E. and Descalzi, L.R. (1974) Ependymitis in mumps virus meningitis. Electron microscopical studies of cerebrospinal fluid. *Archives of Neurology*, **30**, 475–9.

Hesseling, S.C., Van Blitterswijk, C.A., Lim, D.J., Demaria, T.F., Bakaletz, L.O. and Grote, J.J. (1994) Effect of endotoxin on cultured rat middle ear epithelium, rat meatal epidermis and human keratinocytes. *American Journal of Otology*, **15**, 762–8.

Heyderman, R.S., Lambert, H.P., O'Sullivan, I., Stuart, J.M., Taylor, B.L. and Wall, R.A. (2003) Early management of suspected bacterial meningitis and meningococcal septicaemia in adults. *Journal of Infection*, **46**, 75–7.

Heydon, G.M. (1929) Creeping eruption or larva migrans in North Queensland and a note on the worm *Gnathostoma spinigerum* (Owen). *Medical Journal of Australia*, **1**, 588–91.

Hicks, T., Fowler, K., Richardson, M., Dahle, A., Adams, L. and Pass, R. (1993) Congenital cytomegalovirus infection and neonatal auditory screening. *Journal of Pediatrics*, **123**, 779–82.

Hickson, F.S. (2002) Behavioural tests of hearing, in *Paediatric Audiological Medicine* (ed. V.E. Newton), Whurr, London, pp. 91–112.

Hill, J.A., Polgar, K. and Anderson, D.J. (1995) T-helper 1-type immunity to trophoblast in women with recurrent spontaneous abortion. *Journal of the American Medical Association*, **273**, 1933–6.

Hindley, P. (2000) Child and adolescent psychiatry, in *Mental Health and Deafness* (eds P. Hindley and N. Kitson), Whurr, London, pp. 42–74.

Hirst, R.A., Kadioglu, A., O'Callaghan, C. and Andrew, P.W. (2004) The role of pneumolysin in pneumococcal pneumonia and meningitis. *Clinical and Experimental Immunology*, **138**, 195–201.

Ho, M. (1982) Pathology of cytomegalovirus infection, in *Cytomegalovirus, Biology and Infection: Current Topics in Infectious Disease* (eds W.B. Greenough and T.C. Merigan), Plenum Press, New York, pp. 171–204.

Hoberman, A., Paradise, J.L., Greenberg, D.P., Wald, E.R., Kearney, D.H. and Colborn, D.K. (2005) Penicillin susceptibility of Pneumococcal isolates causing acute otitis media in children. *The Paediatric Infectious Disease Journal*, **24**, 115–20.

Hodgson, A., Smith, T., Gagneux, S., Akumah, I., Adjuik, M., Pluschke, G., Binka, F. and Genton, B. (2001) Survival and sequelae of meningococcal meningitis in Ghana. *International Journal of Epidemiology*, **30**, 1440–6.

Hoffman, R.A. and Cohen, N.L. (1995) Complications of cochlear implant surgery. *Annals of Otology, Rhinology and Laryngology Supplement*, **166**, 420–2.

Hofstetter, P., Ding, D., Powers, N. and Salvi, R.J. (1997) Quantitative relationship of carboplatin dose to magnitude of inner and outer hair cell loss and the reduction in distortion product otoacoustic emission amplitude in chinchillas. *Hearing Research*, **112**, 199–215.

Hogan, H. (2001) *Hearing Rehabilitation for Deafened Adults: A Psychosocial Approach*, Whurr, London.

Holderness, M.R. (1987) Neurological manifestations and toxicities of the antituberculosis drugs. A review. *Medical Toxicology*, **2**, 33–51.

Holding, P.A. and Snow, R.W. (2001) Impact of *Plasmodium falciparum* malaria on performance and learning: review of the evidence. *American Journal of Tropical Medicine and Hygiene*, **64**, 68–75.

Holland, G.N. (1999) Immune recovery uveitis. *Ocular Immunology and Inflammation*, **7**, 215–21.

Home, F. (1765) *An Enquiry into the Nature, Cause, and Cure of the Croup*, Kincaid and Bell, Edinburgh.

Homman-Loudiyi, M., Hultenby, K., Britt, W. and Soderberg-Naucler, C. (2003) Envelopment of human cytomegalovirus occurs by budding into Golgi-derived vacuole compartments positive for gB, Rab 3, trans-golgi network 46, and mannosidase II (erratum appears in *Journal of Virology Archives*, 2003, **77**, 8179). *Journal of Virology*, **77**, 3191–203.

Hosenpud, J.D. (1999) Coronary artery disease after heart transplantation and its relation to cytomegalovirus. *American Heart Journal*, **138**(5 Pt 2), S469–72.

Hotomi, M., Tabata, T., Kakiuchi, H. and Kunimoto, M. (1993) Detection of *Haemophilus influenzae* in middle ear of otitis media with effusion with polymerase chain reaction. *International Journal of Pediatric Otorhinolaryngology*, **27**, 119–26.

Howard, C. (1998) Arenaviruses, Chapter 27 in *Zoonoses: Biology, Clinical Practice, and Public Health Control* (eds S.R. Palmer, Lord Soulsby and D.I.H. Simpson), Open University Press, Oxford.

Hoy, J.F., Marriott, D. and Gottlieb, T. (1996) HIV and non-tuberculous mycobacterial infection. *Medical Journal of Australia*, **164**, 543–5.

Hsiung, G.D., Choi, Y.C. and Bia, F. (1978) Cytomegalovirus infection in guinea pigs. Viremia during acute primary and chronic persistent infection. *Journal of Infectious Diseases*, **138**(2), 191–6.

Huang, E.S. and Pagano, J.S. (1978) Cytomegalovirus DNA and adenocarcinoma of the colon: evidence for latent infection. *Lancet*, **1**, 957–60.

Huang, E.S., Mar, E.C., Boldogh, I. and Basker, J. (1984) The oncogenicity of human cytomegalovirus. *Birth Defects: Original Article Series*, **20**, 193–211.

Hughes, P.A., Magnet, A.D. and Fishbain, J.T. (2003) Eosinophilic meningitis: a case series report and review of the literature. *Military Medicine*, **168**, 817–21.

Hughes III, K.V., Green Jr, J.D., Alvarez, S. and Reimer, R. (1997) Vestibular dysfunction due to cryptococcal meningitis. *Otolaryngology – Head and Neck Surgery*, **116**, 536–40.

Hugosson, S., Carlsson, E., Borg, E., Brorson, L.-O., Langeroth, G. and Olcen, P. (1997) Audiovestibular and neuropsychological outcome of adults who had recovered from childhood bacterial meningitis. *International Paediatric Otorhinolaryngology*, **42**, 149–67.

Hungerbuhler, J.P. and Regli, F. (1978) Cochleovestibular involvement as the first sign of syphilis. *Journal of Neurology*, **219**, 199–204.

Huotilainen, M., Kujala, A., Hotakainen, M., Parkkonen, L., Taulu, S., Simola, J., Nenonen, J. and Karjalainen, R. (2005) Short-term memory functions of the human fetus recorded with magnetoencephalography. *Neuroreport*, **16**, 81–4.

Husain, K., Whitworth, C., Somani, S.M. and Rybak, L.P. (2001) Carboplatin-induced oxidative stress in rat cochlea. *Hearing Research*, **158**, 14–22.

Huynh, B.T. Common ear and hearing problems in Vietnam. *HI Newsletter*, Series No. 47.

Hviid, A. and Melbye, M. (2004) Impact of routine vaccination with a conjugate *Haemophilus influenzae* type b vaccine. *Vaccine*, **22**, 378–82.

Hydén, D. (1996) Mumps labyrinthitis, endolymphatic hydrops and sudden deafness in succession in the same ear. *Otorhinolaryngology*, **58**, 338–42.

Hydén, D., Ödkvist, L.M. and Kylén, P. (1979) Vestibular symptoms in mumps deafness. *Acta Otolaryngologica Supplement*, **360**, 182–3.

Hyson, R.L. and Rudy, J.W. (1987) Ontogenetic change in the analysis of sound frequency in the human rat. *Developmental Psychobiology*, **20**, 189–207.

Ikeda, K., Oshima, T., Hidaka, H. and Takasaka, T. (1997) Molecular and clinical implications of loop diuretic ototoxicity. *Hearing Research*, **107**, 1–8.

Illing, R.-J. (2004) Maturation and plasticity of the central auditory system. *Acta Otolaryngologica Supplement*, **552**, 6–10.

Ingall, D., Sanchez, P.J. and Musher, D.M. (1995) Syphilis, in *Infectious Diseases of the Fetus and Newborn Infant*, 4th edn (eds J.S. Remington and J.O. Klein), WB Saunders, Philadelphia, pp. 529–64.

Ishida, K., Kubota, T., Matsuda, S., Sugaya, H., Manabe, M. and Yoshimura, K. (2003) A human case of gnathostomiasis nipponica confirmed indirectly by finding infective larvae in leftover largemouth bass meat. *Journal of Parasitology*, **89**, 407–9.

Ismail, Y. and Arsura, E.L. (1993) Eosinophilic meningitis. *Western Journal of Medicine*, **159**, 623.

Ito, M., Go, T., Okuno, T. and Mikawa, M. (1991) Chronic mumps virus encephalitis. *Pediatric Neurology*, **7**, 467–70.

Ito, N., Kokubo, Y., Narita, Y., Naito, Y. and Kuzuhara, S. (1996) A case of agamma-globulinemia with chronic enteroviral meningomyelitis. *Rinsho Shinkeigaku*, **36**, 306–11.

Iwata, N.K., Hayashi, T., Numaga, J., Yamamichi, N., Sakurai, M. and Kanazawa, I. (2002) Fits and deafness. *Lancet Neurology*, **1**, 387–8.

Jackler, R.K., Luxford, W.M., Schindler, R.A. and McKerrow, W.S. (1987) Cochlear patency problems in cochlear implantation. *Laryngoscope*, **97**, 801–5.

Jackson, A.D. and Fisch, L. (1958) Deafness following maternal rubella; results of a prospective investigation. *Lancet*, **2**, 1241–4.

Jacobs, M.R., Dagan, R., Appelbaum, P.C. and Burch, D.J. (1998) Prevalence of antimi-crobial-resistant pathogens in middle ear fluid: multinational study of 917 children with acute otitis media. *Antimicrobial Agents and Chemotherapy*, **42**, 589–95.

Jacobson, M.A. and Mills, J. (1988) Serious cytomegalovirus disease in the acquired immunodeficiency syndrome (AIDS). *Annals of Internal Medicine*, **108**, 585–94.

Jacobson, M.A., Stanley, H., Holtzer, C., Margolis, T.P. and Cunningham, E.T. (2000) Natural history and outcome of new AIDS-related cytomegalovirus retinitis diag-nosed in the era of highly active antiretroviral therapy. *Clinical Infectious Diseases*, **30**, 231–3.

Jaffe, B.F. (1970) Sudden deafness – a local manifestation of systemic disorders: fat emboli, hypercoagulation and infections. *Laryngoscope*, **80**, 788–801.

Jahn, G., Stenglein, S., Riegler, S., Einsele, H. and Sinzger, C. (1999) Human cytomegalovirus infection of immature dendritic cells and macrophages. *Intervirology*, **42**, 365–72.

James, A.L. and Papsin, B.C. (2004) Cochlear implant surgery at 12 months of age or younger. *Laryngoscope*, **114**, 2191–5.

Jarupant, W., Sithinamsuwan, P., Udommongkol, C., Reuarrom, K., Nidhinandana, S. and Suwantamee, J. (2004) Spinal cord compression and bilateral sensory neural hearing loss: an unusual manifestation of neurocysticercosis. *Journal of the Medical Association of Thailand*, **87**, 1244–9.

Jarvis, M.A., Wang, C.E., Meyers, H.L., Smith, P.P., Corless, C.L., Henderson, G.J., Viera, J., Britt, W.J. and Nelson, J.A. (1999) Human cytomegalovirus infection of Caco-2 cells occurs at the basolateral membrane and is differentiation state dependent. *Journal of Virology*, **73**, 4552–60.

Jastreboff, P.J., Hansen, R., Sasaki, P.G. and Sasaki, C.T. (1986) Differential uptake of salicylate in serum, cerebrospinal fluid and perilymph. *Archives of Otolaryngology – Head and Neck Surgery*, **112**, 1050–3.

Jeffery, N. and Spoor, F. (2004) Prenatal growth and development of the modern human labyrinth. *Journal of Anatomy*, **204**, 71–92.

Jelinek, T., Ziegler, M. and Loscher, T. (1994) Gnathostomiasis nach Aufenthalt in Thailand (Gnathostomiasis after a stay in Thailand). *Deutsche Medizinische Wochenschrift*, **119**, 1618–22.

Jenner, W. (1849) On typhoid and typhus fevers – an attempt to determine the ques-tion of their identity or non-identity, by an analysis of their symptoms, and the appearances found after death in 66 fatal cases observed at the London Fever Hos-pital from January 1847–February 1849. *Monthly Journal of Medical Sciences*, **9**, 663–80.

Jensema, C. (1975) Children in educational programs for the hearing impaired whose impairment was caused by mumps. *Journal of Speech and Hearing Disorders*, **40**, 164–9.

Jirásek, A., Stárek, M., Dolezalová, B. and Hlava, J. (1981) Experimental encephalitis Induced by various strains of mumps virus. *Acta Neuropathologica (Berlin)*, **1981**(Suppl. VII), 145–6.

Jitendra, P., Bhatia, M.L., Prasad, B.G., Dayal, D. and Jain, P.C. (1974) Deafness among the urban community: an epidemiological survey at Lucknow (UP). *Indian Journal of Medical Research*, **62**, 6.

Johansson, B., Tecle, T. and Örvell, C. (2002) Proposed criteria for classification of new genotypes of mumps virus. *Scandinavian Journal of Infectious Diseases*, **34**, 355–7.

Johnson, R.T. (1968) Mumps virus encephalitis in the hamster. *Journal of Neuropathology and Experimental Neurology*, **27**, 80–95.

Johnson, R.T. (1975) Hydrocephalus and viral infections. *Developmental Medicine and Child Neurology*, **17**, 807–16.

Johnson, R.T. and Johnson, K.P. (1968) Hydrocephalus following viral infection: the pathology of aqueductal stenosis developing after experimental mumps virus infection. *Journal of Neuropathology and Experimental Neurology*, **27**, 591–606.

Johnson, M.H., Hasenstab, M.S., Seicshnaydre, M.A. and Williams, G.H. (1995) CT of postmeningitic deafness: observations and predictive value for cochlear implants in children. *American Journal of Neuroradiology*, **16**, 103–9.

Johnstone, J.A., Ross, C.A.C. and Dunn, M. (1972) Meningitis and encephalitis associated with mumps infection; a 10-year survey. *Archives of Diseases in Childhood*, **47**, 647–51.

Joint Committee on Infant Hearing (1995) Position Statement. *Pediatrics*, **95**, 152–6.

Joint Tuberculosis Committee of the British Thoracic Society (1998) Chemotherapy and management of tuberculosis in the United Kingdom: recommendations 1998. *Thorax*, **53**, 536–48.

Jones, M.E. (1974) Auditory acuity in rural Africans: a selected study. *Central African Journal of Medicine*, **20**, 221–6.

Jones, L., Kyle, J. and Wood, P. (1987) *Words Apart: Losing Your Hearing as an Adult*, Tavistock Publications, London.

Jonjic, S., Pavic, I., Lucin, P., Rukavina, D. and Koszinowski, U.H. (1990) Efficacious control of cytomegalovirus infection after long-term depletion of CD8+ T lymphocytes. *Journal of Virology*, **64**, 5457–64.

Jonjic, S., Pavic, I., Polic, B., Crnkovic, I., Lucia, P. and Kozkinowski, U.H. (1994) Antibodies are not essential for the resolution of primary cytomegalovirus infection but limit dissemination of recurrent virus. *Journal of Experimental Medicine*, **179**, 1713–7.

Jubelt, B. (1984) Enterovirus and mumps virus infections of the nervous system. *Neurology Clinics*, **2**(2), 187–213.

Judd, A., Parry, J., Hickman, M., McDonald, T., Jordan, L., Lewis, K., Contreras, M., Dusheiko, G., Foster, G., Gill, N., Kemp, K., Main, J., Murray-Lyon, I. and Nelson, M. (2003) Evaluation of a modified commercial assay in detecting antibody to hepatitis C virus in oral fluids and dried blood spots. *Journal of Medical Virology*, **71**, 49–55.

Julkunen, I., Koskiniemi, M., Lehtokoski-Lehtiniemi, E., Sainio, K. and Vaheri, A. (1985) Chronic mumps virus encephalitis: mumps antibody levels in cerebrospinal fluid. *Journal of Neuroimmunology*, **8**, 167–75.

Kabakus, N., Sydinoglu, H., Yekeler, H. and Arsalan, I.N. (1999) Fatal mumps nephritis and myocarditis. *Journal of Tropical Medicine*, **45**, 358–60.

Kahl, M., Siegel-Axel, D., Stenglein, S., Jahn, G. and Sinzger, C. (2000) Efficient lytic infection of human arterial endothelial cells by human cytomegalovirus strains. *Journal of Virology*, **74**(16), 7628–35.

Kakar, P.K. (1974) Sensorineural deafness and its prevention, in The Commonwealth Foundation Occasional Paper XXXIV, *Problems of Deafness in the Newer World*, Proceedings of a Seminar convened by the Commonwealth Society for the Deaf at the University of Sussex, 9–20 September 1974, pp. 105–6.

Kaltenbach, J.A., Church, M.W., Blakley, B.W., McClasin, D.L. and Burgio, D.L. (1997) Comparison of five agents in protecting the cochlea against effects of cisplatin in the hamster. *Otolaryngology – Head and Neck Surgery*, **117**, 493–500.

Kanda, T. and Igarashi, M. (1969) Ultra-structural changes in vestibular sensory end organs after viomycin sulfate intoxication. *Acta Otolaryngologica*, **68**, 474–88.

Kanegaye, J.T., Soliemanzadeh, P. and Bradley, J.S. (2001) Lumbar puncture in pediatric bacterial meningitis: defining the time interval for recovery of cerebrospinal fluid pathogens after parenteral antibiotic pretreatment. *Pediatrics*, **108**, 1169–74.

Kang'ombe, C.T., Harries, A.D., Ito, K., Clark, T., Nyirenda, T.E., Aldis, W., Nunn, P.P., Semba, R.D. and Salaniponi, F.M. (2004) Long-term outcome in patients registered with tuberculosis in Zomba, Malawi: mortality at 7 years according to initial HIV status and type of TB. *International Journal of Tuberculosis and Lung Disease*, **8**, 829–36.

Kanra, G., Kara, A., Cengiz, A.B., Isik, P., Ceyhan, M. and Atas, A. (2002) Mumps meningoencephalitis effect on hearing. *Pediatric Infectious Disease Journal*, **21**, 1167–9.

Kanzaki, J. and Nomura, Y. (1986) Incidence and prognosis of acute profound deafness in Japan. *Auris Nasus Larynx (Tokyo)*, **13**, 71–7.

Kaplan, S.L., Catlin, F.I., Weaver, T. and Feigin, R.D. (1984) Onset of hearing loss in children with bacterial meningitis. *Pediatrics*, **73**, 575–8.

Karavellas, M.P., Lowder, C.Y., MacDonald, C., Avila Jr, C.P. and Freeman, W.R. (1998) Immune recovery vitritis associated with inactive cytomegalovirus retinitis: a new syndrome. *Archives of Ophthalmology*, **116**, 169–75.

Karimi, M., Asadi-Pooya, A.A., Khademi, B., Asadi-Pooya, K. and Yarmohammadi, H. (2002) Evaluation of the incidence of sensorineural hearing loss in beta-thalassemia major patients under regular chelation therapy with desferrioxamine. *Acta Haematologica*, **108**, 79–83.

Karlsmose, B., Lauritzen, T. and Parving, A. (1999) Prevalence of hearing impairment and subjective hearing problems in a rural Danish population aged 31–50 years. *British Journal of Audiology*, **33**, 395–402.

Karmody, C.S. (1975) Viral labyrinthitis – an experimental study. *Annals of Otology*, **84**, 179–81.

Kassai, T., Cordero del Campillo, M., Euzeby, J., Gaafar, S., Hiepe, Th. and Himonas, C.A. (1988) Standardized Nomenclature of Animal Parasitic Diseases (SNOAPAD). *Veterinary Parasitology*, **29**, 299–326.

Karima, T.M., Bukhari, S.Z., Fatani, M.I., Yasin, K.A.A., Al-Afif, K.A. and Hafiz, F.H. (2003) Clinical and microbiological spectrum of meningococcal disease in adults during Hajj 2000: an implication of quadrivalent vaccination policy. *Journal of Pakistan Medical Association*, **53**, 3–7.

Kastenbauer, S. and Pfister, H.-W. (2003) Pneumococcal meningitis in adults. Spectrum of complications and prognostic factors in a series of 87 cases. *Brain*, **126**, 1015–25.

Kastenbauer, S., Koedel, U. and Pfister, H.W. (1999) Role of peroxynitrite as a mediator of pathophysiological alterations in experimental pneumococcal meningitis. *Journal of Infectious Diseases*, **180**, 1164–70.

Kastenbauer, S., Klein, M., Koedel, U. and Pfister, H.W. (2001) Reactive nitrogen species contribute to blood–labyrinth barrier disruption in suppurative labyrinthitis complicating experimental pneumococcal meningitis in the rat. *Brain Research*, **904**, 208–17.

Katholm, M., Johnsen, N.J., Siim, C. and Willumsen, L. (1991) Bilateral sudden deafness and acute acquired toxoplasmosis. *The Journal of Laryngology and Otology*, **105**, 115–18.

Kay, R., Cheng, A.F. and Tse, C.Y. (1995) *Streptococcus suis* infection in Hong Kong. *Quarterly Journal of Medicine*, **88**, 39–47.

Kayan, A. and Bellman, H. (1990) Bilateral sensorineural hearing loss due to mumps. *British Journal of Clinical Practice*, **44**, 757–9.

Kearns, D.B., Coker, N.J., Pitcock, J.K. and Jenkins, H.A. (1985) Tuberculous petrous apicitis. *Archives of Otolaryngology – Head and Neck Surgery*, **111**, 406–8.

Keithley, E.M., Chen, M.-C. and Linthicum, F. (1998) Clinical diagnoses associated with histologic findings of fibrotic tissue and new bone in the inner ear. *Laryngoscope*, **108**, 87–91.

Keithley, E.M. and Harris, J.P. (1996) Late sequelae of cochlear infection. *Laryngoscope*, **106**, 341–5.

Kemp, D.T., Ryan, S. and Bray, P. (1990) A guide to the effective use of otoacoustic noise immissions. *Ear and Hearing*, **11**, 93–105.

Kesser, B.W., Hashisaki, G.T., Spindel, J.H., Ruth, R.A. and Scheld, W.M. (1999) Time course of hearing loss in an animal model of pneumococcal meningitis. *Otolaryngology – Head and Neck Surgery*, **120**, 628–37.

Khan, A., Handzel, O., Burgess., B.J., Damian, D., Eddington, D.K. and Nadol Jr, J.B. (2005) Is word recognition correlated with the number of surviving spiral ganglion cells and electrode insertion depth in human subjects with cochlear implants? *Laryngoscope*, **115**, 672–7.

Kieseier, B.C., Paul, R., Koedel, U., Seifert, T., Clements, J.M., Gearing, A.J., Pfister, H.W. and Hartung, H.P. (1999) Differential expression of matrix metalloproteinases in bacterial meningitis. *Brain*, **122**, 1579–87.

Kilham, L. and Overman, J.R. (1953) Natural pathogenicity of mumps virus for suckling hamsters on intracerebral inoculation. *Journal of Immunology*, **70**, 147–51.

Kim, H.N., Kim, S.G., Lee, H.K., Ohrr, H., Moon, S.K., Chi, J., Lee, E.H., Park, K., Park, D.J., Lee, J.H. and Yi, S.W. (2000) Incidence of presbycusis of Korean populations in Seoul, Kyunggi and Kangwon provinces. *Journal of Korean Medical Science*, **15**, 580–4.

Kimberlin, D.W., Lin, C.Y., Sanchez, P.T., Demmler, G.J., Dankner, W., Shelton, M., Jacobs, R.F., Vaudry, W., Pass, R.F. *et al.* (2003) Effect of ganciclovir therapy on hearing in symptomatic congenital cytomegalovirus disease involving the central nervous system: a randomized, controlled trial (comment). *Journal of Pediatrics*, **143**, 16–25.

Kinney, C.E. (1953) Hearing impairments in children. *Laryngoscope*, **63**, 220–6.

Kirk, N.T. (1945) Foreword to Mackie *et al.* 1945, in *A Manual of Tropical Medicine*, 1st edn, W.B. Saunders, Philadelphia.

Kisilevsky, B.S., Hains, S.M., Lee, K., Xie, X., Huang, H., Ye, H.H., Zhang, K. and Wang, X. (2003) Effects of experience on fetal voice recognition. *Psychological Science*, **14**, 220–4.

Kisilevsky, B.S., Hains, S.M.J., Jacquet, A.Y., Granier, A.Y., Granier-Deferre, C. and Lecanuet, J.P. (2004) Maturation of fetal responses to music. *Developmental Science*, **7**, 550–9.

Kittiponghansa, S., Tesana, S. and Ritch, R. (1988) Ocular sparganosis: a cause of subconjunctival tumor and deafness. *Tropical Medicine and Parasitology*, **39**, 247–8.

Klebs, T.A.E. (1883) Ueber Diphtherie. *Verhandlung Congress für inneren Medizin*, **2**, 139–54.

Klein, J.O. (2001) Bacterial sepsis and meningitis, in *Infectious Diseases of the Fetus and Newborn Infant* (eds J.S. Remington and J.O. Klein), W.B. Saunders, Philadelphia.

Klein, C., Kimiagar, I., Pollak, L., Gandelman-Marton, R., Itzhaki, A., Milo, R. and Rabey, J.M. (2002) Neurological features of West Nile virus infection during the 2000 outbreak in a regional hospital in Israel. *Journal of Neurological Sciences*, **200**, 63–6.

Klein, M., Koedel, U., Pfister, H.W. and Kastenbauer, S. (2003a) Morphologic correlates of acute and permanent hearing loss during experimental pneumococcal meningitis. *Brain Pathology*, **13**, 123–32.

Klein, M., Koedel, U., Pfister, H.-W. and Kastenbauer, S. (2003b), Meningitis-associated hearing loss: protection by adjunctive antioxidant therapy. *Annals of Neurology*, **54**, 451–8.

Klemm, E. and Wollina, U. (2004) Otosyphilis: report on six cases. *Journal of the European Academy of Dermatology and Venereology*, **18**, 429–34.

Kneen, R., Solomon, T. and Appleton, R. (2002) The role of lumbar puncture in suspected CNS infection – a disappearing skill? *Archives of Disease in Childhood*, **87**, 181–3.

Knight, P. and Swanick, R. (1999) *Raising and Educating a Deaf Child*, Multilingual Matters, Clevedon.

Knox, E.G. (1985) Theoretical aspects of rubella vaccination strategies. *Reviews of Infectious Diseases*, **7**(Suppl. 1), S194–7.

Kobayashi, H., Mizukoshi, K., Watanabe, Y., Nagasaki, T., Ito, M. and Aso, S. (1991) Otoneurological findings in inner ear syphilis. *Acta Otolaryngologia Supplement*, **481**, 551–5.

Kobayashi, T., Rong, Y., Chiba, T., Marcus, D.C., Ohyama, K. and Takasaka, T. (1997) Ototoxic effect of erythromycin on cochlear potentials in the guinea pig. *Annals of Otology, Rhinology and Laryngology*, **106**, 599–603.

Koedel, U. and Pfister, H.W. (1999) Oxidative stress in bacterial meningitis. *Brain Pathology* **9**, 57–67.

Koga, K., Kawashiro, N., Nakayama, T. and Makino, S. (1988) Immunological study on association between mumps and infantile unilateral deafness. *Acta Otolaryngologica Supplement*, **456**, 55–60.

Komanduri, K.V., Donahoe, S.M., Moorhow, J., Schmidt, D.K., Gillespie, G., Ogg, G.S., Roederer, M., Nizon, D.F. and McCune, J.M. (2001a) Direct measurement of CD4+ and CD8+ T-cell responses to CMV in HIV-1-infected subjects. *Virology*, **279**, 459–70.

Komanduri, K.V., Feinberg, J., Hutchins, R.K., Frame, R.D., Schmidt, D.K., Viswanathan, M.N., Lalozgri, J.P. and McCune, J.M. (2001b) Loss of cytomegalovirus-specific CD4+ T cell responses in human immunodeficiency virus type 1-infected patients with high CD4+ T cell counts and recurrent retinitis. *Journal of Infectious Diseases*, **183**, 1285–9.

Komiya, S. and Tachibana, M. (1990) Target sites of polymyxin B ototoxicity. *European Archives of Otorhinolaryngology*, **247**, 129–30.

Koomen, I., Grobbee, D.E., Roord, J.J., Donders, R., Jennekens-Schinkel, A. and van Furth, A.M. (2003) Hearing loss at school age in survivors of bacterial meningitis: assessment, incidence, and prediction. *Pediatrics*, **112**, 1049–53.

Korman, T.M., Turnidge, J.D. and Grayson, M.L. (1997) Neurological complications of chlamydial infections: case report and review. *Clinical Infectious Diseases*, **25**, 847–51.

Koskinen, P.K., Kallio, E.A., Tikkkanen, J.M., Sihvola, R.K., Hayry, P.J. and Lemstrom, K.B. (1999) Cytomegalovirus infection and cardiac allograft vasculopathy. *Transplant Infectious Disease*, **1**, 115–26.

Koskiniemi, M. (1993) CNS manifestations associated with *Mycoplasma pneumoniae* infections: summary of cases at the University of Helsinki and review. *Clinical Infectious Diseases*, **17**(Suppl. 1), S52–7.

Koskiniemi, M., Donner, M. and Pettay, O. (1983) Clinical appearance and outcome in mumps encephalitis in children. *Acta Pædiatrica Scandinavica*, **72**, 603–9.

Kosugi, I.Y., Shinmura, Y., Li, R.Y., Aiba-Masago, S., Baba, S., Miura, K. and Tsutsui, Y. (1998) Murine cytomegalovirus induces apoptosis in non-infected cells of the developing mouse brain and blocks apoptosis in primary neuronal culture. *Acta Neuropathologica*, **96**, 239–47.

Koszinowski, U.H., del Val, M. and Reddehase, M.J. (1990) Cellular and molecular basis of the protective immune response to cytomegalovirus infection. *Current Topics in Microbiology and Immunology*, **154**, 189–220.

Koszinowski, U.H., Reddehase, M.J. and Jonjic, S. (1991) The role of CD4 and CD8 T cells in viral infections. *Current Opinion in Immunology*, **3**, 471–5.

Kotecha, B. and Richardson, G.P. (1994) Ototoxicity *in vitro*: effects of neomycin, gentamicin, dihydrostreptomycin, amikacin, spectinomycin, neamine, spermine and poly-L-lysine. *Hearing Research*, **73**, 173–84.

Kotikoski, M.J., Kleemola, M. and Palmu, A.A. (2004) No evidence of *Mycoplasma pneumoniae* in acute myringitis. *Pediatric Infectious Diseases Journal*, **23**, 465–6.

Kotnis, R. and Simo, R. (2001) Tuberculous meningitis presenting as sensorineural hearing loss. *Journal of Laryngology and Otology*, **115**, 491–2.

Kövamees, J., Rydbeck, R., Örvell, C. and Norrby, E. (1990) Hemagglutinin-neuraminidase (HN) amino acid alterations in neutralization escape mutants of Kilham mumps virus. *Virology Research*, **17**, 119–30.

Kral, A., Hartmann, R., Tillein, J., Heid, S. and Klinke, R. (2001) Delayed maturation and sensitive periods in the auditory cortex. *Audiology and Neurootology*, **6**, 346–62.

Kremlev, S.G., Roberts, R.L. and Palmer, C. (2004) Differential expression of chemokines and chemokine receptors during microglial activation and inhibition. *Journal of Neuroimmunology*, **149**, 1–9.

Kreth, H.W., Kress, L., Kress, H.G., Ott, H.F. and Eckert, G. (1982) Demonstration of primary cytotoxic T cells in venous blood and cerebrospinal fluid of children with mumps meningitis. *Journal of Immunology*, **128**, 2411–15.

Kubba, H., Pearson, J.P. and Birchall, J.P. (2000) The aetiology of otitis media with effusion. *Clinical Otolaryngology*, **25**, 81–94.

Kujala, T., Alho, K. and Naatanen, R. (2000) Cross-modal reorganisation of human cortical functions. *Trends in Neuroscience*, **23**, 115–20.

Kujawa, S.G., Fallon, M. and Bobbin, R.P. (1992) Intracochlear salicylate reduces low-intensity acoustic and cochlear microphonic distortion products. *Hearing Research*, **64**, 73–80.

Kumar, D., Watson, J.M., Charlett, A., Nicholas, S. and Darbyshire, J.H. (1997) Tuberculosis in England and Wales 1993: results of a national survey. *Thorax*, **52**, 1062–7.

Kupers, T.A., Petrich, J.M., Holloway, A.W. and St Geme Jr, J.W. (1970) Depression of tuberculin delayed hypersensitivity by live attenuated mumps virus. *Journal of Pediatrics*, **76**, 716–21.

Kurtz, J.B., Tomlinson, A.H. and Pearson, J. (1982) Mumps isolated from a fetus. *British Medical Journal*, **284**, 471.

Kuruvilla, K.A., Thomas, N., Jesudasan, M.V. and Jana, A.K. (1999) Neonatal group B streptococcal bacteremia in India: ten year experience. *Acta Paediatrica*, **88**, 1031–2.

Kutz, J.W., Simon, L.M., Chennupati, S.K., Giannoni, C.M. and Manolidis, S. (2003) Clinical predictors of hearing loss in children with bacterial meningitis. Poster 302. Annual Meeting of the American Academy of Otolaryngology – Head and Neck Surgery Foundation, Orlando, Florida, 21 September–24 September 2003. *Otolaryngology – Head and Neck Surgery*, **129**, 221–2.

Kwartler, J.A., Linthicum, F.H., Jahn, A.F. and Hawke, M. (1991) Sudden hearing loss due to AIDS-related cryptococcal meningitis – a temporal bone study. *Otolaryngology – Head and Neck Surgery*, **104**, 265–9.

Lacour, M., Maherzi, M., Vienny, H. and Suter, S. (1993) Thrombocytopenia in a case of neonatal mumps infection: evidence for further clinical presentations. *European Journal of Pediatrics*, **152**, 739–41.

Ladd, P. (2003) *Understanding Deaf Culture – In Search of Deafhood*, Multilingual Matters, Clevedon.

Lamb, R.A. and Kolakofsky, D. (2001) Paramyxoviridae: the viruses and their replication, in *Fields Virology* (ed. D.M. Knipe), 4th edn, Lippincott-Raven Publishers, Philadelphia, pp. 1305–40.

Landini, M.P. and LaPlaca, M. (1991) Humoral immune response to human cytomegalovirus proteins: a brief review. *Comparative Immunology Microbiology and Infectious Diseases*, **14**, 97–105.

Lane, H. (1993) *The Mask of Benevolence*. Random House, New York.

Lang, D.J. and Hanshaw, J.B. (1969) Cytomegalovirus infection and the post-perfusion syndrome: recognition of primary infections in four patients. *New England Journal of Medicine*, **280**, 1145–9.

Lang, D.J. and Kummer, J.F. (1975) Cytomegalovirus in semen: observations in selected populations. *Journal of Infectious Diseases*, **132**, 472–3.

Lapéyssonnie, L. (1963) La méningite cérébro-spinale en Afrique. *Bulletin of the World Health Organisation*, **28**(Suppl.), 314–6.

Lataye, R., Campo, P., Pouyatos, B., Cossec, B., Blachere, V. and Morel, G. (2003) Solvent ototoxicity in the rat and guinea pig. *Neurotoxicology and Teratology*, **25**, 39–50.

Laurell, G. and Bagger-Sjoback, D. (1991) Degeneration of the organ of Corti following intravenous administration of cisplatin. *Acta Otolaryngologica*, **111**, 891–8.

Laurell, G. and Engstrom, B. (1989) The ototoxic effect of cisplatin on guinea-pigs in relation to dosage. *Hearing Research*, **38**, 27–34.

Lautermann, J., McLaren, J. and Schacht, J. (1995) Glutathione protection against gentamicin ototoxicity depends on nutritional status. *Hearing Research*, **86**, 15–24.

Lavine-Rebillard, M. and Pujol, R. (1990) Auditory hair cells in human fetuses: synaptogenesis and ciliogenesis. *Journal of Electron Microscopy Technology*, **15**, 115–22.

Lazzarotto, T., Varini, S., Guerra, B., Nicolosi, A., Lanari, M. and Landini, M.P. (2000) Prenatal indicators of congenital cytomegalovirus infection. *Journal of Pediatrics*, **137**, 90–5.

Leach, C.T. and Jenson, H.B. (2002) Measles, in *Paediatric Infectious Diseases; Principles and Practice*, 2nd edn (ed. H.B. Jenson), W.B. Saunders, Baltimore.

Lee, D.J., Gomez-Marin, O. and Lee, H.M. (1996) Prevalence of childhood hearing loss. The Hispanic Health and Nutrition Examination Survey and the National Health and Nutrition Examination Survey II. *American Journal of Epidemiology*, **144**, 442–9.

Lee, S.J. and Harpur, E.S. (1985) Abolition of the negative endocochlear potential as a consequence of the gentamicin-furosemide interaction. *Hearing Research*, **20**, 37–43.

Lee, D.J., Carlson, D.L., Lee, H.M., Ray, L.A. and Markides, K.S. (1991) Hearing loss and hearing aid use in Hispanic adults: results from the Hispanic Health and Nutrition Examination Survey. *American Journal of Public Health*, **81**, 1471–4.

Lee, D.S., Lee, J.S., Oh, S.H., Kim, S.K., Kim, J.W., Chung, J.K., Lee, M.C. and Kim, C.S. (2001a) Cross-modal plasticity and cochlear implants. *Nature*, **409**, 149–50.

Lee, N.Y., Song, J.-H., Kim, S., Peck, K.R., Ahn, K.-M., Lee, S.-I., Yang, Y., Li, J., Chongthaleong, A., Tiengrim, S., Aswapokee, N., Lin, T.-Y., Wu, J.-L., Chiu, C.-H., Lalitha, M.K., Thomas, K., Cherian, T., Perera, J., Yee, T.T., Jamal, F., Warsa, U.C., Van, P.H., Carlos, C.C., Shibl, A.M., Jacobs, M.R. and Appelbaum, P.C. (2001b) Carriage of antibiotic-resistant pneumococci among Asian children: a multinational surveillance by the Asian Network for Surveillance of Resistant Pathogens (ANSORP). *Clinical Infectious Diseases*, **32**, 1463–9.

Leib, S.L., Heimgartner, C., Bifrare, Y.D., Loeffler, J.M. and Täuber, M.G. (2003) Dexamethasone aggravates hippocampal apoptosis and learning deficiency in pneumococcal meningitis in infant rats. *Pediatric Research*, **54**, 353–7.

Leibovici, L., Sharir, T., Kalter-Leibovici, O., Alpert, G. and Epstein, L.M. (1988) An outbreak of measles among young adults. Clinical and laboratory features in 461 patients. *Journal of Adolescent Health Care*, **9**, 203–7.

Lemos, C., Ramirez, R., Ordobas, M., Guibert., D., Sanz., J., Garcia, L. and Martinez Navarro, J.F. (2004) New features of rubella in Spain: the evidence of an outbreak. *European Surveillance*, **9**, 4.

Lemstrom, K., Koskinen, P., Krogerus, L., Daemen, M., Bruggeman, C. and Hayry, P. (1995) Cytomegalovirus antigen expression, endothelial cell proliferation, and intimal thickening in rat cardiac allografts after cytomegalovirus infection. *Circulation*, **92**, 2594–604.

Lemstrom, K., Sihvola, R., Bruggerman, C., Hayry, P. and Koskinen, P. (1997) Cytomegalovirus infection-enhanced cardiac allograft vasculopathy is abolished by DHPG prophylaxis in the rat. *Circulation*, **95**, 2614–16.

Levenbuck, I.S., Nikolayeva, M.A., Chigirinsky, A.E., Ralf, N.M., Kozlov, V.G., Vardanyan, N.V., Sliopushkina, V.G., Kolomiets, O.L., Rukhamina, M.L. and Grigoryeva, L.V. (1979) On the morphological evaluation of the neurovirulence safety of attenuated mumps virus strains in monkeys. *Journal of Biological Standardisation*, **7**, 9–19.

Levi-Montalcini, R. (1949) Development of the acoustico-vestibular centers in the chick embryo in the absence of the afferent root fibers and of descending fiber tracts. *Journal of Comparative Neurology*, **91**, 209–42.

Levitt, L.P., Kinde, S.W. and Gates, E.H. (1970) Central nervous system mumps: a review of 64 cases. *Neurology*, **20**, 829–34.

Lewallen, S., White, V.A., Whitten, R.O., Gardiner, J., Hoar, B., Lindley, J., Lochhead, J., McCormick, A., Wade, K., Tembo, M., Mwenechanyana, J., Molyneux, M.E. and Taylor, T.E. (2000) Clinical-histopathological correlation of the abnormal retinal vessels in cerebral malaria. *Archives of Ophthalmology*, **118**, 924–8.

Lewensohn-Fuchs, I., Osterwall, P., Forsgren, M. and Malm, G. (2003) Detection of herpes simplex virus DNA in dried blood spots making a retrospective diagnosis possible. *Journal of Clinical Virology*, **27**, 210–16.

Li, C.R., Greenberg, P.D., Gilbert, M.J., Goodrich, J.M. and Riddell, S.R. (1994) Recovery of HLA-restricted cytomegalovirus (CMV specific T-cell responses after allogeneic bone marrow transplant: correlation with CMV disease and effect of ganciclovir prophylaxis. *Blood*, **83**, 1971–9.

Libby, P. (2002) Inflammation in atherosclerosis. *Nature*, **420**, 868–74.

Liljestrand, G. (1962) The prize in physiology and medicine: microbiology and serology, in *Nobel: The Man and His Prizes* (eds H. Schück, R. Sohlman, A. Österling, G. Liljestrand, A. Westgren, M. Siegbahn, A. Schou and N.K. Ståhle), Elsevier, Amsterdam, pp. 184–211.

Lim, D.J. (1984) The development and structure of otoconia, in *Ultrastructural Atlas of the Inner Ear* (eds E. Friedmann and J. Ballantyne), Butterworths, London, pp. 245–9.

Lin, H., Mosmann, T.R., Guilbert, L., Tuntipopipat, S. and Wegmann, T.G. (1993) Synthesis of T helper 2-type cytokines at the maternal–fetal interface. *Journal of Immunology*, **151**, 4562–73.

Lindemann, H.H. (1969) Regional differences in sensitivity of the vestibular sensory epithelia to ototoxic antibiotics. *Acta Otolaryngologica*, **67**, 177–89.

Lindo, J.F., Waugh, C., Hall, J., Cunningham-Myrie, C., Ashley, D., Eberhard, M.L., Sullivan, J.J., Bishop, H.S., Robinson, D.G., Holtz, T. and Robinson, R.D. (2002) Enzootic *Angiostrongylus cantonensis* in rats and snails after an outbreak of human eosinophilic meningitis, Jamaica. *Emerging Infectious Diseases*, **8**, 324–6.

Lindo, J.F., Escoffery, C.T., Reid, B., Codrington, G., Cunningham-Myrie, C. and Eberhard, M.L. (2004) Fatal autochthonous eosinophilic meningitis in a Jamaican child caused by *Angiostrongylus cantonensis. American Journal of Tropical Medicine and Hygiene*, **70**, 425–8.

Lindsay, J.R. (1973) Histopathology of deafness due to postnatal viral disease. *Archives of Otolaryngology*, **98**, 258–64.

Lindsay, J.R., Davey, P.R. and Ward, H. (1960) Inner ear pathology in deafness due to mumps. *Annals of Otolaryngology*, **69**, 918–35.

Lindsay, J. and Harrison, R.S. (1954) The pathology of rubella deafness. *Journal of Laryngology and Otolaryngology*, **68**, 461–4.

Lindsay, J.R. and Hemenway, W.G. (1954) Inner ear pathology due to measles. *Annals of Otology, Rhinology and Laryngology*, **63**, 754–71.

Lindsay, J.R., Caruthers, D.G., Hemenway, W.G. and Harrison, S. (1953) Inner ear pathology following maternal rubella. *Annals of Otololgy, Rhinology and Laryngology*, **62**, 1201–18.

Lingappa, J.R., Al-Rabeah, A.M., Hajjeh, R., Mustafa, T., Fatani, A., Al-Bassam, T., Badukhan, A., Turkistani, A., Makki, S., Al-Hamdan, N., Al-Jeffri, M., Al Mazrou, Y., Perkins, B.A., Popovic, T., Mayer, L.W. and Rosenstein, N.E. (2003) Serogroup W-135 meningococcal disease during the Hajj, 2000. *Emerging Infectious Diseases*, **9**, 665–71.

Linstrom, C.J., Pincus, R.L., Leavitt, E.B. and Urbina, M.C. (1993) Otologic neurotologic manifestations of HIV related disease. *Otolaryngology – Head and Neck Surgery*, **108**, 680–7.

Lippe, W.R. and Rubel, E.W. (1985) Ontology of tonotopic organisation of brain stem auditory nuclei in the chicken: implications for the development of the place principle. *Journal of Comparative Neurology*, **237**, 273–89.

Little, P., Bridges, A., Guragain, R., Friedman, D., Prasad, R. and Weir, N. (1993) Hearing impairment and ear pathology in Nepal. *The Journal of Laryngology and Otology*, **107**, 395–400.

Little, J.P., Gardner, G., Acker, J.D. and Land, M.A. (1995) Otosyphilis in a patient with human immunodeficiency virus: internal auditory canal gumma. *Otolaryngology – Head and Neck Surgery*, **112**, 488–92.

Liu, J., Marcus, D.C. and Kobayashi, T. (1996) Inhibitory effect of erythromycin on ion transport by stria vascularis and vestibular dark cells. *Acta Otolaryngologica*, **116**, 572–5.

Liu, X., Xu, L., Zhang, S. and Xu, Y. (1993) Prevalence and aetiology of profound deafness in the general population of Sichuan, China. *The Journal of Laryngology and Otology*, **107**, 990–3.

Liu, X.Z., Xu, L.R., Hu, Y., Hu, Y., Nance, W.E., Sismani, S.A., Zhang, S.L. and Xu, Y. (2001) Epidemiological studies on hearing impairment with reference to genetic factors in Sichuan, China. *Annals of Otology, Rhinology and Laryngology*, **110**, 356–63.

Lodhi, S., Weiner, N.D., Mechigian, I. and Schacht, J. (1980) Ototoxicity of aminoglycosides correlated with their action on monomolecular films of polyphosphoinositides. *Biochemistry and Pharmacology*, **29**, 597–601.

Logigian, E.L., Kaplan, R.F. and Steere, A.C. (1990) Chronic neurologic manifestations of Lyme disease. *New England Journal of Medicine*, **323**, 1438–44.

Lolov, S.R., Encheva, V.I., Kyurkchiev, S.D., Edrev, G.E. and Kehayov, I.R. (2001) Antimeasles immunoglobulin G in sera of patients with otosclerosis is lower than in healthy people. *Otology and Neurotology*, **22**, 766–70.

Long, G.R., Tubis, A. and Jones, K. (1986) Changes in spontaneous and evoked otoacoustic emissions and corresponding psychoacoustic threshold microstructures induced by aspirin consumption, in *Peripheral Auditory Mechanisms* (eds J.G. Allen, J.L. Hall, A. Hubbard, S.T. Neely and A. Tubis), Springer-Verlag, New York, pp. 213–20.

Lopez, I., Honrubia, V., Lee, S.C., Schoeman, G. and Beykirch, K. (1997) Quantification of the process of hair cell loss and recovery in the chinchilla crista ampullaris after gentamicin treatment. *International Journal of Developmental Neuroscience*, **15**, 447–61.

Lo Re III, V. and Gluckman, S.J. (2003) Eosinophilic meningitis. *American Journal of Medicine*, **114**, 217–23.

Löve, A., Rydbeck, R., Ljungdahl, A., Kristensson, K. and Norrby, E. (1986a) Selection of mutants of mumps virus with altered structure and pathogenicity by passage *in vivo*. *Microbiology and Pathology*, **1**, 149–58.

326 REFERENCES

Löve, A., Rydbeck, R., Utter, G., Örvell, C., Kristensson, K. and Norrby, E. (1986b) Monoclonal antibodies against the fusion protein are protective in necrotizing mumps meningoencephalitis. *Journal of Virology*, **58**, 220–2.

Low, K. (2002) Cryptococcal meningitis: implications for the otologist. *ORL Journal of Oto-Rhino-Laryngology and its Related Specialties*, **64**, 35–7.

Lowell, S.H. and Paparella, M.M. (1977) Presbycusis: what is it? *Laryngoscope*, **87**, 1710–17.

Lulu, A.R., Araj, G.F., Khateeb, M.I., Mustafa, M.Y., Yusuf, A.R. and Fenech, F.F. (1988) Human brucellosis in Kuwait: a prospective study of 400 cases. *Quarterly Journal of Medicine*, **66**, 39–54.

Luterman, D. (1999) Counselling families with a hearing impaired child. *Otolaryngologic Clinics of North America*, **32**, 1037–50.

McAlpine, D. and Johnstone, B.M. (1990) The ototoxic mechanism of cisplatin. *Hearing Research*, **47**, 191–204.

MacArthur, A., Gloyd, S., Perdigao, P., Noya, A., Sacarlal, J. and Kreiss, J. (2001) Characteristics of drug resistance and HIV among tuberculosis patients in Mozambique. *International Journal of Tuberculosis and Lung Disease*, **5**, 894–902.

McBride, P. (1882) *Diseases Which Affect the Ear*, Edinburgh Medical Journal.

McBride, P. (1884) *A Guide to the Study of Ear Disease*, Johnston, Edinburgh.

McCarthy, M., Jubelt, B., Fay, D. and Johnson, R.T. (1980) Comparative studies of five strains of mumps virus *in vitro* and in neonatal hamsters: evaluation of growth, cytopathogenicity and neurovirulence. *Journal of Medical Virology*, **5**, 1–15.

McCracken, G.J., Shinefield, H.R., Cobb, K., Rausen, A.R., Dische, R. and Eichenwald, H.F. (1969) Congenital cytomegalic inclusion disease. A longitudinal study of 20 patients. *American Journal of Disease in Childhood*, **117**, 522–39.

Macdonald, M.R., Harrison, R.V., Wake, M., Bliss, B. and Macdonald, R.E. (1994) Ototoxicity of carboplatin: comparing animal and clinical models at the Hospital for Sick Children. *Journal of Otolaryngology*, **23**, 151–9.

McDougall, A.C. (1996) Leprosy. Chapter 5 in *The Wellcome Trust Illustrated History of Tropical Diseases* (ed. F.E.G. Cox), Wellcome Trust, London, pp. 60–71.

McEllistrem, M.C., Adams, J., Mason, E.O. and Wald, E.R. (2003) Epidemiology of acute otitis media caused by *Streptococcus pneumoniae* before and after licensure of the 7-valent pneumococcal protein conjugate vaccine. *Journal of Infectious Diseases*, **188**(11), 1679–84.

McGee, T., Wolters, C., Stein, L., Kraus, N., Johnson, D., Boyer, K., Mets, M., Roizen, N., Beckman, J., Meier, P., Swisher, C., Holfels, E., Withers, S., Patel, D. and McLeod, R. (1992) Absence of sensorineural hearing loss in treated infants and children with congenital toxoplasmosis. *Otolaryngology – Head and Neck Surgery*, **106**, 75–80.

McGhan, L.J. and Merchant, S.N. (2003) Erythromycin ototoxicity. *Otology and Neurotology*, **24**, 701–2.

McGregor, I.A. (1996) Malaria, Chapter 22 in *The Wellcome Trust Illustrated History of Tropical Diseases* (ed. F.E.G. Cox), Wellcome Trust, London, pp. 230–47.

McIntyre, P.B., Berkey, C.S., King, S.M., Schaad, U.B., Kilipi, T., Kanra, G.Y. and Perez, C.M. (1997) Dexamethasone as adjunctive therapy in bacterial meningitis. A meta-analysis of randomized clinical trials since 1988. *Journal of the American Medical Association*, **278**, 925–31.

McKenna, M.J. (1997) Measles, mumps and sensorineural hearing loss. *Annals of New York Academy of Sciences*, **830**, 291–8.

McKenna, M.J., Kristiansen, A.G. and Haines, J. (1996) Polymerase chain reaction amplification of a measles virus sequence from human temporal bone sections with active otosclerosis. *American Journal of Otology*, **17**, 827–30.

McKenna, M.J. and Mills, B.G. (1990) Ultrastructural and immunochemical evidence for measles virus in active otosclerosis. *Acta Otolaryngologica Supplement*, **470**, 130–40.

Mackenzie, I. (2002) Hearing impairment in Asia: Final Report of Four Country Survey. Unpublished Consultant's Report, World Health Organization, Geneva.

McLaughlin, J.C. (1994) *Medical Embryology*, Addison-Wesley, New York.

McLaughlin, J. (2002) Developmental anatomy of the ear, in *Paediatric Audiological Medicine* (ed. V.E. Newton), Whurr, London, pp. 1–14.

McLean, D.M., Larke, R.P.B., Cobb, C., Griffis, E.D. and Hackett, S.M.R. (1967) Mumps and enteroviral meningitis in Toronto 1966. *Canadian Medical Association Journal*, **96**, 1355–61.

McLeod, R., Boyer, K. and the Toxoplasmosis Study Groups and Collaborators (2000) Management of, and outcome for, the newborn infant with congenital toxoplasmosis, in *Congenital Toxoplasmosis* (eds P. Ambroise-Thomas and E. Petersen), Springer-Verlag, France, pp. 121–30.

McPherson, B.D. and Holborow, C.A. (1988) School screening for hearing loss in developing countries. *Scandinavian Audiology Supplement*, **28**, 103–9.

McPherson, B. and Swart, S.M. (1997) Childhood hearing loss in sub-Saharan Africa: a review and recommendations. *International Journal of Pediatric Otorhinolaryngology*, **40**, 1–18.

McVoy, M.A. and Adler, S.P. (1989) Immunologic evidence for frequent age-related cytomegalovirus reactivation in seropositive immunocompetent individuals. *Journal of Infectious Diseases*, **160**, 1–10.

Madsen, L.W., Svensmark, B., Elvestad, K. and Jensen, H.E. (2001) Otitis interna is a frequent sequela to *Streptococcus suis* meningitis in pigs. *Veterinary Pathology*, **38**, 190–5.

Mafong, D.D., Shin, E.J. and Lalwani, A.K. (2002) Use of laboratory evaluation and radiologic imaging in the diagnostic evaluation of children with sensorineural hearing loss. *The Laryngoscope*, **112**, 1–7.

Maidji, E., Percivalle, E., Gerna, G., Fisher, S. and Pereira, L. (2002) Transmission of human cytomegalovirus from infected uterine microvascular endothelial cells to differentiating/invasive placental cytotrophoblasts. *Virology*, **304**, 53–69.

Maitland, S. (1994) *Home Truths*, Hodder and Stoughton (Sceptre), London.

Mann, I. (1966) *Culture, Race, Climate and Eye Disease: An Introduction to the Study of Geographical Ophthalmology*, Charles C. Thomas, Springfield, Illinois.

Manson, P. (1898) *Tropical Diseases*, Cassell, London.

Marcus, D.C. and Marcus, N.Y. (1989) Transepithelial electrical responses to Cl$^-$ of non-sensory region of gerbil utricle. *Biochimica Biophysica Acta*, **987**, 56–62.

Margolis, G., Kilham, L. and Baringer, J.R. (1974) A new look at mumps encephalitis: inclusion bodies and cytopathic effects. *Journal of Neurology and Experimental Neuropathology*, **53**, 13–28.

Margono, S.S., Idris, K.N. and Brodjonegoro, M.S. (1978) Another case of human gnathostomiasis in Indonesia. *Southeast Asian Journal of Tropical Medicine and Public Health*, **9**, 406–8.

Markowitz, L.E., Tomasi, A., Sirotkin, B.I., Carr, R.W., Davis, R.M., Preblud, S.R. and Orenstein, W.A. (1987) Measles hospitalisations, United States, 1977–1984: comparison with national survey data. *American Journal of Public Health*, **77**, 866–8.

Marschak, A. (1931) Über 50 Fälle von einseitiger Taubheit, davon 7 angeboren. *Journal of Laryngology, Rhinology, Otology*, **21**, 145.

Marschark, M. (1993) *The Psychological Development of Deaf Children*, Oxford University Press, Oxford.

Marschark, M. (1997) *Raising and Educating a Deaf Child*, Oxford University Press, Oxford.

Marschark, M. (2000) Education and development of deaf children – or is it development and education?, in *The Deaf Child in the Family and at School: Essays in Honour of Kathryn P. Meadow-Orlans* (eds P.E. Spencer, C. Eerting and M. Marschark), Oxford University Press, Oxford, pp. 275–92.

Martelius, T., Scholz, M., Krogerus, L., Hockerstedt, K., Loginov, R., Bruggerman, C., Cinati Jr, J., Doerr, H.W. and Lautenschlager, I. (1999) Antiviral and immunomodulatory effects of desferrioxamine in cytomegalovirus-infected rat liver allografts with rejection. *Transplantation*, **68**, 1753–61.

Martin, J.A. (1982) Aetiological factors relating to childhood deafness in the European community. *Audiology*, **21**, 149–58.

Martin, G.K., Lonsbury-Martin, B.L., Probst, R. and Coats, A.C. (1988) Spontaneous otoacoustic emissions in a nonhuman primate. 1. Basic features and relations to other emissions. *Hearing Research*, **33**, 49–68.

Masala, W., Meloni, F., Gallisai, D., Careddu, M., Secchi, G., Cuccuru, G.B., Loriga, V. and Salvo, G. (1988) Can deferoxamine be considered an ototoxic drug? *Scandinavian Audiology Supplement*, **30**, 237–8.

Mata Castro, N., Yebra Bango, M., Tutor de Ureta, P., Villarreal Garcia-Lomas, M. and Garcia Lopez, F. (2000) Hearing loss and human immunodeficiency virus infection. Study of 30 patients (article in Spanish). *Revista Clinica Espanola*, **200**, 271–4.

Mathers, C., Smith, A. and Concha, M. (2005) Global burden of adult-onset hearing loss in the year 2000 (paper in preparation). Accessed on 29 August 2004 at http://www3.who.int/whosis/burden/gbd2000docs/Hearing%20loss.zip.

Mathers, C.D., Vos, T., Lopez, A.D. and Ezzati, M. (2001) *National Burden of Disease Studies: A Practical Guide. Global Program on Evidence for Health Policy*, World Health Organization, Geneva, 2001.

Mathers, C., Stein, C., Maffat, D., Rao, C., Inoue, M., Tomijiina, N., Bernard, C., Lopez, A. and Murray, C. (2002) Global Burden of Disease 2000: Version 2, Methods and Results. Global Programme on Evidence for Health Policy. Discussion paper 50. WHO, Geneva, October 2002. Accessed on 29 August 2004 at http://www3.who.int/whosis/discussion_papers/zip/paper50.zip.

Mathers, C.D., Bernard, C., Moesgaard Iburg, K., Inoue, M., Ma Fat, D., Shibuya, K., Stein, C., Tomijima, N. and Xu, H. (2004) Global Burden of Disease in 2002: data sources, methods and results. Global Programme on Evidence for Health Policy. Discussion paper 54. WHO, Geneva, 2003 (revised 2004). Accessed on 29 August 2004 at http://www3.who.int/whosis/burden/gbd2000docs/Dp54.zip.

Matkin, N.D., Diefendorf, A.O. and Erenberg, A. (1998) Children: HIV/AIDS and hearing loss. *Seminars in Hearing*, **19**, 143–53.

Matshushima, J., Shepherd, R.K., Seldon, L., Xu, S.A. and Clark, G.M. (1991) Electrical stimulation of the auditory nerve in deaf kittens. Effects on cochlear nuclei. *Hearing Research*, **56**, 133–42.

Matz, G.J. (1976) The ototoxic effects of ethacrynic acid in man and animals. *Laryngoscope*, **86**, 1065–86.

Matz, G.J. and Naunton, R.F. (1968) Ototoxicity of chloroquine. *Archives of Otolaryngology*, **88**, 370–2.

Maxon, A.B. and Hochberg, I. (1982) Development of psychoacoustic behaviour: sensitivity and discrimination. *Ear and Hearing*, **3**, 301–8.

Mayatepek, E., Grauer, M., Hansch, G.M. and Sonntag, H.G. (1993) Deafness, complement deficiencies and immunoglobulin status in patients with meningococcal diseases due to uncommon serogroups. *Pediatric Infectious Disease Journal*, **12**, 808–11.

Mayer, C. and Akamatsu, T. (1999) Bilingual–bicultural models of literacy education for deaf students: considering the claims. *Journal of Deaf Studies and Deaf Education*, **4**, 1–8.

Mayer, C. and Wells, G. (1996) Can a linguistic interdependence theory support a bilingual–bicultural model of literacy education for deaf students? *Journal of Deaf Studies and Deaf Education*, **1**, 93–107.

McBride, P. A. (1884) *Guide to the Study of Ear Disease*. Johnston, Edinburgh.

Medawar, P.B. (1961) *The Uniqueness of the Individual*, Basic Books, New York.

Medearis, D.N. (1982) CMV immunity: imperfect but protective. *New England Journal of Medicine*, **306**, 985–6.

Meier, J.L. and Stinski, M.F. (1996) Regulation of human cytomegalovirus immediate–early gene expression. *Intervirology*, **39**, 331–42.

Meissner, H.C., Strebel, P.M. and Orenstein, W.A. (2004) Measles vaccines and the potential for worldwide eradication of measles. *Pediatrics*, **114**, 1065–9.

Meli, D.N., Christen, S., Leib, S.L. and Taüber, M.G. (2002) Current concepts in the pathogenesis of meningitis caused by *Streptococcus pneumoniae*. *Current Opinion in Infectious Diseases*, **15**, 253–7.

Meli, D.N., Kummer, J., Joss, P.C. and Leib, S.L. (2003) Doxycycline improves survival and reduces neuronal injury in experimental pneumococcal meningitis. Abstract B-326-2003. Interscience Conference on *Antimicrobial Agents and Chemotherapy*, Chicago.

Menard, A., Dos Santos, G., Dekumyoy, P., Ranque, S., Delmont, J., Danis, M., Bricaire, F. and Caumes, E. (2003) Imported cutaneous gnathostomiasis: report of five cases. *Transactions of the Royal Society of Tropical Medicine and Hygiene*, **97**, 200–2.

Menger, D.J. and Tange, R.A. (2003) The aetiology of otosclerosis: a review of the literature. *Clinical Otolaryngology*, **28**, 112–20.

Mentel, R., Kaftan, H., Wegner, U., Reissmann, A. and Gurtler, L. (2004) Are enterovirus infections a co-factor in sudden hearing loss? *Journal of Medical Virology*, **72**, 625–9.

Merchant, S.N. and Gopen, Q. (1996) A human temporal bone study of acute bacterial meningogenic labyrinthitis. *American Journal of Otology*, **17**, 375–85.

Meyer, H.M., Johnson, R.T., Crawford, I.P., Dascomb, H.E. and Rogers, N.G. (1960) Central nervous system syndromes of 'viral' etiology. A study of 713 cases. *American Journal of Medicine*, **29**, 334–47.

Meynard, J.L., El Amrani, M., Meyohas, M.C., Fligny, I., Gozlan, J., Rozenbaum, W., Roullet, E. and Frottier, J. (1997) Two cases of cytomegalovirus infection revealed by hearing loss in HIV infected patients. *Biomedicine and Pharmacotherapeutics*, **51**, 461–3.

Michaels, L. (1987) *Ear, Nose and Throat Histopathology*, Springer, Berlin, Heidelberg.

Michaels, M.G., Greenberg, D.P., Sabo, D.C. and Wald, E.R. (2003) Treatment of children with congenital cytomegalovirus infection with ganciclovir. *Pediatric Infectious Disease Journal*, **22**, 504–9.

Michel, G.F. and Tyler, A.N. (2005) Critical period: a history of the transition from questions of when, to what, to how. *Developmental Psychobiology*, **46**, 156–62.

Miller, E. (1990) Rubella reinfection. *Archives of Disease in Childhood*, **65**, 820–1.

Miller, D.M., Cebulla, C.M. and Sedmak, D.D. (2002) Human cytomegalovirus inhibition of major histocompatibility complex transcription and interferon signal transduction. *Current Topics in Microbiology and Immunology*, **269**, 153–70.

Miller, E., Cradock-Watson, J.E. and Pollock, T.M. (1982) Consequences of confirmed maternal rubella at successive stages of pregnancy. *Lancet*, **2**, 781–4.

Miller, H.G., Stanton, J.B. and Gibbons, J.L. (1956) Parainfectious encephamyelitis and related syndromes. *Quarterly Journal of Medicine*, **25**, 427–505.

Miller, E., Waight, P.A., Vurdien, J.E., White, J.M., Jones, G., Miller, B.H., Tookey, P.A. and Peckham, C.S. (1991) Rubella surveillance to December 1990: a joint report from the PHLS and National Congenital Rubella Surveillance Programme. *Communicable Diseases Report* (*London English Review*), **1**, R33–7.

Miller, E., Waight, P., Gay, N., Ramsay, M., Vurdien, J., Morgan-Capner, P., Hesketh, L., Brown, D., Tookey, P. and Peckham, C. (1997) The epidemiology of rubella in England and Wales before and after the 1994 measles and rubella vaccination campaign. Fourth report from the PHLS and the National Congenital Rubella Surveillance Programme. *Communicable Diseases Report Weekly*, **7**, R26–32.

Mills, B.G. and Singer, F.R. (1976) Nuclear inclusions in Paget's disease of bone. *Science*, **194**, 201–2.

Mills, B.G., Singer, F.R., Weiner, L.P., Suffin, S.C., Stabile, E. and Holst, P. (1984) Evidence for both respiratory syncytial virus and measles virus antigens in the osteoclasts of patients with Paget's disease of bone. *Clinical Orthopaedics*, **183**, 303–11.

Milner Jr, D.A., Dzamalala, C.P., Liomba, N.G., Molyneux, M.E. and Taylor, T.E. (2005) Sampling of supraorbital brain tissue after death: improving on the clinical diagnosis of cerebral malaria. *Journal of Infectious Diseases*, **191**, 805–8.

Minamishima, I., Ueda, K., Minematsu, T., Minamishima, Y., Umemoto, M., Take, H. and Kuraya, K. (1994) Role of breast milk in acquisition of cytomegalovirus infection. *Current Topics in Microbiology and Immunology*, **38**, 549–52.

Ministry of Health (2002) Health Statistics abstract 2002, in *Burden of Disease and Health Utilization Statistics*, Vol. 1, Ministry of Health, Dar es Salaam, Tanzania.

Minja, B.M. (1998) Aetiology of deafness among children at the Buguruni school for the deaf in Dar es Salaam, Tanzania. *International Paediatric Otorhinolaryngology*, **42**, 225–31.

Mishell, J.H. and Applebaum, E.L. (1990) Ramsay–Hunt syndrome in a patient with HIV infection. *Otolaryngology – Head and Neck Surgery*, **102**, 177–9.

Mitchell, T.E., Psarros, C., Pegg, P., Rennie, M. and Gibson, W.P.R. (2000) Performance after cochlear implantation: a comparison of children deafened by meningitis and congenitally deaf children. *Journal of Laryngology and Otology*, **114**, 33–7.

Mizushima, N. and Murakami, Y. (1986) Deafness following mumps: the possible pathogenesis and incidence of deafness. *Auris Nasus Larynx (Tokyo)*, **13** (Suppl. I), S55–7.

MMWR (2005) Elimination of rubella and congenital rubella syndrome – United States, 1969–2004. *Morbidity and Mortality Weekly Report (MMWR)*, **54**, 279–82.

Mocarski Jr, E.S. (2002) Immunomodulation by cytomegaloviruses: manipulative strategies beyond evasion. *Trends in Microbiology*, **10**, 332–9.

Mocarski, E.S. and Tan Courcelle, C. (2001) Cytomegaloviruses and their replication, in *Fields Virology* (eds D.M.K. Howley and P.M. Howley), Vol. 2, Lippincott Williams and Wilkins, Philadelphia, pp. 2629–73.

Molyneux, E.M., Walsh, A.L., Forsyth, H., Tembo, M., Mwenechanya, J., Kayira, K., Bwanaisa, L., Njobvu, A., Rogerson, S. and Malenga, G. (2002) Dexamethasone treatment in childhood bacterial meningitis in Malawi: a randomised controlled trial. *Lancet*, **360**, 211–18.

Montagnier, L. (2002) A history of HIV discovery. *Science*, **298**, 1727–8.

Monte, S., Fenwick, J.D. and Monteiro, E.F. (1997) Irreversible ototoxicity associated with zalcitabine. *International Journal of Sexually Transmitted Diseases and AIDS*, **8**, 201–2.

Montes, M., Cilla, G., Artieda, J., Vincente, D. and Basterretxea, M. (2002) Mumps outbreak in vaccinated children in Gipuzkoa (Basque Country), Spain. *Epidemiology and Infection*, **129**, 551–6.

Montoya, J.G. and Liesenfeld, O. (2004) Toxoplasmosis. *Lancet*, **363**, 1965–76.

Moon, C.M. and Fifer, W.P. (2000) Evidence of transnatal auditory learning. *Journal of Perinatology*, **20**, S37–44.

Moore, D.A.J., McCrodden, J., DeKumyoy, P. and Chiodini, P.L. (2003) Gnathostomiasis: an emerging imported disease. *Emerging Infectious Diseases*, **9**, 647–50. Available from URL: http://www.cdc.gov/ncidod/EID/vol9no6/02-0625.htm.

Moos, S. and Steinbrügge, H. (1883) Histologische Befunde an 6 Schläfenbeinem dreier an Diphtherie verstorbener Kinder. *Zeitschrift für Ohrenheilkunde*, **12**, 229–36.

Morales, W.J., Dickey, S.S., Bornick, P. and Lim, D.V. (1999) Change in antibiotic resistance of group B streptococcus: impact on intrapartum management. *American Journal of Obstetrics and Gynecology*, **181**, 310–14.

Morata, T.C. (1998) Assessing occupational hearing loss: beyond noise exposures. *Scandinavian Audiology*, **27**(Suppl. 48), 111–16.

Morishima, T., Miyazu, M., Ozaki, T., Isomua, S. and Suzuki, S. (1980) Local immunity in mumps meningitis. *American Journal of Diseases in Childhood*, **134**, 1060–4.

Morizono, T. and Johnstone, B.M. (1975) Ototoxicity of chloramphenicol ear drops with propylene glycol as solvent. *Medical Journal of Australia*, **2**, 634–8.

Morgan-Capner, P. and Crowcroft, N.S. (2002) Guidelines on the management of, and exposure to, rash illness in pregnancy (including consideration of relevant antibody screening programmes in pregnancy). *Communicable Diseases and Public Health*, **5**, 59–71.

Morgan-Capner, P., Miller, E., Vurdien, J.E. and Ramsay, M.E. (1991) Outcome of pregnancy after maternal reinfection with rubella. *Communicable Diseases Report (London English Review)*, **1**, R57–9.

Morgan-Jones, R. (2001) *Hearing Differently: The Impact of Hearing Impairment on Family Life*. Whurr, London.

Moro, D., Lloyd, M.L., Smith, A.L., Shellam, G.R. and Lawson, M.A. (1999) Murine viruses in an island population of introduced house mice and endemic short-tailed mice in Western Australia. *Journal of Wildlife Diseases*, **35**, 301–10.

Morris, M.S. and Prasad, S. (1990) Otologic disease in the acquired immunodeficiency syndrome. *Ear, Nose and Throat Journal*, **69**, 451–3.

Morris, D.J., Sims, D., Chiswick, M., Das, V.K. and Newton, V.E. (1994) Symptomatic congenital cytomegalovirus infection after maternal recurrent infection. *Pediatric Infectious Diseases Journal*, **13**, 61–4.

Morrison, A.W. and Booth, J.B. (1970) Sudden deafness: an otological emergency. *British Journal of Hospital Medicine*, 287–98.

Moscatello, A.L., Worden, D.L, Nadelman, R.B., Womser, G. and Lucente, F. (1991) Otolaryngologic aspects of Lyme disease. *Laryngoscope*, **101**, 592–5.

Moscicki, E.K., Elkins, E.F., Baum, H.M. and Mcnamara, P.M. (1985) Hearing loss in the elderly: an epidemiologic study of the Framingham Heart Study Cohort. *Ear and Hearing*, **6**, 184–90.

Moss, W.J., Clements, C.J. and Halsey, N.A. (2003) Immunization of children at risk of infection with human immunodeficiency virus. *Bulletin of the World Health Organization*, **81**, 61–70.

Mount, R.J., Harrison, R.V., Stanton, S.G. and Nagasawa, A. (1991) Correlation of cochlear pathology with auditory brainstem and cortical responses in cats with high frequency hearing loss. *Scanning Microscopy*, **5**, 1105–12.

Muhaimeed, H.A. (1996) Prevalence of sensorineural hearing loss due to toxoplasmosis in Saudi children: a hospital based study. *International Journal of Pediatric Otorhinolaryngology*, **34**, 1–8.

Mukherjee, D.K. (1979) Chloroquine ototoxicity: a reversible phenomenon? *Journal of Laryngology and Otology*, **93**, 809–15.

Mulheran, M. (1999) The effects of quinine on cochlear nerve fibre activity in the guinea pig. *Hearing Research*, **134**, 145–52.

Mulheran, M. and Degg, C. (1997) Comparison of distortion product OAE generation between a patient group requiring frequent gentamicin therapy and control subjects. *British Journal of Audiology*, **31**, 5–9.

Mulherin, D., Fahy, J., Grant, W., Keogan, M., Kavanagh, B. and Fitzgerald, M. (1991) Aminoglycoside induced ototoxicity inpatients with cystic fibrosis. *Irish Journal of Medical Science*, **160**, 173–5.

Munoz, A., Schrager, L.K., Bacellur, H., Speizer, I., Vermund, S.H., Detels, R., Saah, A.J., Kingsley, L.A., Seminara, D. and Phair, J.P. (1993) Trends in the incidence of outcomes defining acquired immunodeficiency syndrome (AIDS) in the Multicenter AIDS Cohort Study: 1985–1991. *American Journal of Epidemiology*, **137**, 423–38.

Murph, J.R., Bale Jr, J.F., Murray, J.C., Stinski, M.F. and Perlman, S. (1986) Cytomegalovirus transmission in a Midwest day care center: possible relationship to child care practices. *Journal of Pediatrics*, **109**, 35–9.

Murray, C. and Lopez, A.D. (eds) (1996) *The Global Burden of Disease: A Comprehensive Assessment of Mortality and Disability from Diseases, Injuries and Risk Factors in 1990 and Projected to 2020*, Global Burden of Disease and Injury Series, Vol. 1, Harvard University Press, Cambridge.

Murray, C. and Lopez, A.D. (1997) Mortality by cause for eight regions of the world: Global Burden of Disease Study. *Lancet*, **349**, 1269–76.

Mutimer, H.P., Akatsuka, Y., Manley, T., Chuang, E.L., Boeckh, M., Harrington, R., Jones, T. and Riddell, S.R. (2002) Association between immune recovery uveitis and a diverse intraocular cytomegalovirus-specific cytotoxic T cell response. *Journal of Infectious Diseases*, **186**, 701–5.

Mwaba, P., Maboshe, M., Chintu, C., Squire, B., Nyirenda, S., Sunkutu, R. and Zumla, A. (2003) The relentless spread of tuberculosis in Zambia – trends over the past 37 years (1964–2000). *South African Medical Journal; Suid-Afrikaanse Tydskrif Vir Geneeskunde*, **93**, 149–52.

Mylonakis, E., Hohmann, E.L. and Calderwood, S.B. (1998) Central nervous system infection with *Listeria* monocytogenes: 33 years' experience at a general hospital and review of 776 episodes from the literature. *Medicine*, **77**, 313–36.

Nabarro, D. (1954) *Congenital Syphilis*, Edward Arnold, London.

Nabe-Nielsen, J. and Walter, B. (1988) Unilateral total deafness as a complication of the measles–mumps–rubella vaccination. *Scandinavian Audiology Supplement*, **30**, 69–70.

Nabili, V., Brodie, H.A., Neverov, N.I. and Tinling, S.P. (1999) Chronology of labyrinthitis ossificans induced by *Streptococcus pneumoniae* meningitis. *Laryngoscope*, **109**, 931–5.

Naiditch, M.J. and Bower, A.G. (1954) Diphtheria. A study of 1,433 cases observed during a ten-year period at the Los Angeles County Hospital. *American Journal of Medicine*, **17**, 225–45.

Nakahara, H., Zhang, L.I. and Merzenich, M.M. (2004) Specialisation of primary auditory cortex processing by sound exposure in the 'critical period'. *Proceedings of the National Academy of Sciences*, **101**, 7170–4.

Nakayama, M., Miura, H. and Kamei, T. (1991) Investigation of vestibular damage by antituberculous drugs. *Acta Otolaryngologica Supplement*, **481**, 481–5.

Nardone, A., Pebody, R.G., van den Hof, S., Levy-Bruhl, D., Plesner, A.M., Rota, M.C. *et al.* (2003) Sero-epidemiology of mumps in Western Europe. *Epidemiology and Infection*, **131**, 691–701.

Nathan, L., Bohman, V.R., Sanchez, P.J., Leos, N.K., Twickler, D.M. and Wendel Jr, G.D. (1997) *In utero* infection with *Treponema pallidum* in early pregnancy. *Prenatal Diagnosis*, **17**, 119–23.

Nau, R. and Brück, W. (2002) Neuronal injury in bacterial meningitis: mechanisms and implications for therapy. *Trends in Neurosciences*, **25**, 38–45.

Nau, R., Wellmer, A., Soto, A., Koch, K., Schneider, O., Schmidt, H., Gerber, J., Michel, U. and Brück, W. (1999) Rifampicin reduces early mortality in experimental *Streptococcus pneumoniae* meningitis. *Journal of Infectious Diseases*, **179**, 1557–60.

Nawa, Y. (1991) Historical review and current status of gnathostomiasis in Asia. *Southeast Asian Journal of Tropical Medicine and Public Health*, **22** (Suppl.), 217–19.

Nell, M.J., Op't Hof, B.M., Koerten, H.K. and Grote, J.J. (1999) Effect of endotoxin on cultured human middle ear epithelium. *ORL – Otolaryngology and Related Species*, **61**, 201–5.

Neuwelt, E.A., Brummett, R.E., Remsen, L.G., Kroll, R.A., Pagel, M.A., McCormick, C.I., Guitjens, S. and Muldoon, L.L. (1996) *In vitro* and animal studies of sodium thiosulphate as a potential chemoprotectant against carboplatin-induced ototoxicity. *Cancer Research*, **56**, 706–9.

Newcomb, W.W., Homa, F.L., Thomsen, D.R., Trus, B.L., Cheng, N., Steven, A., Booy, F. and Brown, A.C. (1999) Assembly of the herpes simplex virus procapsid from purified components and identification of small complexes containing the major capsid and scaffolding proteins. *Journal of Virology*, **73**, 4239–50.

Newton, V. (2001) Adverse perinatal conditions and the inner ear. *Seminars in Neonatology*, **6**, 543–51.

Newton, C.R.J.C. and Warrell, D.A. (1998) Neurological manifestations of falciparum malaria. *Annals of Neurology*, **43**, 695–702.

Ng, V.L., Yajko, D.M. and Hadley, W.K. (1997) Extrapulmonary pneumocystosis. *Clinical Microbiology Reviews*, **10**, 401–18.

Ni, J., Bowles, N.E., Kim, Y.H., Demmler, G., Kearnery, D., Bricker, J.T. and Towbin, J.A. (1997) Viral infection of the myocardium in endocardial fibroblastosis. Molecular evidence for the role of mumps virus as an etiologic agent. *Circulation*, **95**, 133–9.

Nicoll, A., Lynn, R., Rahi, J., Verity, C. and Haines, L. (2000) Public health outputs from the British Paediatric Surveillance Unit and similar clinician-based systems. *Journal of the Royal Society of Medicine*, **93**, 580–5.

Niedermeyer, H.P., Arnold, W., Neubert, W.J. and Hoeffler, H. (1994) Evidence for measles virus RNA in otosclerotic tissue. *ORL – Journal of Otolaryngology and Its Related Specialties*, **56**, 130–2.

Niedermeyer, H.P., Arnold, W., Neubert, W.J. and Sedlmeier, R. (2000) Persistent measles virus infection as a possible cause of otosclerosis: state of the art. *Ear, Nose and Throat Journal*, **79**, 552–4; 556; 558.

Niedermeyer, H.P., Arnold, W., Schuster, M., Baumann, C., Kramer, J., Neubert, W.J. and Sedlmeier, R. (2001a) Persistent measles infection and otosclerosis. *Annals of Otology, Rhinology and Laryngology*, **110**, 897–903.

Niedermeyer, H.P., Arnold, W., Schwub, D., Wiest, I. and Sedlmeier, R. (2001b) Shift of the distributiuon of age in patients with otosclerosis. *Acta Otolaryngologica*, **121**, 197–9.

Nielsen, H.U.K., Konradsen, H.B., Lous, J. and Frimodt-Moller, N. (2004) Nasopharyngeal pathogens in children with acute otitis media in a low-antibiotic use country. *International Journal of Pediatric Otorhinolaryngology*, **68**, 1149–55.

Niskar, A.S., Kieszak, S.M., Holmes, A., Esteban, E., Rubin, C. and Brody, D.J. (1998) Prevalence of hearing loss among children 6 to 19 years of age: the Third National Health and Nutrition Examination Survey. *Journal of the American Medical Association*, **279**, 1071–5.

Nojd, J., Tecle, T., Samuelsson, A. and Orvell, C. (2001) Mumps virus neutralizing antibodies do not protect against reinfection with a heterologous mumps genotype. *Vaccine*, **19**, 1727–31.

Nomura, Y., Harada, T., Sakata, H. and Sugiura, A. (1988) Sudden deafness and asymptomatic mumps. *Acta Otolaryngologica (Stockholm) Supplement*, **456**, 9–11.

Nomura, Y., Nagakura, K., Kagei, N., Tsutsumi, Y., Araki, K. and Sugawara, M. (2000) Gnathostomiasis possibly caused by *Gnathostoma malaysiae*. *Tokai Journal of Experimental and Clinical Medicine*, **25**, 1–6.

Nontasut, P., Bussaratid, V., Chullawichit, S., Charoensook, N. and Visetsuk, K. (2000) Comparison of ivermectin and albendazole treatment for gnathostomiasis. *Southeast Asian Journal of Tropical Medicine and Public Health*, **31**, 374–7.

Norman, J.M. (ed) *Morton's Medical Bibliography*, 5th edn, Scolar Press, Aldershot, UK.

Nowaks, D.A., Boehmer, R. and Fuchs, H.-H. (2003) A retrospective clinical, laboratory and outcome analysis in 43 cases of acute aseptic meningitis. *European Journal of Neurology*, **10**, 271–80.

Nussinovitch, M., Volovitz, B. and Varsano, I. (1995) Complications of mumps requiring hospitalization in children. *European Journal of Pediatrics*, **154**, 732–4.

Nwawolo, C.C. (2003) The WHO Ear and Hearing Disorders Survey Protocol: Practical Challenges in its Use in a Developing Country (Nigeria), in *Informal Consultation on Epidemiology of Deafness and Hearing Impairment in Developing Countries and Update of the WHO Protocol*, World Health Organization, Geneva, March 2003.

Nye, S.W., Tangchai, P., Sundarakiti, S. and Punyagupta, S. (1970) Lesions of the brain in eosinophilic meningitis. *Archives of Pathology and Laboratory Medicine*, **89**, 9–19.

Obiako, M.N. (1985) Chloroquine ototoxicity: an iatrogenic problem. *Materia Medica Polona*, **17**, 195–7.

O'Connor, S., Taylor, C., Campbell, L.A., Epstein, S. and Libby, P. (2001) Potential infectious etiologies of atherosclerosis: a multifactorial perspective. *Emerging Infectious Diseases*, **7**, 780–8.

Odio, C.M., Faingezicht, I., Paris, M., Nassar, M., Baltodano, A., Rogers, J., Sáez-Llorens, X., Olsen, K.D. and McCracken Jr, G.H. (1991) The beneficial effects of early dexamethasone administration in infants and children with bacterial meningitis. *New England Journal of Medicine*, **324**, 1525–31.

Office for National Statistics (2001) *Abortion Statistics*, Medical Series AB 26, Office for National Statistics.

Ogaro, F.O., Orinda, V.A., Onyango, F.E. and Black, R.E. (1993) Effect of vitamin A on diarrhoeal and respiratory complications of measles. *Tropical Geographical Medicine*, **45**, 283–6.

Ogata, H., Oka, K. and Mitsudome, A. (1992) Hydrocephalus due to acute aqueductal stenosis following mumps infection: report of a case and review of the literature. *Brain Development*, **14**, 417–9.

Oghalai, J.S., Ramirez, A.L., Hegarty, J.L. and Jackler, R.K. (2004) Chronic pachymeningitis presenting as asymmetric sensorineural hearing loss. *Otology and Neurotology*, **25**, 616–21.

Ohashi, Y. and Nakai, Y. (1991) Current concepts of mucociliary dysfunction in otitis media with effusion. *Acta Otolaryngologica (Stockholm)*, **486**, 149–51.

Okada, T., Kato, I., Miho, I., Minami, S., Kinoshita, H., Akao, I., Kenmochi, M., Miyabe, S. and Takeyama, I. (1996) Acute sensorineural hearing loss caused by *Mycoplasma pneumoniae*. *Acta Otolaryngologica*, **522**(Suppl.), 22–5.

Okamoto, M., Shitara, T., Nakayama, M., Takamiya, H., Nishiyama, K., Ono, Y. and Sano, H. (1994) Sudden deafness accompanied by asymptomatic mumps. *Acta Otolaryngologica Supplement*, **514**, 45–8.

Oldfelt, V. (1949) Sequelae of mumps meningoencephalitis. *Acta Medica Scandinavica*, **134**, 405.

Oliver, D., He, D.Z., Klocker, N., Ludwig, J., Schulte, U., Waldegger, S., Ruppersberg, J.P., Dallos, P. and Fakler, B. (2001) Intracellular anions as the voltage sensor of prestin, the outer hair cell motor protein. *Science*, **292**, 2340–3.

Olivieri, N.F., Buncic, J.R., Chew, E., Gallant, T., Harrison, R.V., Keenan, N., Logan, W., Mitchell, D., Ricci, G. and Skarf, B. (1986) Visual and auditory neurotoxicity in patients receiving subcutaneous deferioxamine infusions. *New England Journal of Medicine*, **314**, 869–73.

Olsho, L.W., Koch, E.G. and Halpin, C.F. (1987) Level and age effects in infant frequency discrimination. *Journal of the Acoustic Society of America*, **71**, 509–11.

Orloff, S.L., Streblow, D.N., Soderberg-Naucler, C., Yin, Q., Kreklywich, C., Corless, C.L., Smith, P.A., Loomes, C.B., Miles, L.K., Cook, J.W., Bruggeman, C.A., Nelson, J.A. and Wagner, C.R. (2002) Elimination of donor-specific alloreactivity prevents cytomegalovirus-accelerated chronic rejection in rat small bowel and heart transplants. *Transplantation*, **73**, 679–88.

Ormerod, F.C. and Shillingford, A.A. (1961) *Survey of Deafness in Africa: Preliminary Report on a Visit to East and West Africa*, Unpublished Report to the Colonial Office and Nuffield Trust, London.

Örvell, C. (1984) The reactions of monoclonal antibodies with structural proteins of mumps virus. *Journal of Immunoloy*, **132**, 2622–9.

Örvell, C., Tecle, T. and Johansson, B. (2002) Mumps virus – an underestimated viral pathogen. *Current Topics in Virology*, **2**, 101–13.

O'Shea, S., Woodward, S., Best, J.M., Banatvala, J.E., Holzel, H. and Dudgeon, J.A. (1988) Rubella vacination: persistence of antibodies for 10–21 years. *Lancet*, **2**(8616), 909.

Osuntokun, B.O. (1983) Malaria and the nervous system. *African Journal of Medicine and Medical Sciences*, **12**, 165–72.

Owen, R. (1836) *Gnathostoma spinigerum* n.sp. *Proceedings of the Royal Society of London*, Part **4**, 123–6.

Ozkutlu, S., Soylemezoglu, O., Calikoblu, A.S., Kale, G. and Karaaslan, E. (1989) Fatal mumps myocarditis. *Japanese Heart Journal*, **30**, 109–14.

Padden, C. and Humphries, T. (1988) *Deafness in America: Voices from a Culture*, Harvard University Press, London.

Paganini, H., Gonzalez, F., Santander, C., Casimir, L., Berberian, G. and Rosanova, M. (2000) Tuberculous meningitis in children: clinical features and outcome in 40 cases. *Scandinavian Journal of Infectious Diseases*, **32**, 41–5.

Pai, M., Flores, L.L., Pai, N., Hubbard, A., Riley, L.W. and Colford, J.M. (2003) Diagnostic accuracy of nucleic acid amplification tests for tuberculous meningitis: a systematic review and meta-analysis. *Lancet Infectious Diseases*, **3**, 633–43.

Palmer, S.R., Soulsby, Lord and Simpson, D.I.H. (1998) *Zoonoses: Biology, Clinical Practice, and Public Health Control*, Open University Press, Oxford.

Palmu, A.A., Herva, E., Savolainen, H., Karma, P., Makela, P.H. and Kilpi, T.M. (2004) Association of clinical signs and symptoms with bacterial findings in acute otitis media. *Clinical Infectious Diseases*, **38**, 234–42.

Panagiotopoulos, T. and Georgakopoulou, P. (2004) Epidemiology of rubella and congenital rubella syndrome in Greece, 1994–2003. *Eurosurveillance Monthly*, **9**, 15–16.

Pantev, C., Ross, B., Fujioka, T., Trainor, L.J., Schulte, M.M. and Schulz, M. (2003) Music and learning-induced cortical plasticity. *Annals of the New York Academy of Sciences*, **999**, 438–50.

Paparella, M.M. and Schachern, P.A. (1991) Sensorineural hearing loss in children – nongenetic, in *Otolaryngology* (eds M. Paparella, D.A. Shumrick, J.L. Gluckman and W.L. Meyerhoff), Vol. II, 3rd edn, W.B. Saunders, Philadelphia, pp. 1561–78.

Paradise, J.L., Rockette, H.E., Colborn, D.K., Bernard, B.S., Smith, C.G., Kurs-Lasky, M. *et al.* (1997) Otitis media in 2235 Pittsburg infants: prevalence and risk factors during the first two years of life. *Pediatrics*, **99**, 318–33.

Parent du Chatelet, I., Traore, Y., Gessner, B.D., Antignac, A., Naccro, B., Njanpop-Lafourcade, B.M., Ouedraogo, M.S., Tiendrebeogo, S.R., Varon, E. and Taha, M.K. (2005) Bacterial meningitis in Burkina Faso: surveillance using field-based polymerase chain reaction testing. *Clinical Infectious Diseases*, **40**, 17–25.

Parney, I.F., Johnson, E.S. and Allen, P.B.R. (1997) 'Idiopathic' cranial hypertrophic pachymeningitis responsive to antituberculous therapy: case report. *Neurosurgery*, **41**, 965–71.

Parry, J.V., Mortimer, P.P., Perry, K.R., Pillay, D., Zuckerman, M. and Health Protection Agency HIV Laboratory Diagnosis Forum (2003) Towards error-free HIV diagnosis: guidelines on laboratory practice. *Communicable Disease Public Health*, **6**, 334–50.

Parving, A. (1993) Epidemiology of hearing loss and aetiological diagnosis of hearing impairment in childhood. *International Journal of Pediatric Otorhinolaryngology*, **5**, 151–65.

Parving, A., Biering-Sorensen, M., Bech, B., Christensen, B. and Sorensen, M.S. (1997) Hearing in the elderly greater than 80 years of age: prevalence of problems and sensitivity. *Scandinavian Audiology*, **26**, 99–106.

Paschoal, R.C., Hirata, M.H., Hirata, R.C., Melhem, M.S.C., Dias, A.L.T. and Paula, C.R. (2004) Neurocryptococcosis: diagnosis by PCR method. *Revista do Instituto de Medicina Tropical de Sao Paulo*, **46**, 203–7.

Pascolini, D. and Smith, A. (2005) *Available Data on Deafness and Hearing Impairment*, World Health Organization, Geneva (in preparation).

Pass, R.F. and Hutto, C. (1986) Group day care and cytomegaloviral infections of mothers and children. *Reviews of Infectious Diseases*, **8**, 599–605.

Pass, R.F., Long, W.K., Whitley, R.J., Soong, S.J., Diethelm, A.G., Reynolds, D.W. and Alford Jr, C.A. (1978) Productive infection with cytomegalovirus and herpes simplex virus in renal transplant recipients: role of source of kidney. *Journal of Infectious Diseases*, **137**, 556–63.

Pass, R.F., Stagno, S., Britt, W.J. and Alford, C.A. (1983) Specific cell mediated immunity and the natural history of congenital infection with cytomegalovirus. *Journal of Infectious Diseases*, **148**, 953–61.

Pass, R.F., Sohh, Y.M. *et al.* (1991) Increased rate of congenital cytomegalovirus infection in offspring of young adolescents. *Pediatric Research*, **29**, 181A.

Pass, R.F., Duliege, A.M., Boppana, S., Sekulovich, R., Percell, S., Britt, W. and Burke, R.L. (1999) A subunit cytomegalovirus vaccine based on recombinant envelope glycoprotein B and a new adjuvant. *Journal of Infectious Diseases*, **180**, 970–5.

Patel, V.B., Padayatchi, N., Bhigjee, A.I., Allen, J., Bhagwan, B., Moodley, A.A. and Mthiyane, T. (2004) Multidrug-resistant tuberculous meningitis in KwaZulu-Natal, South Africa. *Clinical Infectious Diseases*, **38**, 851–6.

Pearson, A., Jacobson, A., van Calcar, R. and Sauter, R. (1973) *The Development of the Ear*. American Academy of Ophthalmology and Otolaryngology, Rochester, Minnesota.

Peckham, C.S., Martin, J.A.M., Marshall, W.C. and Dudgeon, J.A. (1979) Congenital rubella deafness: a preventable disease. *Lancet*, **1**(8110), 258–61.

Peckham, C.S., Chin, K.S., Coleman, J.C., Henderson, K., Hurley, R. and Preece, P.M. (1983) Cytomegalovirus infection in pregnancy: preliminary findings from a prospective study. *Lancet*, **1**, 1352–5.

Peckham, C.S., Stark, O., Dudgeon, J.A., Martin, J.A. and Hawkins, G. (1987) Congenital cytomegalovirus infection: a cause of sensorineural hearing loss. *Archives of Disease in Childhood*, **62**, 1233–7.

Peckham, C., Tookey, P., Logan, S. and Giaquinto, C. (2001) Screening options for prevention of congenital cytomegalovirus infection. *Journal of Medical Screening*, **8**(3), 119–24.

Peeling, R.W. and Ye, H. (2004) Diagnostic tools for preventing and managing maternal and congenital syphilis: an overview. *Bulletin of the World Health Organization*, **82**, 439–46.

Peltola, H., Patja, A., Leinikki, P., Valle, M., Davidkin, I. and Paunio, M. (1998) No evidence for measles, mumps, and rubella vaccine-associated inflammatory bowel disease or autism in a 14-year prospective study. *Lancet*, **351**, 1327–8.

Permin, P.M. (1957) Histological studies of the guinea pig labyrinth following prolonged administration of quinine. *Acta Otolaryngologica (Stockholm)*, **47**(2), 167–71.

Petersen, L.R. and Marfin, A.A. (2002) West Nile virus: a primer for the clinician. *Annals of Internal Medicine*, **137**, 173–9.

Phelps, P.D., King, A. and Michaels, L. (1994) Cochlear dysplasia and meningitis. *American Journal of Otology*, **15**, 551–7.

Pichichero, M.E. and Pichichero, C.L. (1995) Persistent acute otitis media: 1. Causative pathogens. *Paediatric Infectious Disease Journal*, **14**, 178–83.

Pike, D.A. and Bosher, S.K. (1980) The time course of the strial changes produced by intravenous furosemide. *Hearing Research*, **3**, 79–89.

Pirvola, U., Xing-Qun, L., Virkkala, J., Saarma, M., Murakata, C., Camoratto, A.M., Walton, K.M. and Ylikoski, J. (2000) Rescue of hearing, auditory hair cells, and neurons by CEP-1347/KT7515, an inhibitor of c-Jun N-terminal kinase activation. *Journal of Neuroscience*, **20**, 43–50.

Plachter, B., Sinzger, C. and Jahn, G. (1996) Cell types involved in replication and distribution of human cytomegalovirus. *Advances in Virus Research*, **46**, 195–261.

Platt, R. (Lord). (1972) *Private and Controversial*. Cassell, London.

Plotkin, S.A. (1999) Vaccination against cytomegalovirus, the changeling demon. *Pediatric Infectious Disease Journal*, **18**, 313–25; quiz 326.

Plotkin, S.A., Starr, S.E., Friedman, H.M., Brayman, K., Harris, S., Jackson, S., Tustin, N.B., Grossman, R., Dafoe, D. and Barker, C. (1991) Effect of Towne live virus vaccine on cytomegalovirus disease after renal transplant. A controlled trial. *Annals of Internal Medicine*, **114**, 525–31.

Podsiadly, E., Chmielewski, T. and Tylewska-Wierzbanowska, S. (2003) *Bartonella henselae* and *Borrelia burgdorferi* infections of the central nervous system. *Annals of the New York Academy of Science*, **990**, 404–6.

Poggio, G.P., Rodriguez, C., Cisterna, D., Freire, M.C. and Cello, J. (2000) Nested PCR for rapid detection of mumps virus in cerebrospinal fluid of patients with neurological diseases. *Journal of Clinical Microbiology*, **38**, 274–8.

Pongponratn, E., Turner, G.D., Day, N.P., Phu, N.H., Simpson, J.A., Stepniewska, K., Mai, N.T., Viriyavejakul, P., Looareesuwan, S., Hien, T.T., Ferguson, D.J. and White, N.J. (2003) An ultrastructural study of the brain in fatal *Plasmodium falciparum* malaria. *American Journal of Tropical Medicine and Hygiene*, **69**, 345–59.

Popelka, M., Cruickshanks, K., Wiley, T., Tweed, T., Klein, B. and Klein, R. (1998) Low prevalence of hearing aid use among older adults with hearing loss: the epidemiology of hearing loss study. *Journal of the American Geriatrics Society*, **46**, 1075–8.

Popelka, M., Cruickshanks, K., Wiley, T., Tweed, T., Klein, B., Klein, R. and Nodahl, D. (2000) Moderate alcohol consumption and hearing loss: a protective effect. *Journal of the American Geriatrics Society*, **48**, 1273–8.

Porciv, P. and Brindles, B.J. (1984) Eosinophilic meningitis. *Medical Journal of Australia*, **141**, 319.

Porritt, R.J., Mercer, J.L. and Munro, R. (2003) Ultrasound-enhanced latex immuno-agglutination test (USELAT) for detection of capsular polysaccharide antigen of *Neisseria meningitidis* from CSF and plasma. *Pathology*, **35**, 61–4.

Portegies, P., Solod, L., Cinque, P., Chaudhuri, A., Begovac, J., Everall, I., Weber, T., Bojar, M., Martinez-Martin, P. and Kennedy, P.G.E. (2004) Guidelines for the diagnosis and management of neurological complications of HIV infection. *European Journal of Neurology*, **11**, 297–304.

Porter, J.B., Jaswon, M.S., Huehns, E.R., East, C.A. and Hazell, J.W. (1989) Desferrioxamine ototoxicity: evaluation of risk factors in thalassaemic patients and guidelines for safe dosage. *British Journal of Haematology*, **73**, 403–9.

Post, J.C. (2001) Direct evidence of bacterial biofilms in otitis media. *The Laryngoscope*, **111**, 2083–94.

Post, J.C., Preston, R.A., Aul, J.J., Larkins-Pettigrew, M., Rydquist-White, J., Anderson, K.W. *et al.* (1995) Molecular analysis of bacterial pathogens in otitis media with effusion. *Journal of the American Medical Association*, **273**, 1598–604.

Post, J.C., Stoodley, P., Hall-Stoodley, L. and Ehrlich, G.D. (2004) The role of biofilms in otolaryngologic infections. *Current Opinion in Otolaryngology – Head and Neck Surgery*, **12**, 185–90.

Potasman, I., Davidovitch, M., Tal, Y., Tal, J., Zelnik, N. and Jaffe, M. (1995) Congenital toxoplasmosis: a significant cause of neurological morbidity in Israel? *Clinical Infectious Diseases*, **20**, 259–62.

Pottumarthy, S., Fritsche, T.R., Sader, H.S., Stilwell, M.G. and Jones, R.N. (2005) Susceptibility patterns of *Streptococcus pneumoniae* isolates in North America (2002–2003): contemporary *in vitro* activities of amoxycillin/clavulanate and 15 other antimicrobial agents. *International Journal of Antimicrobial Agents*, **25**, 282–9.

Powers, S., Gregory, S. and Thoutenhoofd, E.D. (1998) *The Educational Achievements of Deaf Children – A Literature Review*, Department for Education and Science, London.

Prada, J.L., Torre-Cisneros, J., Kindelan, J.M., Jurado, R., Villanueva, J.L., Navarro, M. and Linares, M.J. (letter) (1996) Deafness and blindness in a HIV positive patient with cryptococcal meningitis. *Post Graduate Medical Journal*, **72**, 575.

Prasansuk, S. (1974) A case of neuro-otological gnathostomiasis. *Transactions of the Royal Society of Tropical Medicine and Hygiene*, **68**, 200.

Prasansuk, S. (2000) Incidence/prevalence of sensorineural hearing impairment in Thailand and Southeast Asia. *Audiology*, **39**(4), 207–11.

Prasansuk, S. and Hinchcliffe, R. (1975) Gnathostomiasis: a case of otological interest. *Archives of Otolaryngology*, **101**, 254–8.

Preece, P.M., Tookey, P., Ades, A. and Peckham, C.S. (1986) Congenital cytomegalovirus infection: predisposing maternal factors. *Journal of Epidemiology and Community Health*, **40**, 205–9.

Prescott, C.A. and Kibel, MA. (1991) Ear and hearing disorders in rural grade 2 (Sub B) schoolchildren in the western Cape. *South African Medical Journal*, **79**, 90–3.

Prezant, T.R., Agapian, J.V., Bohlman, M.C., Bu, X., Oztas, S., Qiu, W.Q., Arnos, K.S., Cortopassi, G.A., Jaber, L. and Rotter, J.I. (1993) Mitochondrial ribosomal RNA mutation associated with both antibiotic-induced and non-syndromic deafness. *Nature Genetics*, **4**, 289–94.

Prince, A.M., Szumuness, W., Millian, J.J. and David, D.S. (1971) A serologic study of cytomegalovirus infections associated with blood transfusions. *New England Journal of Medicine*, **284**, 1125–31.

Public Health Laboratory Service, Public Health Medicine Environmental Group, Scottish Centre for Infection and Environmental Health (2002) Guidelines for public health management of meningococcal disease in the UK. *Communicable Disease and Public Health*, **5**, 187–204.

Puel, J.-L., Bobbin, R.P. and Fallon, M. (1990) Salicylate, mefenamate, meclofenamate, and quinine on cochlear potentials. *Otolaryngology – Head and Neck Surgery*, **102**, 66–73.

Puel, J.-L., Bledsoe, S.C., Bobbin, R.P., Ceasar, G. and Fallon, M. (1989) Comparative actions of salicylate on the amphibian lateral line and guinea pig cochlea. *Comparative Biochemistry and Physiology*, **C93**, 73–80.

Puente, S., Garate, T., Grobusch, M.P., Janitschke, K., Bru, F., Rodriguez, M. and Gonzalez-Lahoz, J.M. (2002) Two cases of imported gnathostomiasis in Spanish women. *European Journal of Clinical Microbiology and Infectious Diseases*, **21**, 617–20.

Pugh, R.N., Akinosi, B., Pooransingh, S., Kumar, J., Grant, S., Lively, E., Linnane, J. and Ramaiah, S. (2002) An outbreak of mumps in the metropolitan area of Walsall, UK. *International Journal of Infectious Diseases*, **6**, 283–7.

Pujol, R. (1986) Periods of sensitivity to antibiotic treatment. *Acta Otolaryngologica (Stockholm) Supplement*, **429**, 29–33.

Pujol, R. and Lavigne-Rebillard, M. (2004) Development and plasticity of the human auditory system, in *Textbook of Audiological Medicine* (eds L.M. Luxon, J.M. Furman, A. Martini and D. Stephens), Martin Dunitz, London.

Punyagupta, S., Juttijudata, P. and Bunnag, T. (1975) Eosinophilic meningitis in Thailand: clinical studies of 484 typical cases probably caused by *Angiostrongylus cantonensis*. *American Journal of Tropical Medicine and Hygiene*, **24**, 921–31.

Punyagupta, S., Juttijudata, P., Bunnag, T. and Comer, D.S. (1968) Two fatal cases of eosinophilic myeloencephalitis, a newly recognised disease, caused by *Gnathostoma spinigerum*. *Transactions of the Royal Society of Tropical Medicine and Hygiene*, **62**, 801–9.

Qazi, S.A., Khan, M.A., Mughal, N., Ahmad, M., Joomro, B., Sakata, Y., Kuriya, N., Matsuishi, T., Abbas, K.A. and Yamashita, F. (1996) Dexamethasone and bacterial meningitis in Pakistan. *Archives of Disease in Childhood*, **75**, 482–8.

Quagliarello, V.J., Long, W.J. and Scheld, W.M. (1986) Morphologic alterations of the blood–brain barrier with experimental meningitis in the rat. Temporal sequence and role of encapsulation. *Journal of Clinical Investigation*, **77**, 1084–95.

Quaranta, A., Assennato, G. and Sallustio, V. (1996) Epidemiology of hearing problems among adults in Italy. *Scandinavian Audiology Supplementum*, **42**, 9–13.

Quinnan Jr, G.V., Kirmani, N., Rook, A.H., Manischewsitz, J.F., Jackson, L., Moreschi, G., Santos, C.W., Saraf, R. and Burns, W.H. (1982) Cytotoxic t cells in cytomegalovirus infection: HLA-restricted T-lymphocyte and non-T-lymphocyte cytotoxic responses correlate with recovery from cytomegalovirus infection in bone-marrow-transplant recipients. *New England Journal of Medicine*, **307**, 7–13.

Rabinstein, A., Jerry, J., Saraf-Lavi, E., Sklar, E. and Bradley, W.G. (2001) Sudden sensorineural hearing loss associated with herpes simplex virus type 1 infection. *Neurology*, **56**, 571–2.

Rafila, A., Marin, M., Pistol, A., Nicolaiciuc, D., Lupulescu, E., Uzicanin, A. and Reef, S. (2004) A large rubella outbreak, Romania – 2003. *Eurosurveillance Monthly*, **9**, 7–8.

Rahko, T., Baer, M., Virolainen, E. and Karma, P. (1984) Audiological and vestibular findings in 219 cases of meningitis. *European Archives of Oto-Rhino-Laryngology*, **240**, 15–20.

Rapp, M., Messerle, M., Lucin, P. and Koszinowski, U.H. (1993) *In vivo* protection studies with MCMV glycoproteins gB and gH expressed by vaccinia virus, in *Multi-disciplinary Approach to Understanding Cytomegalovirus Disease* (eds S. Michelson and S.A. Plotkin), Excerpta Medica, Amsterdam, pp. 327–32.

Rappaport, J.M., Bhatt, S.M., Burkard, R.F., Merchant, S.N. and Nadol Jr, J.B. (1999a) Prevention of hearing loss in experimental pneumococcal meningitis by administration of dexamethasone and ketorolac. *Journal of Infectious Diseases*, **179**, 264–8.

Rappaport, J.M., Bhatt, S.M., Kimura, R.S., Lauretano, A.M. and Levine, R.A. (1999b) Electron microscopic temporal bone histopathology in experimental pneumococcal meningitis. *Annals of Otology. Rhinology and Laryngology*, **108**, 537–47.

Rappelli, P., Are, R., Casu, G., Fiori, P.L., Cappuccinelli, P. and Aceti, A. (1998) Development of a nested PCR for detection of *Cryptococcus neoformans* in cerebrospinal fluid. *Journal of Clinical Microbiology*, **36**, 3438–40.

Rarey, K. (1990) Otologic pathophysiology in patients with human immunodeficiency virus. *American Journal of Otolaryology*, **11**, 366–9.

Rarey, K.E. and Davis, L.E. (1993) Temporal bone histopathology 14 years after cytomegalic inclusion disease: a case study. *Laryngoscope*, **103**, 904–9.

Rasmussen, F. (1969) The ototoxic effect of streptomycin and dihydrostreptomycin on the foetus. *Scandinavian Journal of Respiratory Diseases*, **50**, 61–7.

Ravi, R., Somani, S.M. and Rybak, L.P. (1995) Mechanism of cisplatin ototoxicity: antioxidant system. *Pharmacology and Toxicology*, **76**, 386–94.

Ray, B., Roy, T.S., Wadhwa, S. and Roy, K.K. (2005) Development of the human fetal cochlear nerve: a morphometric study. *Hearing Research*, **202**, 74–86.

Read, A.P. (2000) Hereditary deafness: lessons for developmental studies and genetic diagnosis. *European Journal of Pediatrics*, **159**(Suppl. 3), S232–5.

Read, W. (2002) Vogt–Koyanagi–Harada disease. *Ophthalmology Clinics of North America*, **15**, 333–41.

Reaney, E.A., Tohani, V.K., Devine, M.J., Smithson, R.D. and Smyth, B. (2001) Mumps outbreak among young people in Northern Ireland. *Communicable Disease and Public Health*, **4**, 311–15.

Reddehase, M.J., Balthesen, M., Rapp, M., Janjic, S., Pavic, I. and Koszinowsky, U.H. (1994) The conditions of primary infection define the load of latent viral genome in organs and the risk of recurrent cytomegalovirus disease. *Journal of Experimental Medicine*, **179**(1), 185–93.

Reefhuis, J., Honein, M.A., Whitney, C.G., Chamany, S., Mann, E.A., Biernath, K.R., Broder, K., Manning, S., Avashia, S., Victor, M., Costa, P., Devine, O., Graham, A. and Boyle, C. (2003) Risk of bacterial meningitis in children with cochlear implants. *New England Journal of Medicine*, **349**, 435–45.

Reinert, P., Soubeyrand, B. and Gauchoux, R. (2003) 35 year measles, mumps rubella vaccination assessment in France. *Archives of Pediatrics*, **10**, 948–54.

Remington, J.S., McLeod, R., Thulliez, P. and Desmonts, G. (2001) Toxoplasmosis, in *Infectious Diseases of the Fetus and Newborn Infant* (eds J.S. Remington and J.O. Klein), 5th edn, W.B. Saunders, Philadelphia, pp. 140–267.

Reuben, D.B.H.L. (1998) Hearing loss in community-dwelling older persons: national prevalence data and identification using simple questions. *Journal of the American Geriatrics Society*, **46**(8), 1008–11.

Reuben, D.B.H.L. (1999) Prognostic value of sensory impairment in older persons. *Journal of the American Geriatrics Society*, **47**, 930–5.

Reusser, P., Riddell, S.R., Meyers, J.D. and Greenberg, P.D. (1991) Cytotoxic T-lymphocyte response to cytomegalovirus after human allogeneic bone marrow transplantation: pattern of recovery and correlation with cytomegalovirus infection and disease. *Blood*, **78**, 1373–80.

Reusser, P., Attenhofer, R., Hebart, H., Helg, C., Chapuis, B. and Einsele, H. (1997) Cytomegalovirus specific T-cell immunity in recipients of autologous peripheral blood stem cell or bone marrow transplants. *Blood*, **89**, 3873–9.

Revello, M.G. and Gerna, G. (2002) Diagnosis and management of human cytomegalovirus infection in the mother, fetus, and newborn infant. *Clinical Microbiology Reviews*, **15**, 680–715.

Revello, M.G., Zavattoni, M., Furione, M., Baldanti, F. and Gerna, G. (1999) Quantification of human cytomegalovirus DNA in amniotic fluid of mothers of congenitally infected fetuses. *Journal of Clinical Microbiology*, **37**, 3350–2.

Revuelta, R., Soto-Hernandez, J.L., Vales, L.O. and Gonzalez, R.H. (2003) Cerebellopontine angle cysticercus and concurrent vascular compression in a case of trigeminal neuralgia. *Clinical Neurology and Neurosurgery*, **106**, 19–22.

Reynolds, D.W., Stagno, S., Stubbs, K.G., Dahle, A.J., Livingston, M.M., Saxon, S.S. and Alford, C.A. (1974) Inapparent congenital cytomegalovirus infection with elevated cord IgM levels: causal relationship with auditory and mental deficiency. *New England Journal of Medicine*, **209**, 291–6.

Richardson, M.P., Reid, A., Tarlow, M.J. and Rudd, P.T. (1997a) Hearing loss during bacterial meningitis. *Archives of Disease in Childhood*, **76**, 134–8.

Richardson, M.P., Reid, A., Williamson, T.J., Tartlow, M.J. and Rudd, P.T. (1997b) Acute otitis media and otitis media with effusion in children with bacterial meningitis. *The Journal of Laryngology and Otology*, **111**, 913–16.

Richardson, M.P., Williamson, T.J., Reid, A., Tarlow, M.J. and Rudd, P.T. (1998) Otoacoustic emissions as a screening test for hearing impairment in children recovering from acute bacterial meningitis. *Pediatrics*, **102**, 1364–68.

Richens, J. (1996) Typhoid, Chapter 2 in *The Wellcome Trust Illustrated History of Tropical Diseases* (ed. F.E.G. Cox), Wellcome Trust, London.

Riddell, S.R., Watanabe, K.S., Godrich, J.M., Li, C.R., Agha, M.E. and Greenberg, P.D. (1992) Restoration of viral immunity in immunodeficient humans by the adoptive transfer of T cell clones. *Science*, **257**, 238–41.

Riddell, S.R., Gilbert, M.J., Li, C.R., Walter, B.A. and Greenberg, P.D. (1993) Reconstitution of protective CD8+ cytotoxic T lymphocyte responses to human cytomegalovirus in immunodeficient humans by the adoptive transfer of T cell clones. in *Multidisciplinary Approach to Understanding Cytomegalovirus Disease* (eds S. Michelson and S.A. Plotkin), Elsevier Science, Amsterdam, pp. 155–64.

Rifkind, D. (1965) Cytomegalovirus infection after renal transplantation. *Archives of Internal Medicine*, **116**, 554–8.

Rima, B.K. (1999) Measles virus, in *Encyclopedia of the Life Sciences*, Macmillan Reference Ltd, Stockton Press, Article number 418 (CD ROM only).

Rima, B.K., Gassen, U., Helfrich, M.H. and Ralston, S.H. (2002) The pro and con of measles virus in Paget's disease: con. *Journal of Bone and Mineral Research*, **17**(12), 2290–2; author reply 2293.

Rinne, T., Bronstein, A.M., Rudge, P., Gresty, M.A. and Luxon, L.M. (1998) Bilateral loss of vestibular function: clinical findings in 53 patients. *Journal of Neurology*, **245**, 314–21.

Ritter, B.S. (1958) Mumps meningoencephalitis in children. *Journal of Pediatrics*, **52**, 424–33.

Rivera, L.B., Boppana, S.B., Fowler, K.B., Britt, W.J., Stagno, S. and Pass, R.F. (2002) Predictors of hearing loss in children with symptomatic congenital cytomegalovirus infection. *Pediatrics*, **110**, 762–7.

Roald, B., Storvold, G., Mair, I.W. and Mjoen, S. (1992) Respiratory tract viruses in otosclerotic lesions. An immunohistochemical study. *Acta Otolaryngologica*, **112**, 334–8.

Roberts, D.B. (1980) The etiology of bullous myringitis and the role of mycoplasmas in ear disease: a review. *Pediatrics*, **65**, 761–6.

Robertson, I.D. and Blackmore, D.K. (1989) Occupational exposure to *Streptococcus suis* type 2. *Epidemiology and Infection*, **103**, 157–64.

Robertson, S.A., Seamark, R.F., Guilbert, L.J. and Wegmann, T.G. (1994) The role of cytokines in gestation. *Clinical Reviews in Immunology*, **14**, 239–92.

Robertson, S.E., Featherstone, D.A., Gacic-Dobo, M. and Hersh, B.S. (2003) Rubella and congenital rubella syndrome: global update. *Revista Panamericana de Salud Publica*, **14**, 306–15.

Robinson, K. (1987) *Children of Silence*, Penguin Books, London.

Robinson, P.J. and Chopra, S. (1989) Antibiotic prophylaxis in cochlear implantation: current practice. *Journal of Otolaryngology Supplement*, **18**, 20–1.

Rojas-Molina, N., Pedraza-Sachez, S., Torres-Bibiano, B., Meza-Martinez, H. and Escobar-Gutierrez, A. (1999) Gnathostomosis, an emerging foodborne zoonotic disease in Acapulco, Mexico. *Emerging Infectious Diseases*, **5**, 264–6.

Roosa, D.B., St, J. (1880) *A Practical Treatise on Diseases of the Ear. Including the Anatomy of the Organ*, 4th edn, W Wood and Company, New York.

Rosenfeld, R.M. (1998) Amusing parents while nature cures otitis media with effusion. *International Journal of Pediatric Otorhinolaryngology*, **43**, 189–92.

Rosenstein, N.E., Perkins, B.A., Stephens, D.S., Popovic, T. and Hughes, J.M. (2001) Medical progress: meningococcal disease. *New England Journal of Medicine*, **344**, 1378–88.

Rowson, K.E., Hinchcliffe, R. and Gamble, D.R. (1975) A virological and epidemiological study of patients with acute hearing loss. *Lancet*, **1**(7905), 471–3.

Rozina, E.E. and Hilgenfeldt, M. (1985) Comparative study on the neurovirulence of different vaccine strains of parotitis virus in monkeys. *Acta Virologica*, **29**, 225–30.

Rozina, E.E., Kaptsova, T.I., Sharova. O.K., Nikolaeva, M.A. and Nesterova, T.P. (1984) Study of mumps virus invasiveness in monkeys. *Acta Virologica*, **28**, 107–13.

Ru, de J.A. and Grote, J.J. (2004) Otitis media with effusion: disease or defense? A review of the literature. *International Journal of Pediatric Otorhinolaryngology*, **68**, 331–9.

Rubin, R. (2002) Clinical approach to infection in the compromised host, in *Infection in the Organ Transplant Recipient* (eds R. Rubin and L.S. Young), Kluwer Academic Press, New York, pp. 573–679.

Rubin, S.A., Pletnikov, M. and Carbone, K.M. (1998) Comparison of the neurovirulence of a vaccine and a wild-type mumps virus strain in the developing rat brain. *Journal of Virology*, **72**, 8037–42.

Rubin, S.A., Pletnikov, M., Taffs, R., Snoy, P.J., Kobasa, D., Brown, E.G., Wright, K.E. *et al.* (2000) Clinical approach to infection in the compromised host. *Journal of Virology*, **74**, 5382–4.

Ruggero, M.A. and Rich, N.C. (1991) Furosemide alters organ of Corti mechanics: evidence for feedback of outer hair cells upon the basilar membrane. *Journal of Neuroscience*, **11**, 1057–67.

Russell, P.F. (1955) *Man's Mastery of Malaria*, Open University Press, London.

Russell, R.R. and Donald, J.C. (1958) The neurological complications of mumps. *British Medical Journal*, **30**, 27–30.

Ryals, B., Westbrook, E. and Schacht, J. (1997) Morphological evidence of ototoxicity of the iron chelator deferoxamine. *Hearing Research*, **112**, 44–8.

Rybak, L.P. and Kelly, T. (2003) Ototoxicity: bioprotective mechanisms. *Current Opinion in Otolaryngology – Head and Neck Surgery*, **11**, 328–33.

Rybak, L.P., Ravi, R. and Somani, S.M. (1995) Mechanisms of protection by diethyldithiocarbamate against cisplatin ototoxicity: antioxidant system. *Fundamental Applications of Toxicology*, **26**, 293–300.

Rybak, L.P., Whitworth, C. and Scott, V. (1991) Comparative acute ototoxicity of loop diuretic compounds. *European Archives of Otorhinolaryngology*, **248**, 353–7.

Saag, M.S., Graybill, R.J., Larsen, R.A., Pappas, P.G., Perfect, J.R., Powderly, W.G., Sobel, J.D. and Dismukes, W.E. (2000) Practice guidelines for the management of cryptococcal disease. Infectious Diseases Society of America. *Clinical Infectious Diseases*, **30**, 710–18.

Sade, J. (1994) The nasopharynx, Eustachian tube and otitis media. *The Journal of Laryngology and Otology*, **108**, 95–100.

Saederup, N. and Mocarski Jr, E.S. (2002) Fatal attraction: cytomegalovirus-encoded chemokine homologs. *Current Topics in Microbiology and Immunology*, **269**, 235–56.

Saederup, N., Lin, Y.C., Dairaghi, D.J., Schall, T.J. and Mocarski, E.S. (1999) Cytomegalovirus-encoded beta chemokine promotes monocyte-associated viremia in the host. *Proceedings of the National Academy of Sciences of the United States of America*, **96**, 10881–6.

Saederup, N., Aguirre, S.A., Sparer, T.E., Bouley, D.M. and Mocarski, E.S. (2001) Murine cytomegalovirus CC chemokine homolog MCK-2 (m131-129) is a determinant of dissemination that increases inflammation at initial sites of infection. *Journal of Virology*, **75**, 9966–76.

Saito, T., Saito, H., Saito, K., Wakui, S., Manabe, Y. and Tsuda, G. (1989) Ototoxicity of carboplatin in guinea pigs. *Auris Nasus Larynx*, **16**, 13–21.

Saito, H., Takahashi, Y., Harata, S. *et al.* (1996) Isolation and characterization of mumps virus strains in a mumps outbreak with a high incidence of aseptic meningitis. *Microbioloy and Immunology*, **40**, 271–5.

Saitoh, A., Pong, A., Waecker Jr, N.J., Leake, J.A.D., Nespeca, M.P. and Bradley, J.S. (2005) Prediction of neurological sequelae in childhood tuberculous meningitis: a review of 20 cases and proposal of a novel scoring system. *Pediatric Infectious Disease Journal* **24**, 207–12.

Saksirisampant, W., Kulkaew, K., Nuchprayoon, S., Yentakham, S. and Wiwanitkit, V. (2002) A survey of the infective larvae of *Gnathostoma spinigerum* in swamp eels bought in a local market in Bangkok, Thailand. *Annals of Tropical Medicine and Parasitology*, **96**, 191–5.

Salazar-Mather, T.P., Hamilton, T.A. and Biron, C.A. (2000) A chemokine-to-cytokine-to-chemokine cascade critical in antiviral defense. *Journal of Clinical Investigation*, **105**, 985–93.

Salmon, L.F.W. (1974) Some thoughts about preventing deafness in Malawi, in *The Commonwealth Foundation*. Occasional Paper XXXIV. Problems of Deafness in the Newer World. Proceedings of a Seminar convened by the Commonwealth Society for the Deaf at the University of Sussex, 9–20 September 1974, pp. 103–5.

Saloojee, H., Velaphi, S., Goga, Y., Afadapa, N., Steen, R. and Lincetto, O. (2004) The prevention and management of congenital syphilis: an overview and recommendations. *Bulletin of the World Health Organization*, **82**, 424–30.

Samarasinghe, S., Perera, B.J. and Ratnasena, B.G. (2002) First two cases of gnathostomiasis in Sri Lanka. *Ceylon Medical Journal*, **47**, 96–7.

Samuel, C.E. (2001) Antiviral actions of interferons. *Clinical Microbiology Reviews*, **14**, 778–809.

Sanchez, V., Greis, K.D., Sztul, E. and Britt, W.J. (2000) Accumulation of virion tegument and envelopeproteins in a stable cytoplasmic compartment during human cytomegalovirus replication. Characterization of a potential site of virus assembly. *Journal of Virology*, **74**, 975–86.

Sando, I., Harada, T., Loehr, A. and Sobel, J.H. (1977) Sudden deafness. Histopathologic correlations in temporal bone. *Annals of Otology*, **86**, 269–79.

Saraf-Lavi, E. and Sklar, E.M.L. (2001) Enhancement of the eighth cranial nerve and labyrinth on MR imaging in sudden sensorineural hearing loss associated with human herpesvirus 1 infection: case report. *American Journal of Neuroradiology*, **22**, 1380–2.

Sarnat, H.B. (1995) Ependymal reactions to injury: a review. *Journal of Neuropathology and Experimental Neurology*, **54**, 1–15.

Saunders, W.H. and Lippy, W.H. (1959) Sudden deafness and Bell's palsy: a common cause. *Annals of Otology, Rhinology and Laryngology*, **68**, 830–7.

Sawada, M. (1979) Electrocochleography of ears with mumps deafness. *Archives of Otolaryngology*, **105**, 475–8.

Sawanyawisuth, K., Tiamkao, S., Kanpittaya, J., Dekumyoy, P. and Jitpimolmard, S. (2004) MR imaging findings in cerebrospinal gnathostomiasis. *American Journal of Neuroradiology*, **25**, 446–9.

Scarpidis, U., Madnani, D., Shoemaker, C., Fletcher, C.H., Kojima, K., Eshragi, A.A., Staecker, H., Lefebvre, P., Malgrange, B., Balkany, T.J. and van de Water, T.R. (2003) Arrest of apoptosis in auditory neurons: implications for sensorineural preservation in cochlear implantation. *Otology and Neurotology*, **24**, 409–17.

Schattner, A., Halperin, D., Wolf, D. and Zimhony, O. (2003) Enteroviruses and sudden deafness. *Canadian Medical Association Journal*, **168**, 1421–3.

Scheld, W.M., Koedel, U. and Nathan, B. (2002) Pathophysiology of bacterial meningitis: mechanism(s) of neuronal injury. *Journal of Infectious Diseases*, **186**(Suppl. 2), S225–33.

Schlottmann, A., Kleemann, D., Kranz, K. and Schmal, G. (1996) Sudden deafness and increased toxoplasmosis IgM titer. *Laryngorhinootologie*, **75**, 687–90.

Schmitz, H., Kohler, B., Laue, T., Drosten, C., Veldkamp, P.J., Gunther, S., Emmerich, P., Geisen, H.P., Fleischer, K., Beersma, M.F. and Hoerauf, A. (2002) Monitoring of clinical and laboratory data in two cases of imported Lassa fever. *Microbes and Infection*, **4**, 43–50.

Schoeman, J.F., Van Zyl, L.E., Laubscher, J.A. and Donald, P.R. (1997) Effect of corticosteroids on intracranial pressure, computed tomographic findings, and clinical outcome in young children with tuberculous meningitis. *Pediatrics*, **99**, 226–31.

Schoeman, J., Wait, J., Burger, M., van Zyl, F., Fertig, G., van Rensburg, A.J., Springer, P. and Donald, P. (2002) Long-term followup of childhood tuberculous meningitis. *Developmental Medicine and Child Neurology*, **44**, 522–6.

Schönweiler, B., Held, M. and Schönweiler, R. (2001) Endocochleäre Schwerhörigkeit nach Infektion mit Mycoplasma pneumoniae. *Laryngo-Rhino-Otologie*, **80**, 127–31.

Schopfer, K., Lauber, E. and Krech, U. (1978) Congenital cytomegalovirus infection in newborn infants of mothers infected before pregnancy. *Archives of Diseases in Childhood*, **53**, 536–9.

Schoppel, K., Kropff, B., Schmidt, C., Vornhagen, R. and Mach, M. (1997) The humoral immune response against human cytomegalovirus is characterized by a delayed synthesis of glycoprotein-specific antibodies. *Journal of Infectious Diseases*, **175**, 533–44.

Schoppel, K., Schmidt, C., Einsele, H., Hebart, H. and Mach, M. (1998) Kinetics of the antibody response against human cytomegalovirus-specific proteins in allogeneic bone marrow transplant recipients. *Journal of Infectious Diseases*, **178**, 1233–43.

Schrag, S.J., Zywicki, S., Farley, M.M., Reingold, A.L., Harrison, L.H., Lefkowitz, L.B., Hadler, J.L., Danila, R., Cieslak, P.R. and Schuchat, A. (2000) Group B streptococcal disease in the era of intrapartum antibiotic prophylaxis. *New England Journal of Medicine*, **342**, 15–20.

Schuchat, A., Robinson, K., Wenger, J.D., Harrison, L.H., Farley, M, Reingold, A.L., Lefkowitz, L. and Perkins, B.A. (1997) Bacterial meningitis in the United States in 1995. *New England Journal of Medicine*, **337**, 970–6.

Schuknecht, H.F. and Donovan, E.D. (1986) The pathology of idiopathic sudden sensorineural hearing loss. *Archives of Otorhinolaryngology*, **243**, 1–15.

Schuknecht, H.F., Suzuka, Y. and Zimmermann, C. (1990) Delayed endolymphatic hydrops and its relationship to Meniere's disease. *Annals of Otology, Rhinology and Laryngology*, **99**, 843–53.

Schwab, J. and Ryan, M. (2004) Varicella zoster virus meningitis in a previously immunized child. *Pediatrics*, **114**, e273–4.

Schwartze, H. (1892) *Handbuch der Ohrenheilkunde*, Vogel, Leipzig.

Schwendemann, G., Wlinsky, J.S., Hatzidimitriou, G., Merz, D.C. and Waxham, M.N. (1982) Post-embedding immunocytochemical localization of paramyxovirus antigens by light and electron microscopy. *Journal of Histochemistry and Cytochemistry*, **30**, 1313–19.

Seely, D.R., Gloyd, S.S., Wright, A.D. and Norton, S.J. (1995) Hearing loss prevalence and risk factors among Sierra Leonean children. *Archives of Otolaryngology – Head and Neck Surgery*, **121**, 853–8.

Senanayake, S.N., Pryor, D.S., Walker, J. and Pam Konecny, P. (2003) First report of human angiostrongyliasis acquired in Sydney. *Medical Journal of Australia*, **179**, 430–1.

Sha, S.H. and Schacht, J. (1999) Salicylate attenuates gentamicin-induced ototoxicity. *Laboratory Investigation*, **79**, 807–13.

Sha, S.H., Taylor, R., Forge, A. and Schacht, J. (2001) Differential vulnerability of basal and apical hair cells is based on intrinsic susceptibility to free radicals. *Hearing Research*, **155**, 1–8.

Shafinoori, S., Ginocchio, C.C., Greenberg, A.J., Yeoman, E., Cheddie, M. and Rubin, L.G. (2005) Impact of pneumococcal conjugate vaccine and the severity of winter influenza-like illnesses on invasive pneumococcal infections in children and adults. *Pediatric Infectious Disease Journal*, **24**, 10–16.

Sharma, A., Dorman, M.F. and Spahr, A.J. (2002) A sensitive period for the development of the central auditory system in children with cochlear implants: implications for age of implantation. *Ear and Hearing*, **23**, 532–9.

Shehata, W.E., Brownell, W.E. and Dieler, R. (1991) Effects of salicylate on shape, electromotility and membrane characteristics of isolated outer hair cells from guinea pig cochlea. *Acta Otolaryngologica*, **111**, 707–18.

Shehata, M.A., el-Arini, F. and Zeid, S.A. (1970) Eighth cranial nerve affection in leprosy. *International Journal of Leprosy and Other Mycobacterial Diseases*, **38**, 164–9.

Shen, C.Y., Ho, M.S., Chang, S.F., Yen, M.S., Ng, H.T., Huang, E.S. and Wu, C.W. (1993) High rate of concurrent genital infections with human cytomegalovirus and human papillomaviruses in cervical cancer patients. *Journal of Infectious Diseases*, **168**, 449–52.

Shepard, C.W., Rosenstein, N.E., Fischer, M. and Active Bacterial Core Surveillance Team (2003) Neonatal meningococcal disease in the United States, 1990 to 1999. *Pediatric Infectious Disease Journal*, **22**, 418–22.

Shepherd, R.K. and Hardie, N.A. (2001) Deafness-induced changes in the auditory pathway: implications for cochlear implants. *Audiology and Neurootology*, **6**, 305–18.

Shingadia, D. and Novelli, V. (2003) Diagnosis and treatment of tuberculosis in children. *Lancet Infectious Diseases*, **3**, 624–32.

Shirane, M. and Harrison, R.V. (1987) A study of the ototoxicity of deferoxamine in chinchilla. *Journal of Otolaryngology*, **16**, 334–9.

Shotland, L.I., Mastrioanni, M.A., Choo, D.L., Szymko-Bennett, Y.M., Dally, L.G., Pikus, A.T., Sledjeski, K. and Marques, A. (2003) Audiologic manifestations of patients with post-treatment Lyme disease syndrome. *Ear and Hearing*, **24**, 508–17.

Simon, T., Hero, B., Dupuis, W., Selle, B. and Berthold, F. (2002) The incidence of hearing impairment after successful treatment of neuroblastoma. *Klinische Pediatrie*, **214**, 149–52.

Singh, A.E. and Romanowski, B. (1999) Syphilis: review with emphasis on clinical epidemiologic and some biologic features. *Clinical Microbiology Reviews*, **12**, 187–209.

Singh, A.P., Chandra, M.R., Dayal, D., Chandra, R. and Bhushan, V. (1980) Prevalence of deafness in a rural population of Lucknow District. *Indian Journal of Public Health*, **24**, 23–51.

Singh, T.R., Agrawal, S.K., Bajaj, A.K. and Singh, R.K. (1984) Evaluation of audiovestibular status in leprosy. *Indian Journal of Leprosy*, **56**, 24–9.

Sinzger, C. and Jahn, G. (1996) Human cytomegalovirus cell tropism and pathogenesis. *Intervirology*, **39**, 302–19.

Sinzger, C., Plachter, B., Stenglein, S. and Jahn, G. (1993) Immunohistochemical detection of viral antigens in smooth muscle, stromal, and epithelial cells from acute human cytomegalovirus gastritis. *Journal of Infectious Diseases*, **167**, 1427–32.

Sinzger, C., Grefte, A., Plachter, B., Gouw, A.S., The, T.H. and Jahn, G. (1995) Fibroblasts, epithelial cells, endothelial cells and smooth muscle cells are major targets of human cytomegalovirus infection in lung and gastrointestinal tissues. *Journal of General Virology*, **76**(Pt 4), 741–50.

Sinzger, C., Schmidt, K., Knapp, J., Kahl, M., Beck, R., Walman, J., Hebart, H., Einsele, H. and Jahn, G. (1999) Modification of human cytomegalovirus tropism through propagation *in vitro* is associated with changes in the viral genome. *Journal of General Virology*, **80**, 2867–77.

Skinner, L.J., Beurg, M., Mitchell, T.J., Darrouzet, V., Aran, J.M. and Dulon, D. (2004) Intracochlear perfusion of pneumolysin, a pneumococcal protein, rapidly abolishes auditory potentials in the Guinea pig cochlea. *Acta Otolaryngologia*, **124**, 1000–7.

Slevogt, H., Grobusch, M.P. and Suttorp, N. (2003) Gnathostomiasis without eosinophilia led to a 5-year delay in diagnosis. *Journal of Travel Medicine*, **10**, 196.

Slom, T.J., Cortese, M.M., Gerber, S.I., Jones, R.C., Holtz, T.H., Lopez, A.S., Zambrano, C.H., Sufit, R.L., Sakolvaree, Y., Chaicumpa, W., Herwaldt, B.L. and Johnson, S. (2002) An outbreak of eosinophilic meningitis caused by *Angiostrongylus cantonensis* in travelers returning from the Caribbean. *New England Journal of Medicine*, **346**, 668–75.

Sloyer, H.L., Howie, V.M., Ploussard, J.H., Bradac, J., Habercorn, M. and Ogra, P.L. (1977) Immune response to acute otitis media in children. III. Implications of viral antibody in middle ear fluid. *Journal of Immunology*, **118**, 248–50.

Smeeth, L., Cook, C., Fombonne, E., Heavey, L., Rodrigues, L.C., Smith, P.G. and Hall, A.J. (2004) MMR vaccination and pervasive developmental disorders: a case-control study. *Lancet*, **364**, 963–9.

Smith, M.E. and Canalis, R.F. (1989) Otologic manifestations of AIDS: the otosyphilis connection. *Laryngoscope*, **99**, 365–72.

Smith, G.A. and Gussen, R. (1976) Inner ear pathologic features following mumps infection. *Archives of Otolaryngology*, **102**, 108–11.

Smith, A.W., Bradley, A.K., Wall, R.A., McPherson, B., Secka, A., Dunn, D.T. and Greenwood, B.M. (1988) Sequelae of epidemic meningococcal meningitis in Africa. *Transactions of the Royal Society of Tropical Medicine and Hygiene*, **82**, 312–20.

Smolders, J.W. (1999) Functional recovery in the avian ear after hair cell regeneration. *Audiology and Neurootology*, **4**, 286–302.

Snedeker, J.D., Kaplan, S.L., Dodge, P.R., Holmes, S.J. and Feigin, R.D. (1990) Subdural effusion and its relationship with neurologic sequelae of bacterial meningitis in infancy: a prospective study. *Pediatrics*, **86**, 163–70.

Snow, J.R. and Telian, S.A. (1991) Sudden deafness, in *Otolaryngology* (eds M. Paparella, D.A. Shumrick, J.L. Gluckman and W.L. Meyerhoff), Vol. II, 3rd edn, W.B. Saunders, Philadelphia, pp. 1619–28.

Sobanski, M.A., Vince, R., Biagini, G.A., Cousins, C., Guiver, M., Gray, S.J., Kaczmarski, E.B. and Coakley, W.T. (2002) Ultrasound enhanced detection of individual meningococcal serogroups by latex immunoassay. *Journal of Clinical Pathology*, **55**, 37–40.

Sobol, S.E., Samadi, D.S. and Wetmore, R.F. (2004) Actinomycosis of the temporal bone: a report of a case. *Ear, Nose and Throat Journal*, **83**, 327–9.

SOCA (1992) SOCA Research Group and AIDS Clinical Trials Group: Studies of ocular complications of AIDS. Foscarnet-Ganciclovir cytomegalovirus retinitis trial: 2. Mortality. *New England Journal of Medicine*, **326**, 213–20.

Soderberg-Naucler, C. and Emery, V.C. (2001) Viral infections and their impact on chronic renal allograft dysfunction. *Transplantation*, **71**(Suppl. 11), SS24–30.

Soderberg-Naucler, C., Fish, K.N. and Nelson, J.A. (1997) Reactivation of latent human cytomegalovirus by allogeneic stimulation of blood cells from healthy donors. *Cell*, **91**, 119–26.

Sohmer, H. and Freeman, S. (2001) The pathway for the transmission of external sounds into the fetal inner ear. *Journal of Basic Clinical Physiology and Pharmacology*, **12**, 91–9.

Sohmer, H., Perez, R., Sichel, J.Y., Priner, R. and Freeman, S. (2001) The pathway enabling external sounds to reach and excite the fetal inner ear. *Audiology and Neurootology*, **6**, 109–16.

Sohn, Y.M., Oh, M.K., Balcarck, K.B., Cloud, G.A. and Pass, R.F. (1991) Cytomegalovirus infection in sexually active adolescents. *Journal of Infectious Diseases*, **163**, 460–3.

Song, B.-B., Anderson, D.J. and Schacht, J. (1997) Protection from gentamicin ototoxicity by iron chelators in guinea pig *in vivo*. *Journal of Pharmacology and Experimental Therapeutics*, **282**, 369–77.

Song, J.H., Lee, N.Y., Ichiyama, S., Yoshida, R., Hirakata, Y., Fu, W., Chongthaleong, A., Aswapokee, N., Chiu, C.H., Lalitha, M.K., Thomas, K., Perera, J., Yee, T.T., Jamal, F., Warsa, U.C., Vinh, B.X., Jacobs, M.R., Appelbaum, P.C., Pai, C.H. *et al.* (1999) Spread of drug-resistant *Streptococcus pneumoniae* in Asian countries: Asian Network for Surveillance of Resistant Pathogens (ANSORP) Study. *Clinical Infectious Diseases*, **28**, 1206–11.

Sonne, J.E., Zeifer, B. and Linstrom, C. (2002) Manifestations of otosyphilis as visualized with computed tomography. *Otology and Neurology*, **23**, 806–7.

Sorasuchart, A., Khunadorn, N. and Edmeads, J. (1968) Parasitic diseases of the nervous system in Thailand. *Canadian Medical Association Journal*, **98**, 859–67.

Sorlie, P.D., Nieto, F.J., Adam, E., Folsom, A.R., Shahar, E. and Massing, M. (2000) A prospective study of cytomegalovirus, herpes simplex virus 1, and coronary heart disease: the atherosclerosis risk in communities (ARIC) study. *Archives of Internal Medicine*, **160**, 2027–32.

Soucek, S. and Michaels, L. (1996) The ear in the acquired immunodeficiency syndrome. II. Clinical and audiological investigations. *American Journal of Otology*, **17**, 35–9.

Spector, S.A., Hirata, K.K. and Newman, T.R. (1984) Identification of multiple cytomegalovirus strains in homosexual men with acquired immunodeficiency syndrome. *Journal of Infectious Diseases*, **150**, 953–6.

Spector, S.A., Hsia, K., Crager, M., Pilcher, M., Cabral, S. and Stempien, M.J. (1999) Cytomegalovirus (CMV) DNA load is an independent predictor of CMV disease and survival in advanced AIDS. *Journal of Virology*, **73**, 7027–30.

Speir, E., Modali, R., Huang, E.S., Leon, M.B., Shawl, F., Finkel, T. and Epstein, S.E. (1994) Potential role of human cytomegalovirus and p53 interaction in coronary restenosis. *Science*, **265**, 391–4.

Speir, E., Shibutani, T., Yu, Z.X., Ferrans, V. and Epstein, S.E. (1996) Role of reactive oxygen intermediates in cytomegalovirus gene expression and in the response of human smooth muscle cells to viral infection. *Circulation Research*, **79**, 1143–52.

Spencer, J.V., Lockridge, K.M., Barry, P.A., Lin, G., Tsang, M., Penfold, M.E. and Schall, T.J. (2002) Potent immunosuppressive activities of cytomegalovirus-encoded interleukin-10. *Journal of Virology*, **76**, 1285–92.

Stagno, S., Reynolds, D.W., Tsiantos, A., Fucillo, D.A., Long, W. and Alford, C.A. (1975a) Cervical cytomegalovirus excretion in pregnant and nonpregnant women: suppression in early gestation. *Journal of Infectious Disease*, **131**, 522–7.

Stagno, S., Reynolds, D.W., Tsiantos, A., Fucillo, D.A., Long, W. and Alford, C.A. (1975b) Comparative serial virologic and serologic studies of symptomatic and subclinical congenitally and natally acquired cytomegalovirus infections. *Journal of Infectious Disease*, **132**, 568–77.

Stagno, S., Reynolds, D.W., Amos, C.S., Dahle, A.J., McCollister, F.P., Mohindra, I., Ennocilla, R. and Alford, C.A. (1977a) Auditory and visual defects resulting from symptomatic and subclinical congenital cytomegaloviral and toxoplasma infections. *Journal of Pediatrics*, **59**, 669–78.

Stagno, S., Reynolds, D.W., Huang, E.S., Thames, S.D., Smith, R.J. and Alford, C.A. (1977b) Congenital cytomegalovirus infection: occurrence in an immune population. *New England Journal of Medicine*, **296**, 1254–8.

Stagno, S., Reynolds, D.W., Pass, R.F. and Alford, C.A. (1980) Breast milk and the risk of cytomegalovirus infection. *New England Journal of Medicine*, **302**, 1073–6.

Stagno, S., Pass, R.F., Dworsky, M.E., Henderson, R.E., Moore, E.G., Walton, P.D. and Alford, C.A. (1982) Congenital cytomegalovirus infection: the relative importance of primary and recurrent maternal infection. *New England Journal of Medicine*, **306**, 945–9.

Stagno, S., Pass, R.F., Cloud, G., Britt, W.J., Henderson, R.E., Walton, P.D., Veren, D.A., Page, F. and Alford, C.A. (1986) Primary cytomegalovirus infection in pregnancy. Incidence, transmission to fetus, and clinical outcome. *Journal of the American Medical Association*, **256**, 1904–8.

Stals, F.S. (1999) Animal models for cytomegalovirus infection: rat CMV, in *Handbook of Animal Models of Infection* (eds O. Zak and M. Sande), Academic Press, London, pp. 943–50.

Starr, S.E., Tolpin, M.D., Friedman, H.M., Paucker, K. and Plotkin, S.A. (1979) Impaired cellular immunity to cytomegalovirus in congenitally infected children and their mothers. *Journal of Infectious Diseases*, **140**, 500–5.

Statement, N.C. (1993) Early identification of hearing impairment in infants and young children, Washington, DC. *National Institutes of Health*, **11**, 1–24.

Steffens, H.P., Kurz, S., Holrappels, R. and Reddehase, M.J. (1998) Preemptive CD8 T-cell immunotherapy of acute cytomegalovirus infection prevents lethal disease, limits the burden of latent viral genomes, and reduces the risk of virus recurrence. *Journal of Virology*, **72**, 1797–804.

Stern, H. (1984) Live cytomegalovirus vaccinaton of healthy volunteers: eight-year follow-up studies, in *CMV: Pathogenesis and Prevention of Human Infection* (eds S.A. Plotkin, S. Michelson, J.S. Pagano and F. Rapp), Alan R. Liss, New York, pp. 263–9.

Stevens, J.P., Eames, M., Kent, A., Halket, S., Holt, D. and Harvey, D. (2003) Longterm outcome of neonatal meningitis. *Archives of Disease in Childhood Fetal and Neonatal Edition*, **88**, F179–84.

Stewart, B.J.A. and Prabhu, P.U. (1993) Reports of sensorineural deafness after measles, mumps, and rubella immunisation. *Archives of Diseases in Childhood*, **69**, 153–4.

Stewart, I., Stewart, L., Skowronski, D., Westerberg, B.D., Bernauer, M., Mudurikwa, L., Chitunhu, J. and Shoniwa, C. (1998) The prevalence of hearing impairment in primary schools in Manicaland. Report from The Rotary Hearing Health Care Program in Zimbabwe (unpublished).

Stokes, J. (1970) Recent advances in immunization against viral diseases. *Annals of Internal Medicine*, **73**, 829–40.

Stokroos, R.J. and Albers, F.W.J. (1996) The etiology of idiopathic sudden sensorineural hearing loss. A review of the literature. *Acta Otolaryngologica (Belgium)*, **50**, 69–76.

Stockroos, R.J., Albers, F.W.J. and Schirm, J. (1998) The etiology of idiopathic sudden sensorineural hearing loss: experimental herpes simplex virus infection of the inner ear. *American Journal of Otology*, **19**, 447–52.

Stoll, B.J., Hansen, N., Fanaroff, A.A., Wright, L.L., Carlo, W.A., Ehrenkranz, R.A., Lemons, J.A., Donovan, E.F., Stark, A.R., Tyson, J.E., Oh, W., Bauer, C.R., Korones, S.B., Shankaran, S., Laptook, A.R., Stevenson, D.K., Papile, L.A. and Poole, W.K. (2004) To tap or not to tap: high likelihood of meningitis without sepsis among very low birth weight infants. *Pediatrics*, **113**, 1181–6.

Stone, J.S., Oesterle, E.C. and Rubel, E.W. (1998) Recent insights into regeneration of auditory and vestibular hair cells. *Current Opinion in Neurology*, **11**, 17–24.

Strauss, M. (1990) Human cytomegalovirus labyrinthitis. *American Journal of Otolaryngology*, **11**, 292–8.

Strauss, M. and Davis, G.L. (1973) Viral disease of the labyrinth. I. Review of the literature and discussion of the role of cytomegalovirus in congenital deafness. *Annals of Otology, Rhinology and Laryngology*, **82**, 577–83.

Stray-Pedersen, B. (1993) Toxoplasmosis in pregnancy, in *Infectious Diseases. Challenges for the 1990s* (ed. G.L. Gilbert), Ballière's Clinical Obstetrics and Gynaecology, London Baillière Tindall, London, Vol. 7(1), pp. 107–37.

Stray-Pedersen, B. (2003) Toxoplasma gondii-epidemiology, in *Parasites of the Colder Climate* (eds H. Akuuffo, E. Linder, I. Ljungstrom and M. Wahlgren), Taylor and Francis, London and New York, pp. 149–55.

Stray-Pedersen, B. and Foulon, W. (2000) Effect of treatment of the infected pregnant woman and her fetus, in *Congenital Toxoplasmosis* (eds P. Ambroise-Thomas and E. Petersen), Springer-Verlag, France, pp. 121–30.

Streblow, D.N., Orloff, S.L. and Nelson, J.A. (2001) Do pathogens accelerate atherosclerosis? *Journal of Nutrition*, **131**, 2798S–804S.

Streblow, D.N., Kreklywich, C., Yin, Q., De La Melena, V.T., Corless, C.L., Smith, P.A., Brakehill, C., Cook, J.W., Vink, C., Bruggeman, C.A., Nelson, J.A. and Orloff, S.L. (2003) Cytomegalovirus-mediated upregulation of chemokine expression correlates with the acceleration of chronic rejection in rat heart transplants. *Journal of Virology*, **77**, 2182–94.

Streppel, M., Richling, F., Roth, B., Walger, M., von Wedel, H. and Eckel, H.E. (1998) Epidemiology and etiology of acquired hearing disorders in childhood in the Cologne area. *International Journal of Paediatric Otorhinolaryngology*, **44**, 235–43.

Strussberg, S., Winter, S., Friedman, A., Benderly, A., Kahana, D. and Freundlich, E. (1969) Notes on mumps meningoencephalitis: some features of 199 cases in children. *Clinical Pediatrics*, **8**, 373–4.

Stypulkowski, P.H. (1990) Mechanisms of salicylate ototoxicity. *Hearing Research*, **46**, 113–45.

Sugiura, S., Yoshikawa, T., Nishiyama, Y., Morishita, Y., Sato, E., Hattori, T. and Nakashima, T. (2003) Detection of human cytomegalovirus DNA in perilymph of patients with sensorineural hearing loss using real-time PCR. *Journal of Medical Virology*, **69**, 72–5.

Sugiura, S., Yoshikawa, T., Nishiyama, Y., Morishita, Y., Sato, E., Beppu, R., Hattori, T. and Nakashima, T. (2004) Detection of herpesvirus DNAs in perilymph obtained from patients with sensorineural hearing loss by real-time polymerase chain reaction. *Laryngoscope*, **114**, 2235–8.

Sullivan, T.D., LaScolea, L.J. and Neter, E. (1982) Relationship between the magnitude of bacteremia in children and the clinical disease. *Pediatrics*, **69**, 699–702.

Sullivan, V., Biron, K.K., Talarico, C., Stanat, S.C., Davis, M., Pozzi, L.M. and Coen, D.M. (1993) A point mutation in the human cytomegalovirus DNA polymerase gene confers resistance to ganciclovir and phosphonylmethoxyalkyl derivatives. *Antimicrobial Agents and Chemotherapy*, **37**, 19–25.

Sutherland, H., Griggs, M. and Young, A.M. (2003) Deaf adults and family intervention projects. In *Deafness and Education in the UK: Research Perspectives* (eds C. Gallaway and A.M. Young), Whurr, London.

Sutton, D.V., Derkay, C.S., Darrow, D.H. and Strasneck, B. (2000) Resistant bacteria in middle ear fluid at the time of tympanostomy tube surgery. *Annals of Otology Rhinology, Laryngology*, **109**(1), 24–9.

Suzuki, K., Murtuza, B., Suzuki, N., Khan, M., Karieda, Y. and Yacoub, M.H. (2002) Human cytomegalovirus immediate-early protein IE2-86, but not IE1-72, causes graft coronary arteriopathy in the transplanted rat heart. *Circulation*, **106** (12 Suppl. 1), 1158–62.

Swartz, M.N. (2004) Bacterial meningitis – a view of the past 90 years. *New England Journal of Medicine*, **351**, 1826–8.

Sykes, H. (1984) The ototoxicity of chloroquine phosphate in the guinea pig. *British Journal of Audiology*, **18**, 59–69.

Szabo, C. (1998) Role of poly(ADP-ribose)synthetase in inflammation. *European Journal of Pharmacology*, **350**, 1–19.

Taha, M.K., Parent Du Chatelet, I., Schlumberger, M., Sanou, I., Djibo, S., de Chabalier, F. and Alonso, J.M. (2002) *Neisseria meningitidis* serogroups W135 and A were equally prevalent among meningitis cases occurring at the end of the 2001 epidemics in Burkina Faso and Niger. *Journal of Clinical Microbiology*, **40**, 1083–4.

Takano, T., Takikita, S. and Shimada, M. (1999) Experimental mumps virus-induced hydrocephalus: viral neurotropism and neuronal maturity. *NeuroReport*, **10**, 2215–21.

Takeuchi, K., Tanabayashi, K., Hishiyama, M. and Yamada, A. (1996) The mumps virus SH protein is a membrane protein and not essential for virus growth. *Virology*, **225**, 156–62.

Takikita, S., Takano, T., Narita, T., Takikita, M., Ohno, M. and Shimada, M. (2001) Neuronal apoptosis mediated by IL-1β expression in viral encephalitis caused by a neuroadapted strain of the mumps virus (Kilham strain) in hamsters. *Experimental Neurology*, **172**, 47–59.

Tan, K.K., Manickam, W.D. and Cardosa, M.J. (1992) Mumps encephalomyelitis. *Singapore Medical Journal*, **33**, 525–6.

Tanaka, K., Fukuda, S., Suenaga, T. and Terayama, Y. (1988a) Experimental mumps virus-induced labyrinthitis: immunohistochemical and ultrastructural studies. *Acta Otolaryngologica Supplement*, **456**, 98–105.

Tanaka, K., Fukuda, S., Terayama, Y., Toriayam, M., Ishidoy, J., Ito, Y. and Sugiura, A. (1988b) Experimental mumps labyrinthitis in monkeys (*Macaca irus*) – immunohistochemical and ultrastructural studies. *Auris Nasus Larynx*, **15**, 89–96.

Tangchai, P., Nye, S.W. and Beaver, P.C. (1967) Eosinophilic meningoencephalitis caused by angiostrongyliasis in Thailand. Autopsy report. *American Journal of Tropical Medicine and Hygiene*, **16**, 454–61.

Tange, R.A., Dreschler, W.A., Claessen, F.A. and Perenboom, R.M. (1997) Ototoxic reactions of quinine in healthy persons and patients with *Plasmodium falciparum* infection. *Auris Nasus Larynx*, **24**, 131–6.

Tarkkanen, J. and Aho, J. (1966) Unilateral deafness in children. *Acta Otolaryngologica*, **61**, 270–8.

Tarlow, M.J., Comis, S.D. and Osborne, M.P. (1991) Endotoxin induced damage to the cochlea of guinea pigs. *Archives of Disease in Childhood*, **66**, 181–4.

Tashima, C.K. (1969) CSF pleocytosis after mumps. *New England Journal of Medicine*, **280**, 1362.

Tasker, A., Dettmar, P.W., Panetti, M., Koufman, J.A., Birchall, J.P. and Pearson, J.P. (2002) Reflux of gastric juice and glue ear in children. *Lancet*, **359**, 493–5.

Taylor, R. and Forge, A. (2005) Developmental biology: life after deaf for hair cells? *Science*, **307**, 1056–8.

Taylor, F.B. and Toreson, W.E. (1963) Primary mumps meningo-encephalitis. *Archives of Internal Medicine*, **112**, 216–21.

Taylor, H.G., Michaels, R., Mazur, P., Bauer, R. and Liden, C. (1984) Intellectual, neurophysiological and achievement outcomes in children six to eight years after recovery from *Haemophilus influenzae* meningitis. *Pediatrics*, **74**, 198–205.

Taylor, B., Miller, E., Lingam, R., Andrews, N., Simmons, A. and Stowe, J. (2002) Measles, mumps, and rubella vaccination and bowel problems or developmental regression in children with autism: population study. *British Medical Journal*, **324**, 393–6.

Tecle, T., Mickiene, M., Johansson, B., Lindquist, L. and Örvell, C. (2002) Molecular characterization of two mumps virus genotypes circulating during an epidemic in Lithuania from 1998 to 2000. *Archives of Virology*, **147**, 243–53.

ter Meulen, J., Lenz, O., Koivogui, L., Magassouba, N., Kaushik, S.K., Lewis, R. and Aldis, W. (2001) Short communication: Lassa fever in Sierra Leone: UN peacekeepers are at risk. *Tropical Medicine and International Health*, **6**, 83–4.

Therien, J.M., Worwa, C.T., Mattia, F.R. and dReregnier, R.A. (2004) Altered pathways for auditory discrimination and recognition memory in preterm infants. *Developmental Medicine and Child Neurology*, **46**, 816–24.

Thobois, S., Broussolle, E., Aimard, G. and Chazot, G. (1996) L'ingestion du poisson cru: une cause de méningite á éosinophiles due á *Angiostrongylus cantonensis* après un voyage á Tahiti (Ingestion of raw fish: a cause of eosinophilic meningitis caused by *Angiostrongylus cantonensis* after a trip to Tahiti). *Presse Médicale*, **25**, 508.

Thomas, A.J. (1984) *Acquired Hearing Loss: Psychological and Psychosocial Implications*, Academic Press, London.

Thomas, A.J. and Herbst, K.G. (1980) Social and psychological implications of acquired deafness in adults of employment age. *British Journal of Audiology*, **14**, 76–85.

Thomas, H.I., Morgan-Capner, P., Enders, G., O'Shea, S., Caldicott, D. and Best, J.M. (1992) Persistence of specific IgM and low avidity specific IgG1 following primary rubella. *Journal of Virological Methods*, **39**, 149–55.

Thomas, R., Kameswaran, M., Murugan, V. and Okafar, B.C. (1993) Sensorineural hearing loss in neurobrucellosis. *Journal of Laryngology and Otology*, **107**, 1034–6.

Thompson, N.P., Montgomery, S.M., Pounder, R.E. and Wakefield, A.J. (1995) Is measles vaccination a risk factor for inflammatory bowel disease? *Lancet*, **345**, 1071–4.

Thwaites, G., Chau, T.T.H., Mai, N.T.H., Drobniewski, F., McAdam, K. and Farrar, J. (2000) Neurological aspects of tropical disease: tuberculous meningitis. *Journal of Neurology, Neurosurgery and Psychiatry*, **68**, 289–99.

Thwaites, G.E., Bang, N.D., Dung, N.H., Quy, H.T., Oanh, D.T.T., Thoa, N.T.C., Hien, N.Q., Thuc, N.T., Hai, N.N., Lan, N.T.N., Lan, N.N., Duc, N.H., Tuan, V.N., Hiep, C.H., Chau, T.T.H., Mai, P.P., Dung, N.T., Stepniewska, K., White, N.J., Hien, T.T. and Farrar, J.J. (2004) Dexamethasone for the treatment of tuberculous meningitis in adolescents and adults. *New England Journal of Medicine*, **351**, 1741–51.

Tieri, L., Masi, R., Ducci, M. and Marsella, P. (1988) Unilateral sensorineural hearing loss in children. *Scandinavian Audiology Supplement*, **30**, 33–6.

Timmons, G.G. and Johnson, K.P. (1970) Aqueductal stenosis and hydrocephalus after mumps encephalitis. *New England Journal of Medicine*, **27**, 1505–7.

Timon, C.I. and Walsh, M.A. (1989) Sudden sensorineural hearing loss as a presentation of HIV infection. *The Journal of Laryngology and Otology*, **103**, 1071–2.

Tookey, P. (2004) Rubella in England, Scotland and Wales. *Eurosurveillance Monthly*, **9**, 21–2.

Tookey, P.A., Cortina-Borja, M. and Peckham, C.S. (2002) Rubella susceptibility among pregnant women in North London, 1996–1999. *Journal of Public Health Medicine*, **24**, 211–6.

Tookey, P.A., Molyneaux, P. and Helms, P. (2000) UK case of congenital rubella can be linked to Greek cases. *British Medical Journal*, **321**, 766–7.

Tookey, P.A. and Peckham, C.S. (1999) Surveillance of congenital rubella in Great Britain, 1971–96. *British Medical Journal*, **318**, 769–70.

Tookey, P.A., Johnson, C., Ades, A.E. and Peckham, C.S. (1988) Racial differences in rubella immunity among pregnant women. *Public Health*, **102**, 57–62.

Topcu, I., Cüreoğlu, S., Yaramiş, A., Tekin, M., Oktay, F., Osma, U., Meric, F. and Katar, S. (2002) Evaluation of brainstem auditory evoked response audiometry findings in children with tuberculous meningitis at admission. *Auris Nasus Larynx*, **29**, 11–4.

Topley, J.M., Bamber, S., Coovadia, H.M. and Corr, P.D. (1998) Tuberculous meningitis and co-infection with HIV. *Annals of Tropical Paediatrics*, **18**, 261–6.

Townsend, G.C. and Scheld, W.M. (1993) Adjunctive therapy for bacterial meningitis: rationale for use, current status, and prospects for the future. *Clinical Infectious Diseases*, **17** (Suppl. 2), S537–49.

Townsend, J.J., Baringer, J.R., Wolinsky, J.S., Malamud, N., Mednick, J.P., Panitch, H.S., Scott, R.A., Oshiro, L. and Cremer, N.E. (1975) Progressive rubella panencephalitis. Late onset after congenital rubella. *New England Journal of Medicine*, **292**, 990–3.

Toynbee, J. (1868) *The Diseases of the Ear: Their Nature, Diagnosis, and Treatment*, H.K. Lewis, London.

Tran Ba Huy, P., Bernard, P. and Schacht, J. (1986) Kinetics of gentamicin uptake and release in the rat: comparison of inner ear tissues and fluids with other organs. *Journal of Clinical Investigation*, **77**, 1492–500.

Tran Ba Huy, P., Manuel, C., Meulemans, A., Sterkers, O., Wassef, M. and Amiel, C. (1983) Ethacrynic acid facilitates gentamicin entry into endolymph of the rat. *Hearing Research*, **11**, 191–202.

Trehub, S.E., Endman, M.W. and Thorpe, L.A. (1990) Infant's perception of timbre: classification of complex tones by spectral structure. *Journal of Experimental Psychology*, **4**, 300–13.

Trotter, C.L., Ramsay, M.E. and Kaczmarski, E.B. (2002) Meningococcal serogroup C conjugate vaccination in England and Wales: coverage and initial impact of the campaign. *Communicable Disease and Public Health*, **5**, 220–5.

Tsibulevskaya, G., Oburra, H. and Aluoch, J.R. (1996) Sensorineural hearing loss in patients with sickle cell anaemia in Kenya. *East African Medical Journal*, **73**, 471–3.

Tsutsui, Y. (1998) Murine cytomegalovirus for the animal models of congenital cytomegalovirus infection in human. *Nippon Rinsho – Japanese Journal of Clinical Medicine*, **56**, 90–6.

Tsutsumi, H., Chiba, Y., Abo, W., Chiba, S. and Nakao, T. (1980) T-cell-mediated cytotoxic response to mumps virus in humans. *Infection and Immunity*, **30**, 129–34.

Tunkel, A.R., Hartman, B.J., Kaplan, S.L., Kaufman, B.A., Roos, K.L., Scheld, M. and Whitley, R.J. (2004) Practice guidelines for the management of bacterial meningitis. *Clinical Infectious Diseases*, **39**, 1267–84.

Tunstall, M.J., Gale, J.E. and Ashmore, J.F. (1995) Action of salicylate on membrane capacitance of outer hair cells from the guinea-pig cochlea. *Journal of Physiology*, **485** (Pt 3), 739–52.

Tuomanen, E., Hengstler, B., Rich, R., Bray, M., Zak, O. and Tomasz, A. (1987) Nonsteroidal anti-inflammatory agents in the therapy for experimental pneumococcal meningitis. *Journal of Infectious Diseases*, **155**, 985–90.

Tylecote, J.H. (1880) The effect of climate on health and disease. *British Medical Journal*, **1**, 713.

Uimonen, S., Huttunen, K., Jounio-Ervasti, K. and Sorri, M. (1999) Do we know the real need for hearing rehabilitation at the population level? Hearing impairments in the 5- to 75-year-old cross-sectional Finnish population. *British Journal of Audiology*, **33**, 53–9.

Unal, H., Katircioglu, S., Karatay, M.C., Suoglu, Y., Erdamar, B. and Aslan, I. (1998) Sudden total bilateral deafness due to asymptomatic mumps infection. *International Journal of Pediatric Otorhinolaryngology*, **45**(2), 167–9.

Unhanand, M., Mustafa, M.M., McCracken Jr, G.H. and Nelson, J.D. (1993) Gram-negative enteric bacillary meningitis: a twenty-one year experience. *Journal of Pediatrics*, **122**, 15–21.

Usami, S., Abe, S., Tono, T., Komune, S., Kimberling, W.J. and Shinkawa, H. (1998) Isepamicin sulfate-induced sensorineural hearing loss in patients with the 1555 A→G mitochondrial mutation. *Otorhinolaryngology*, **60**, 164–9.

Utz, J.P., Kasel, J.A., Cramblett, H.G., Szwed, C.F. and Parrott, R.H. (1957) Clinical and laboratory studies of mumps. I. Laboratory diagnosis by tissue-culture technics. *New England Journal of Medicine*, **257**, 497–502.

Uus, K. and Davis, A. (2000) Epidemiology of permanent childhood hearing impairment in Estonia, 1985–1990. *Audiology*, **39**, 192–7.

Uzun, C., Koten, M., Adali, M.K., Yorulmaz, F., Yagiz, R. and Karasalihoglu, A.R. (2001) Reversible ototoxic effect of azithromycin and clarithromycin on transiently evoked otoacoustic emissions in guinea pigs. *The Journal of Laryngology and Otology*, **115**, 622–8.

Vaheri, A., Julkunen, I. and Koskiniemi, M.-L. (1982) Chronic encephalitis with specific increase in intrathecal mumps antibodies. *Lancet*, **25**, 685–8.

van Camp, G. (1996) Proceedings of 2nd Meeting of European Working Group on the Genetics of Hearing Impairment, Milan, 11–15 October.

van de Beek, D. and de Gans, J. (2004a) Dexamethasone and pneumococcal meningitis. *Annals of Internal Medicine*, **141**, 327.

van de Beek, D. and de Gans, J. (2004b) Meningitis-associated hearing loss: protection by adjunctive antioxidant therapy. *Annals of Neurology*, **55**, 597–8.

van de Beek, D., de Gans, J., McIntyre, P. and Prasad, K. (2003) *Corticosteroids in Acute Bacterial Meningitis*, The Cochrane Library, John Wiley & Sons, Ltd, Chichester, Issue 4.

van de Beek, D., de Gans, J., Spanjaard, L., Weisfelt, M., Reitsma, J. and Vermeulen, M. (2004) Clinical features and prognostic factors in adults with bacterial meningitis. *New England Journal of Medicine*, **351**, 1849–59.

Vandenbroucke, J.P. (1999) Case reports in an evidence-based world. *Journal of the Royal Society of Medicine*, **92**, 159–63.

van den Pol, A.N., Reuter, J.D. and Santarelli, J.G. (2002) Enhanced cytomegalovirus infection of developing brain independent of the adaptive immune system. *Journal of Virology*, **76**, 8842–54.

van den Pol, A.N., Mocarski, E., Saederup, N., Vieira, J. and Meier, J.J. (1999) Cytomegalovirus cell tropism, replication, and gene transfer in brain. *Journal of Neuroscience*, **19**, 10948–65.

van der Hulst, R.J., Dreschler, R.J. and Urbanus, N.A. (1988) High frequency audiometry in prospective clinical research of ototoxicity due to platinum derivatives. *Annals of Otology Rhinology and Laryngology*, **97**, 133–7.

van de Water, T.R., Lallemend, F., Eshraghi, A.A., Ahsan, S., He, J., Guzman, J., Polak, M., Malgrange, B., Lefebvre, P.P., Staecker, H. and Balkany, T.J. (2004) Caspases, the enemy within, and their role in oxidative stress-induced apoptosis of inner ear sensory cells. *Otology and Neurotology*, **25**, 627–32.

Van Dishoeck, H.A.E. and Bierman, T.A. (1957) Sudden perceptive deafness and viral infection (report of the first one hundred patients). *Annals of Otology, Rhinology and Laryngology*, **66**, 963–80.

van Haeften, R., Palladino, S., Kay, I., Keil, T., Heath, C. and Waterer, G.W. (2003) A quantitative LightCycler PCR to detect *Streptococcus pneumoniae* in blood and CSF. *Diagnostic Microbiology and Infectious Disease*, **47**, 407–14.

van Kempen, M.J.P., Vaneechoutte, M., Claeys, G., Verschraegen, G.L.C., Vermeiren, J. and Dhooge, I.J. (2004) Antibiotic susceptibility of acute otitis media pathogens in otitis-prone Belgian children. *European Journal of Paediatrics*, **163**, 524–9.

Van Lettow, M., Kumwenda, J.J., Harries, A.D., Whalen, C.C., Taha, T.E., Kumwenda, N., Kang'ombe, C. and Semba, R.D. (2004) Malnutrition and the severity of lung disease in adults with pulmonary tuberculosis in Malawi. *International Journal of Tuberculosis and Lung Disease*, **8**, 211–7.

Van Loon, A.M., Cleator, G.M. and Klapper, P.E. (2003) Herpesviruses, in *Infectious Diseases* (eds A. Armstrong and J. Cohen), 2nd edn, Mosby Press, New York and London, pp. 673–89.

Van Naarden, K., Decouflé, P. and Caldwell, K. (1999) Prevalence and characteristics of children with serious hearing impairment in metropolitan Atlanta, 1991–1993. *Pediatrics*, **103**, 570–5.

Vartiainen, E. and Karjalainen, S. (1998) Prevalence and etiology of unilateral sensorineural hearing impairment in a Finnish childhood population. *International Journal of Paediatric Otorhinolaryngology*, **43**, 253–9.

Veenhoven, R., Bogaert, D., Uiterwaal, C., Brouwer, C., Kiezebrink, H., Bruin, J., Ijzerman, E., Hermans, P., de Groot, R., Zegers, B., Kuis, W., Rijkers, G., Schilder, A. and Sanders, E. (2003) Effect of a conjugate pneumococcal vaccine followed by polysaccharide pneumococcal vaccine on recurrent acute otitis media: a randomised study. *The Lancet*, **361**, 2189–95.

Veltri, R.W., Wilson, W.R., Sprinkle, P.M., Rodman, S.M. and Kavesh, D.A. (1981) The implication of viruses in idiopathic sudden hearing loss: primary infection or reactivation of latent viruses? *Otolaryngology – Head and Neck Surgery*, **89**, 137–41.

Vidal, J.E., Sztajnbok, J. and Seguro, A.C. (2003) Eosinophilic meningoencephalitis due to *Toxocara canis*: case report and review of the literature. *American Journal of Tropical Medicine and Hygiene*, **69**, 341–3.

Vienny, H., Despland, P.A., Lutschg, J., Deonna, T., Dutoit-Marco, M.L. and Gander, C. (1984) Early diagnosis and evolution of deafness in childhood bacterial meningitis: a study using brainstem auditory evoked potentials. *Pediatrics*, **73**, 579–86.

Viljoen, D.L., Dent, G.M., Sibanda, A.G., Seymour, M., Chigumo, R., Karikoga, A. and Beighton, P. (1988) Childhood deafness in Zimbabwe. *South African Medicine Journal*, **73**, 286–8.

Viola, L., Chiaretti, A., Castorina, M., Tortorola, L., Piastra, M., Villani, A. *et al.* (1998) Acute hydrocephalus as a consequence of mumps meningoencephalitis. *Pediatric Emergency Care*, **14**, 212–4.

Vochem, M., Hamprecht, K., Jahn, G. and Speer, C.P. (1998) Transmission of cytomegalovirus to preterm infants through breast milk. *Pediatric Infectious Diseases Journal*, **17**, 53–8.

Volterra, V. (1981) Gestures, sign and words at two years: when does communication become language? *Sign Language Studies*, **33**, 351–62.

Vuori, M., Lahikainen, E.A. and Peltonen, T. (1962) Perceptive deafness in connection with mumps: a study of 298 servicemen suffering from mumps. *Acta Otolaryngologica*, **55**, 231–6.

Vyse, A.J., Gay, N.J., White, J.M., Ramsay, M.E., Brown, D.W., Cohen, B.J., Hesketh, L.M., Morgan-Capner, P. and Miller, E. (2002) Evolution of surveillance of measles, mumps, and rubella in England and Wales: providing the platform for evidence-based vaccination policy. *Epidemiology Review*, **24**(2), 125–36.

Waites, K.B. and Talkington, D.F. (2004) *Mycoplasma pneumoniae* and its role as a human pathogen. *Clinical Microbiology Reviews*, **17**, 697–728.

Wald, E.R., Bergman, I., Taylor, H.G., Chiponis, D., Porter, C. and Kubek, K. (1986) Long-term outcome of group B streptococcal meningitis. *Pediatrics*, **77**, 217–21.

Wallon, M., Kodjikian, L., Binquet, C., Garweg, J., Fleury, J., Quantin, C. and Peyron, F. (2004) Long-term ocular prognosis in 327 children with congenital toxoplasmosis. *Pediatrics*, **113**, 1567–72.

Walmus, B.F., Yow, M.D., Lester, J.W., Leeds, L., Thompson, P.K. and Woodward, R.M. (1988) Factors predictive of cytomegalovirus immune status in pregnant women. *Journal of Infectious Diseases*, **157**, 172–7.

Walter, E.A., Greenberg, P.D., Gilbert, M.J., Finch, R.J., Watanabe, K.S., Thomas, E.D. and Riddell, S.R. (1995) Reconstitution of cellular immunity against cytomegalovirus in recipients of allogeneic bone marrow by transfer of T-cell clones from the donor. *New England Journal of Medicine*, **333**, 1038–44.

Wan, K.S. and Weng, W.C. (2004) Eosinophilic meningitis in a child raising snails as pets. *Acta Tropica*, **90**, 51–3.

Waner, J.L., Hopkins, D.R., Weller, T.H. and Allred, E.N. (1977) Cervical excretion of cytomegalovirus: correlation with secretory and humoral antibody. *Journal of Infectious Diseases*, **136**, 805–9.

Wangemann, P. (2002) K(+) cycling and the endocochlear potential. *Hearing Research*, **165**, 1–9.

Wangemann, P., Liu, J. and Marcus, D.C. (1995) Ion transport mechanisms responsible for K$^+$ secretion and the transepithelia voltage across marginal cells of stria vascularis *in vitro*. *Hearing Research*, **84**, 19–29.

Wangemann, P. and Schacht, J. (1996) Homeostatic mechanisms in the cochlea, in *The Cochlea* (eds P. Dallos, A.N. Popper and R.R. Fay), Springer-Verlag, New York, pp. 130–85.

Ward, P.H., Honrubia, V. and Moore, B.S. (1968) Inner ear pathology in deafness due to maternal rubella. *Archives of Otolaryngology*, **87**, 22–8.

Warren, K.S. and Mahmoud, A.A.F. (eds) (1984) *Tropical and Geographical Medicine*, McGraw-Hill, New York.

Wasserman, L. and Haghighi, P. (1992) Otic and ophthalmic pneumocystosis in acquired immunodeficiency syndrome. *Archives of Pathology and Laboratory Medicine*, **116**, 500–3.

Watanabe, K., Jinnouchi, K., Hess, A., Michel, O. and Yagi, T. (2001) Detection of apoptotic change in the lipopolysaccharide (LPS)-treated cochlea of guinea pigs. *Hearing Research*, **158**, 116–22.

Watson, N.K., Bartt, R.E., Houff, S.A., Leurgans, S.E. and Schneck, M.J. (2005) Focal neurological deficits and West Nile virus infection. *Clinical Infectious Diseases*, **40**, e59–e62.

Weber, J.R., Freyer, D., Alexander, C., Schröder, N.W.J., Reiss, A., Küster, C., Pfeil, D., Tuomanen, E.I. and Schumann, R.R. (2003) Recognition of pneumococcal peptidoglycan: an expanded, pivotal role for LPS binding protein. *Immunity*, **19**, 269–79.

Wei, X., Zhao, L., Liu, J., Dodel, R.C., Farlow, M.R. and Du, Y. (2005) Minocycline prevents gentamicin-induced ototoxicity by inhibiting p38 MAP kinase phosphorylation and caspase 3 activation. *Neuroscience*, **131**, 513–21.

Weinstein, L., Shelokov, A., Seltser, L.R. and Winchell, G.D. (1952) A comparison of the clinical features of poliomyelitis in adults and in children. *New England Journal of Medicine*, **246**, 296–302.

Weir, E. and Fishman, D. (2002) Syphilis: have we dropped the ball? *Canadian Medical Association Journal*, **167**(11), 1267–8.

Wellman, M.B., Sommer, D.D. and McKenna, J. (2003) Sensorineural hearing loss in postmeningitic children. *Otology and Neurotology*, **24**, 907–12.

Wellmer, A., Zysk, G. and Gerber, J. (2002) Decreased virulence of a pneumolysin-deficient strain of *Streptococcus pneumoniae* in murine meningitis. *Infection and Immunity*, **70**, 6504–8.

Wendel, G.D. (1988) Gestational and congenital syphilis. *Clinical Perinatology*, **15**, 287–303.

Wendt H. (1874) In H. von Ziemssen (ed.), *Handbuch der Speziellen Pathologic*, Carl Genold's Sohn, Leipzig.

Werner, L.A. and Gray, L. (1998) Behavioural studies of hearing development, in *Early Embryology of the Vertebrate Ear* (eds E.W. Rubel, A.N. Popper and R.R. Fay), Springer-Verlag, New York, pp. 12–79.

Wersäll, J., Lundquist, P.-G. and Björkroth, B. (1969) Ototoxicity of gentamicin. *Journal of Infectious Diseases*, **119**, 410–6.

West, B.A., Brummett, R.E. and Himes, D.L. (1973) Interaction of kanamycin and ethacrynic acid. Severe cochlear damage in guinea pigs. *Archives of Otolaryngology*, **98**, 32–7.

Westmore, G.A., Pickard, B.H. and Stern, H. (1979) Isolation of mumps virus from the inner ear after sudden deafness. *British Medical Journal*, **1**, 14–5.

Wetmore, S.J. and Abramson, M. (1979) Bullous myringitis with sensorineural hearing loss. *Otolaryngology – Head and Neck Surgery*, **87**, 66–70.

Whitcup, S.M., Fortin, E., Lindblad, A.S., Griffiths, P., Metcalf, J.A., Robinson, M.R., Manischewitz, J., Baird, B., Perry, C., Kidd, I.M. *et al.* (1999) Discontinuation of anti-cytomegalovirus therapy in patients with HIV infection and cytomegalovirus retinitis. *Journal of the American Medical Association*, **282**, 1633–7.

White, N.H., Yow, M.D., Demmler, G.J., Norton, H.J., Hoyle, J., Prankard, K., Mishaw, C. and Pokorny, S. (1989) Prevalence of cytomegalovirus antibody in subjects between the ages of 6 and 22 years. *Journal of Infectious Diseases*, **159**, 1013–7.

Whitley, R.J., Hayden, F.G., Reisinger, K.S., Young, N., Dutkowski, R., Ipe, D., Mills, R.G. and Ward, P. (2001) Oral oseltamivir treatment of influenza in children. *Pediatric Infectious Diseases Journal*, **20**, 127–33.

WHO (1959) Zoonoses, Second Report of the Joint WHO/FAO Expert Committee, World Health Organization, Geneva.

WHO (1980) Final report of the Global Commission for the Certification of Smallpox Eradication: The Achievement of Global Eradication of Smallpox. World Health Organization, Geneva.

WHO (1991) Report of the Informal Working Group on Prevention of Deafness and Hearing Impairment Programme Planning, Document WHO/PDH/91.1, World Health Organization, Geneva.

WHO (1995) Prevention of Hearing Impairment, Resolution of the 48th World Health Assembly, (12 May 1995), World Health Organization, Geneva, WHA48.9.

WHO (1997a) Report of the First Informal Consultation on Future Programme Developments for the Prevention of Deafness and Hearing Impairment, World Health Organization, Geneva, 23–24, January 1997, WHO/PDH/97.3.

WHO (1997b) Regional Office For South-East Asia Multicentre Study on the Magnitude and Etiology of Hearing Impairment, Report of a Meeting of Principal Investigators, Colombo, Sri Lanka, 3–5 September 1997.

WHO (1998) Progress towards leprosy elimination. *Weekly Epidemiological Review*, **73**, 153–60.

WHO (1998a) International Workshop on Primary Ear and Hearing Care, Cape Town, South Africa, 12–14 March 1998.

WHO (1998b) *Control of Epidemic Meningococcal Disease*, WHO Practical Guidelines. 2nd edn, World Health Organization, Geneva.

WHO (1998c) Progress towards leprosy elimination. *Weekly Epidemiological Review*, **73**, 153–60.

WHO (1999) WHO Ear and Hearing Disorders Survey: Protocol and Software Package, World Health Organization, Geneva, July 1999, WHO/PBD/PDH/99.8. (This package has been developed for those planning to conduct a population-based survey in a development country.)

WHO (2000a) Report on Global Surveillance of Epidemic-Prone Infectious Diseases, Chapter 5, Meningococcal Disease, pp. 55–61, World Health Organization Department of Communicable Disease Surveillance and Response 2000, WHO/CDS/CSR/ISR/2000.1.

WHO, Department of Vaccines (2000b) Reporting on a meeting on preventing congenital rubella syndrome (CRS): immunization strategies, surveillance needs, World Health Organization, Geneva, 12–14 January 2000, unpublished document WHO/V&B/00.10.

WHO (2001a) BCG in immunization programmes. *Weekly Epidemiological Record*, **76**, 33–9.

WHO (2001b) Global Prevalence and Incidence of Selected Curable Sexually Transmitted Infections, World Health Organization, Geneva.

WHO (2001c) World Health Report 2001, Mental Health: New Understanding, New Hope, World Health Organization, Geneva.

WHO (2001d) Press release: WHO Calls on Private Sector to Provide Affordable Hearing Aids in Developing World, World Health Organization/34, 11 July 2001.

WHO (2001e) International Classification of Functioning, Disability and Health: ICF, World Health Organization, Geneva.

WHO (2003) The Africa Malaria Report, World Health Organization, Geneva.

WHO (2004a) Global Tuberculosis Control – Surveillance, Planning, Financing, World Health Organization Report 2004.

WHO (2004b) World Health Report 2004, World Health Organisation, Geneva.

WHO (2004c) AIDS Epidemic Update, World Health Organization, Geneva.

WHO (2005) Progress towards elimination of measles and prevention of congenital rubella infection in the WHO European Region, 1990–2004. *Weekly Epidemiological Records*, **80**, 66–71.

Wicher, V. and Wicher, K. (2001) Pathogenesis of maternal-fetal syphilis revisited. *Clinical Infectious Diseases*, **33**, 354–63.

Wild, N.J., Sheppard, S., Smithells, R.W., Holzel, H. and Jones, G. (1989) Onset and severity of hearing loss due to congenital rubella infection. *Archives of Diseases in Childhood*, **64**, 1280–3.

Williamson, W.D., Demmler, G.J., Percy, A.K. and Catlin, F.I. (1992) Progressive hearing loss in infants with asymptomatic congenital cytomegalovirus infection. *Pediatrics*, **90**, 862–6.

Wilson, C., Roberts, A. and Stephens, D. (2003) Improving hearing assessment of children post-meningitis. *Archives of Disease in Childhood*, **88**, 976–7.

Wilson, C.B., Remington, J.S., Stagno, S. and Reynolds, D.W. (1980) Developmental of adverse sequelae in children born with subclinical congenital toxoplasmosis. *Pediatrics*, **66**, 767–74.

Wilson, W.R., Vetri, R.W., Laird, N. and Sprinkle, P.M. (1983) Viral and epidemiological studies of idiopathic sudden hearing loss. *Otolaryngology – Head and Neck Surgery*, **91**, 653–8.

Wilson, D.H., Walsh, P.G., Sanchez, L., Davis, A.C., Taylor, A.W., Tucker, G. and Meagher, I. (1999) The epidemiology of hearing impairment in an Australian adult population. *International Journal of Epidemiology*, **28**, 247–52.

Winter, A., Marwick, S., Osborne, M., Comis, S., Stephen, J. and Tarlow, M. (1996) Ultrastructural damage to the organ of Corti during acute experimental *Escherichia coli* and pneumococcal meningitis in guinea pigs. *Acta Otolaryngologia*, **116**, 401–7.

Winter, A.J., Comis, S.D., Osborne, M.P., Tarlow, M.J., Stephen, J., Andrew, P.W., Hill, J. and Mitchell, T.J. (1997) A role for pneumolysin but not neuraminidase in the hearing loss and cochlear damage induced by experimental pneumococcal meningitis in guinea pigs. *Infection and Immunity*, **65**, 4411–8.

Witenberg, G., Jacoby, J. and Stechelmacher, S. (1950) A case of ocular gnathostomiasis. *Ophthalmologia*, **119**, 114–22.

Wittmaack, K. (1904) Beiträge zur Kenntnis der Wirkung des Chinins das Gehörorgan. *Archiv für gesamte Physiologie*, **95**, 209–33; 234–63.

Wittmaack, K. (1907) Weitere Beiträge zur Kenntnis der degenerativen Neuritis und Atrophie des Hörnerven. Atrophie des Hörnerven nach Typhus. *Zeitschrift für Ohrenheilkunde*, **53**, 12–6.

Wittmaack, K. (1919) Ueber die Wirkung des Chinins im Gehörorgan. *Beitr. Anat.*, **12**, 27–43.

Wittmaack, K. (1936) Ueber Chininwirkung im Gehörorgan. *Zeitschrift für Hals-, Nasen und Ohrenheilkunde*, **39**, 211–22.

Wolf, L.R., Otten, E.J. and Spadafora, M.P. (1992) Cinchonism: two case reports and review of acute quinine toxicity and treatment. *Journal of Emergency Medicine*, **10**, 295–301.

Wolinsky, J.S. (1996) Mumps virus, in *Field's Virology* (eds B.N. Fields, D.M. Knipe and P.M. Howley), 3rd edn, Lippincott-Raven Publishers, Philadelphia, pp. 1243–65.

Wolinsky, J.S., Klassen, T. and Baringer, J.R. (1976) Persistence of neuroadapted mumps virus in brains of newborn hamsters after intraperitoneal inoculation. *Journal of Infectious Diseases*, **133**, 260–7.

Wolinsky, J.S. and Stroop, W.G. (1978) Virulence and persistence of three prototype strains of mumps virus in newborn hamsters. *Archives of Virology*, **57**, 355–9.

Wolinsky, J.S., Waxham, M.N. and Server, A.C. (1985) Protective effects of glycoprotein-specific monoclonal antibodies on the course of experimental mumps virus meningoencephalitis. *Journal of Virology*, **53**, 727–34.

Wolinsky, J.S., Barninger, J.R., Margolis, G. and Kilham, L. (1974) Ultrastructure of mumps virus replication in newborn hamster central nervous system. *Laboratory Investigations*, **31**, 403–12.

Woll, B. and Kyle, J.G. (1989) Communication and language development in children of deaf parents, in *The Social and Cognitive Aspects of Normal and Atypical Language Development* (eds S. von Tetzchner, L.S. Siegel and L. Smith), Springer-Verlag, New York.

Wong-Riley, M.T.T., Walsh, S.M., Leake-Jones, P.A. and Merzenich, M.M. (1981) Maintenance of neuronal activity by electrical stimulation of unilaterally deafened cats demonstrable with cytochrome oxidase technique. *Annals of Otology, Rhinology and Laryngology Supplement*, **82**, 30–2.

Woods, C.R. and Englund, J. (1993) Congenital toxoplasmosis presenting with eosinophilic meningitis. *Pediatric Infectious Disease Journal*, **12**, 347–8.

Woodward, J. (1972) Implications for sociolinguistics research among the deaf. *Sign Language Studies*, **1**, 1–7.

Woodward, T.E. and Osterman, J.V. (1984) Rickettsial diseases, Chapter 94 in *Tropical and Geographical Medicine* (eds K.S. Warren and A.A.F. Mahmoud), McGraw-Hill, New York.

Woolf, N.K. (1990) Experimental congenital cytomegalovirus labyrinthitis and sensorineural hearing loss. *American Journal of Otolaryngology*, **11**, 299–303.

Woolf, N.K. (1991) Guinea pig model of congenital CMV-induced hearing loss: a review. *Transplantation Proceedings*, **23**, 32–4.

Woolf, N.K., Harris, J.P., Ryan, A.F., Butler, D.M. and Richman, D.D. (1985) Hearing loss in experimental cytomegalovirus infection of the guinea pig inner ear: prevention by systemic immunity. *Annals of Otology, Rhinology and Laryngology*, **94**, 350–6.

Woolf, N.K., Ochi, J.W., Silva, E.J., Sharp, P.A., Harris, J.P. and Richman, D.D. (1988) Ganciclovir prophylaxis for cochlear pathophysiology during experimental guinea pig cytomegalovirus labyrinthitis. *Antimicrobial Agents and Chemotherapy*, **32**, 865–72.

Woolf, N.K., Koehrn, F.J., Harris, J.P. and Richman, D.D. (1989) Congenital cytomegalovirus labyrinthitis and sensorineural hearing loss in guinea pigs. *Journal of Infectious Diseases*, **160**, 929–37.

Woolley, A.L., Kirk, K.A., Neumann, A.M., McWilliams, S.M., Murray, J., Friend, D. and Wiatrak, B.J. (1999) Risk factors for hearing loss from meningitis in children: the Children's Hospital experience. *Archives of Otolaryngology – Head and Neck Surgery*, **125**, 509–14.

Wreghitt, T.G., Hakim, M., Gray, J.J., Kucia, S., Wallwork, J. and English, T.A. (1988) Cytomegalovirus infections in heart and heart and lung transplant recipients. *Journal of Clinical Pathology*, **41**(6), 660–7.

Wright, C.G. and Schaefer, S.D. (1982) Inner ear histopathology in patients treated with *cis*-platinum. *Laryngoscope*, **92**, 1408–23.

Wright, D. (1969) *Deafness: A Personal Account*, Allen Lane, London.

Wright, A. (1997) Anatomy and ultrastructure of the human ear, in *Scott Brown's Basic Sciences* (ed. M. Gleeson), Butterworth and Heinemann, Oxford.

Wright, A. (1998) Ototoxicity, in *Diseases of the Ear* (eds H. Ludman and A. Wright), 6th edn, Arnold, London, pp. 502–15.

Wright, A. (1999) Bacterial meningitis and deafness. *Clinical Otolaryngology*, **24**, 385–7

Wright, K.E., Dimock, K. and Brown, E.G. (2000) Biological characteristics of genetic variants of Urabe AM9 mumps vaccine virus. *Research in Virology*, **67**, 49–57.

Wu, H.C., Lecain, E., Chiappini, I., Yang, T.H. and Tran Ba Hy, P. (2003) Influence of auditory deprivation upon the tonotopic organisation in the inferior colliculus of a Fos immunocytochemical study in the rat. *European Journal of Neuroscience*, **17**, 2540–52.

Wylie, P.A.L., Stevens, D., Drake III, W., Stuart, J. and Cartwright, K. (1997) Epidemiology and clinical management of meningococcal disease in West Gloucestershire: retrospective, population based study. *British Medical Journal*, **315**, 774–9.

Yagi, M., Harada, T., Yamasoba, T. and Kikuchi, S. (1994) Clinical features of idiopathic bilateral sensorineural hearing loss. *ORL – Journal of Otorhinolaryngology and Its Related Specialties*, **56**, 5–10.

Yakahashi, Y., Teranishi, A., Yamada, Y., Yoshida, Y., Hashimoto, K., Sakamoto, Y. *et al.* (1998) A case of congenital mumps infection complicated with persistent pulmonary hypertension. *American Journal of Perinatology*, **15**, 409–12.

Yamamoto, M., Watanabe, Y. and Mizukoshi, K. (1993) Neurotological findings in patients with acute mumps deafness. *Acta Otolaryngologica Supplement*, **504**, 94–7.

Yamamoto, A.P., Mussi-Pinhata, M.M., Pinto, P.C.G., Figueiredo, L.T.M. and Jorge, S.M. (2001) Congenital cytomegalovirus infection in preterm and full-term newborn infants from a population with a high seroprevalence rate. *Pediatric Infectious Disease Journal*, **20**, 188–92.

Yanagita, N. and Murahashi, K. (1986) A comparative study of mumps deafness and idiopathic profound sudden deafness. *Archives of Otorhinolaryngologica*, **243**, 197–9.

Yapo Ette, H., Koffi, K., Botti, K., Jouvet, A., Effi, A.B. and Honde, M. (2002) Sudden death caused by parasites: postmortem cerebral malaria discoveries in the African endemic zone. *American Journal of Forensic Medicine and Pathology*, **23**, 202–7.

Yeo, S.F. and Wong, B. (2002) Current status of nonculture methods for diagnosis of invasive fungal infections. *Clinical Microbiology Reviews*, **15**, 465–84.

Yogev, R. (2002) Meningitis, in *Pediatric Infectious Diseases. Principles and Practice* (eds H.B. Jenson and R.S. Baltimore), 2nd edn, W.B. Saunders, Philadelphia.

Yokosawa, N., Kubota, T. and Fujji, N. (1998) Poor induction of interferon-induced 2′-5′-oligoadenylate synthetase (2′-5′ AS) in cells persistently infected with mumps virus in caused by a decrease in STAT-1alpha. *Archives of Virology*, **143**, 1985–92.

Yoon, T.H., Paparella, M.M., Schachern, P.A. and Alleva, M. (1990) Histopathology of sudden hearing loss. *Laryngoscopy*, **100**(7), 707–15.

Yoshinago-Itano, C. (2003) From screening to early identification and intervention: discovering predictors to successful outcomes for children with significant hearing loss. *Journal of Deaf Studies and Deaf Education*, **8**, 11–30.

Yoshinaga-Itano, C., Coulter, D. and Thomson, V. (2000) The Colorado Newborn Hearing Screening Project effects on speech and language development for children with hearing loss. *Journal of Perinatology*, **20**, 5132–7.

Young, A.M. (1999) The impact of a cultural linguistic model of deafness on hearing families' adjustment to a deaf child. *Journal of Social Work Practice*, **13**, 157–72.

Young, A.M. (2002) Factors affecting communication choice in the first year of life. *Deafness and Education International*, **4**, 1–12.

Young, A.M. (2003) *Parenting and Deaf Children – A Psychosocial Literature Based Framework*, National Deaf Children's Society, London.

Yurochko, A.D., Hwang, E.S., Rasmussen, L., Keay, S., Pereiro, L. and Huang, E.S. (1997) The human cytomegalovirus UL55 (gB) and UL75 (gH)glycoprotein ligands initiate the rapid activation of Sp1 and NF-kappaB during infection. *Journal of Virology*, **71**, 5051–9.

Zaia, J.A., Forman, S.J., Ting, Y.P., Vanderwal-Urbina, E. and Blume, K.S. (1986) Polypeptide-specific antibody response to human cytomegalovirus after infection in bone marrow transplant recipients. *Journal of Infectious Diseases*, **153**, 780–7.

Zaia, J.A., Gallez-Hawkins, G.M., Tegtmeier, B.R., terVeer, A., Niland, J.C. and Forman, S.J. (1997) Late cytomegalovirus disease in marrow transplantation is predicted by virus load in plasma. *Journal of Infectious Diseases*, **176**, 782–5.

Zakzouk, S. (1997) Epidemiology and etiology of hearing impairment among infants and children in a developing country: Part II. *Journal of Otolaryngology*, **26**, 335–44.

Zakzouk, S.M. (2003) Epidemiological Study of Childhood Hearing Impairment in Saudi Arabia. Informal Consultation on Epidemiology of Deafness and Hearing Impairment in Developing Countries and Update of the WHO Protocol, World Health Organization, Geneva, March 2003.

Zanghellini, F., Emery, V., Boppana, S., Griffiths, P.D. and Pass, R.F. (1998) Virologic characteristics and immune response to cytomegalovirus infection in normal adolescents, Southern Society for Pediatric Research Annual Meeting, New Orleans.

Zeller, J.A., Zunker, P., Witt, K., Schlueter, E. and Deuschl, G. (2002) Unusual presentation of carcinomatous meningitis: case report and review of typical CSF findings.
Neurological Research, **24**, 652–4.

Zeltser, R. and Kurban, A.K. (2004) Syphilis. *Clinics in Dermatology*, **22**, 461–8.

Zemke, D. and Majid, A. (2004) The potential of minocycline for neuroprotection in
human neurologic disease. *Clinical Neuropharmacology*, **27**, 293–8.

Zheng, J., Shen, W., He, D.Z., Long, K.B., Madison, L.D. and Dallos, P. (2000) Prestin is
the motor protein of cochlear outer hair cells. *Nature*, **405**, 149–55.

Zheng, J., Ren, T., Parthasarathi, A. and Nuttall, A.L. (2001) Quinine-induced alterations of electrically evoked otoacoustic emissions and cochlear potentials in guinea
pigs. *Hearing Research*, **154**, 124–34.

Zhou, Y.F., Leon, M.B., Waclawiw, M.A., Popma, J.J., Yu, Z.X., Finkel, T. and Epstein,
S.E. (1996) Association between prior cytomegalovirus infection and the risk of
restenosis after coronary atherectomy (see comments). *New England Journal of
Medicine*, **335**, 624–30.

Zhou, Y.F., Shou, M., Guetta, E., Guzman, R., Unger, E.F., Yu, Z.X., Zhang, J., Finkel,
T. and Epstein, S.E. (1999) Cytomegalovirus infection of rats increases the neointi-
mal response to vascular injury without consistent evidence of direct infection of the
vascular wall. *Circulation*, **100**, 1569–75.

Zhu, J., Quyyumi, A.A., Norman, J.E., Osago, G. and Epstein, S.E. (1999)
Cytomegalovirus in the pathogenesis of atherosclerosis: the role of inflammation as
reflected by elevated C-reactive protein levels. *Journal of the American College of
Cardiology*, **34**, 1738–43.

Zysk, G., Bruck, W., Gerber, J., Bruck, Y., Prange, H.W. and Nau, R. (1996) Anti-
inflammatory treatment influences neuronal apoptotic cell death in the dentate
gyrus in experimental pneumococcal meningitis. *Journal of Neuropathology and
Experimental Neurology*, **55**, 722–8.

INDEX

A

Actinomycosis, 197
Acquired immunodeficiency syndrome (AIDS), 164–8
Adenovirus, 177, 269
Allograft, 69
Amikacin, 168, 243
Aminoglycosides, 239, 242–8, 260
Angiostrongylasis, 199, 218, 230, 231–2
Antibiotic resistance, 174–5, 193, 205–6
Antibody
  in diagnosis, 177, 263–70
  in ear, 137, 140
Antioxidants, 247, 249
Antiretrovirals, 168, 276
Apoptosis, 246
Audiometry,
  high frequency, 244, 248
  pure tone, 121, 243
Auditory brainstem responses, 149–50, 201–2, 213, 267, 270
Auditory cortex, 14–15, 23
Autism, 100, 104, 135
Azithromycin, 168, 253

B

Bacteroides spp., 175, 198
Balance, 1, 167, 239, 243
Bartonella henselae, 194
Biofilm, 175–6
Blood-perilymph barrier, 242, 250
Borrelia burgdorferi, 194, 275
Brain-derived neurotrophic factor, 209
Brill-Zinsser disease, 221, 222
Brucella melitensis, 195
Brucellosis, 195

C

Caspases, 188–9, 246
Cataracts, 99, 262
Cephalosporin, 205
  Cefotaxime, 205
Ceftriaxone, 205
Cerebrospinal fluid (CSF), 115, 119, 123, 203–4
Chlamydia, 195
Chloramphenicol, 254
Chloroquine, 230
Cisplatin (cis-platinum), 188, 248, 249
Citrobacter spp., 190, 193
Cochlea, 8–9, 11, 22–4
Cochlear implant, 26, 27, 30, 210–3, 281
Cochleotoxicity, 239
Cochleovestibular nerve (VIIIth cranial nerve, auditory nerve), 14–15, 23, 123, 160, 163, 166, 184
Cholesteatoma, 180, 198
Chorioretinitis, 74, 146, 147, 169, 262
Clarithromycin, 168, 253
Clindamycin, 147, 188, 193
Communication, 280, 281, 282
Coxsackie virus, 269
Crista, 13, 20, 245
Critical period, 26, 143, 247
Cryptococcus neoformans, 166, 198
CSF (See cerebrospinal fluid)
Cyclooxygenase inhibitors, 209
Cytokines, 134, 161
Cytomegalovirus (CMV)
  clinical features (disease), 67–9
  congenital, 71–4, 79–84, 263–4, 274
  experimental model for, 87–9
  diagnosis of, 263–8, 270

Infection and Hearing Impairment. Edited by V.E. Newton and P.J. Vallely
© 2006 John Wiley & Sons, Ltd

epidemiology, 70–73
hearing, effect on, 79–84
immune response to, 77–9
pathogenesis
    of infection, 76–9
    of hearing loss, 84–9
treatment, 90–91, 276–7
viral properties, 74–6

D
DALY, 31, 40–44
Dexamethasone, 205, 207–8
Desferrioxamine, 254–5
Diphtheria, 223–4
Diuretics, loop, 242, 251–2
Doxycycline, 209, 275

E
Ear
    development of, 17–25, 99, 143
    external, 1–4, 17–19,
    inner, 8–9, 19–24, 100–1, 180–1, 241–2
    middle, 4–8, 19, 180
Eardrum (see also tympanic membrane), 236
Electronystagmography, 213, 245
Encephalitis
    Acute, 109, 116, 135, 146, 169, 231
    post-infectious, 116, 135, 138
Endocochlear potential, 11, 23, 248
Endolymph, 11, 13, 19
Enterobacteriacae, 193
Enteroviruses, 177, 200–01
Epidemic
    HIV/AIDS, 67, 164–5
    Measles, 131
    Meningitis, 191–2
    Mumps, 109
    Rubella, 95, 104, 271
    Tuberculosis, 225–6
    Typhus, 221–2
Epstein-Barr virus, 269
Erythromycin, 163, 193, 205, 242, 253
Escherichia coli, 185, 192, 193, 212
Eustachian tube, 6,19, 168, 171–2

F
Facial nerve (VIIth cranial nerves), 7, 19,
    166–7

Fibrosis, 86, 87, 89, 125, 173, 179, 186, 259
Free radicals, 209, 246–7
Furosemide (Frusemide), 251
Fusobacterium sp, 175

G
Ganciclovir, 90, 276, 277
Gene mutation, 247,
Gentamicin, 243, 255
Glutathione, 208, 247, 249
Gnathostoma spinigerum, 199, 218, 230,
    232–4

H
Haemophilus influenzae, 173–5, 189, 212,
    268, 272
Hair cells
    inner, 10–12, 23, 184–5, 188–9
    outer, 10–13, 23, 184–5
Hearing aid, 30, 235, 281
Hearing impairment (or loss)
    laterality
        bilateral, 30, 80, 100, 120, 195
        unilateral, 30, 100, 110, 120, 195
    onset
        acquired, 33, 42, 57, 80, 82, 93, 100,
            259, 265–8
        congenital, 29, 79–84, 100–01,
            149–51, 163, 258, 263–4
        early, 27, 33, 57
        progressive, 80, 82, 93, 202, 248–9,
            279, 283
        sudden, 110, 163, 268–71
    type
        conductive, 150, 160, 167, 179–80
        retrocochlear, 184, 210,
        sensorineural, 29–30, 93, 99, 138–9,
            143, 149, 153, 158, 164–5, 180,
            183, 184, 192, 195, 199, 200, 201,
            202, 220, 225, 227, 232, 235,
Herpes simplex virus, 169, 177, 200, 264
Human cytomegalovirus (HCMV), (See
    cytomegalovirus)
Human immunodeficiency virus (HIV),
    164–8, 270–1, 275–6

I
Immunisation (See also vaccination),
    102–4, 133, 191, 271–5

Immunocompromised, 67, 68, 90, 133, 146
Immune response
  cell-mediated, 134
  fetal, 161, 264
  humoral, 263
  inner ear, 87, 137, 140, 187
  maternal, 72, 263
Incus, 6, 19
Inflammatory response, 78, 161, 187
Interferons, 78, 119

K

Kaposi's sarcoma,166
Ketrorolac, 209
Klebsiella spp, 193

L

Labyrinth, 8, 20, 23, 100, 124, 138, 142, 160, 180, 184, 224
  ossification of, 186, 210, 211, 215
Labyrinthitis, 84, 86–7, 125, 138, 139, 148, 179, 184, 186, 211, 214
Lassa fever, 219–21
Leprosy, 226–7
Lipopolysaccharides, 187, 189
Listeria monocytogenes, 190, 192, 193, 205, 205

M

Macula, 14, 20, 125, 245
Magnetic resonance, 201
Malaria, 42, 143, 227–229
Malleus, 5, 6, 7, 19
Mastoid, 4, 6, 19, 143, 165, 171, 180, 224
Mastoiditis, 275
Measles
  clinical features, 133
  epidemiology, 131
  hearing, effect on, 135–6
  immune response to, 134, 270
  pathogenesis, 136–42
  viral properties, 128–31
Meninges, 186, 201, 211
Meningitis, 32, 42, 55, 56–59, 180
  Bacterial,

Haemophilus influenzae, 184, 207
  pneumoccocal, 187, 188, 190, 192, 209, 210, 214, 273
  Listeria, 192, 205
  meningococcal, 186, 190–2, 194, 204–7, 213–4, 272–3, 278
  tuberculous, 196–7
  eosinophilia, 199, 230–233
  pachymeningitis, 201
  recurrent, 200, 259
  viral, 199–201
Meningoencephalitis, 98, 116, 120, 124, 166, 200, 201, 230, 275
Microcephaly, 74, 83, 99
Microphthalmia, 99
Middle latency response, 150
Minocycline, 209, 215
Mismatch negativity, 25
MMR, 101–4, 106, 110, 111, 132, 258, 271–2
Mondini defect, 29, 180
Moraxella catarrhalis, 173, 174, 175, 269
Mumps
  clinical features, 114
  epidemiology, 112
  hearing, effect on, 110–112, 120–5
  immune response to, 119–120, 269
  pathogenesis, 114–15
  viral properties, 112–14
Mycobacterium tuberculosis, 168, 197, 226, 268
Mycoplasma pneumoniae, 195

N

Neisseria meningitides, 186, 190, 268, 272
Neurones, 14, 15, 23, 27, 116, 117, 139, 187, 201, 210, 245, 250
Nucleic acid amplification, 98, 115, 176, 264, 269, 270

O

Organ of Corti,
  normal, 10, 12, 22–3
  abnormal, 86, 89, 121, 125, 139, 188, 199, 243, 246, 250, 254
Orientia tsutsugannishi, 222

Ossicles, 4, 5–6, 7, 19, 173, 179
Otitis media, 59–61, 135–6, 137–8, 198, 275
  Acute, 174, 175, 177, 178, 195, 269, 273
  Chronic, 32, 47, 54, 179–80
  chronic suppurative, 179–80
  with effusion, 179
  recurrent, 167, 172, 173
Otoacoustic emissions, 213, 250, 252
Otocyst, 20, 26
Otorrhoea, 176
Otosclerosis, 127, 136, 139–140, 163
Otoscopy, 233
Ototoxicity
  antibiotics
    aminoglycosides, 29, 188, 198, 209, 241, 244, 245, 247, 248, 260
    macrolides, 253
    other, 253, 254
  anti-inflammatories, 250–1
  antimalarials, 229–230, 249–250
  antineoplastic agent, 243, 246, 248–9, 252
  loop diuretics, 251, 252

P

Pandemic
  HIV/AIDS, 235
  rubella, 95, 96
  tuberculosis, 225
Parainfluenza, 177, 269
Paramyxoviruses, 112, 119, 123, 124, 128, 129, 140
Parasite, 143, 145, 146, 148, 229, 230, 231, 235
Parasitemia, 145, 146
Parvovirus, 95, 98
Penicillin, 153, 163, 174, 175, 193, 205, 206
Perilymph, 8, 11, 13, 19, 23, 241, 242, 245, 250, 254
Pinna (or auricle), 1–3, 18
Plasmodium falciparum, 228, 229
Plasticity, 26–8
Pneumocystis carinii, 167, 168
Pneumolysin, 188, 209
Poliovirus, 137
Polymerase, viral, 75, 90, 112, 113

Polymyxin B, 254
Porphyromonas spp, 175
Posturography, dynamic, 245
Prestin, 251
Prevalence, of hearing loss, 34–40, 79, 101, 104, 110, 183, 221, 278
Prevotella spp, 175
Proteus mirabilis, 198
Pseudomonas aeruginosa, 175
Psuedophyllidean cestodes, 235

Q

Quinine, 229–30, 249–50

R

Radicals, free, 246, 247, 249
Ramsey Hunt syndrome, 167
Rash, 95, 97, 102, 133, 137, 158, 159, 162, 221
Rehabilitation, 283, 286
Reissner's membrane, 9, 11, 22, 121, 124, 125
Respiratory syncytial virus, 141, 177, 273
Retinitis, 79
Retinoids, 260
Retrovirals (see antiretrovirals)
Reverse transcriptase PCR
Rickettsia prowazekii, 221–2
Rifampicin, 188, 197, 205–6, 209–10
Rubella
  clinical features, 95, 98
  congenital, 93, 94, 96, 98–100
  epidemiology, 101, 104
  hearing, effect on, 100–1
  viral properties, 95

S

Saccule, 20, 22, 122, 125, 245
Salicylates, 242, 246, 249, 250–1
Salmonella spp, 193, 208
Scala
  media, 8, 9, 11, 189, 245, 248
  tympani, 8, 22, 89, 180, 185, 242
  vestibule, 8, 11, 22, 242
Screening,
  infection, 80, 82, 278
    antenatal, 102, 104, 160
    maternal, 274, 276

neonatal, 277
TORCH, 263
hearing, 74, 204, 213, 258
neonatal, 46, 82, 281
Semicircular canals, 13–14, 20, 185
Seroconversion, 98, 110, 125, 133
Sign language
British, 280
American, 280
Sparganosis, 234–5
Speech, 25, 28, 29, 30, 45, 100, 116, 210,
243, 259, 281,
Spiral ganglion, 14, 23, 84, 86, 89, 125,
139, 186, 189, 210, 245, 250
Stapes, 6, 7, 8, 11, 19, 139
Stapedius, 7, 19
Staphylococcus aureus, 174, 175, 190
Streptomycin, 225, 239, 243, 254
Stria Vascularis, 9, 11, 22, 23, 100, 121–3,
125, 248, 251, 252, 253
Streptococcus
Group B, 190, 192, 193, 202, 204, 206, 209
S. agalactiae, 192
S. pneumoniae, 173, 178, 268, 269, 273
S. suis, 186, 194
S. viridans, 212
Syphilis
clinical features
congenital, 160–3
primary, 157–8
secondary, 158–9
tertiary, 159–60
diagnosis, laboratory, 264, 270
epidemiology, 156–7
hearing, effect on, 153, 155, 158, 160
immune response to, 161
pathogenesis, 159, 160, 163
properties, 155–6
therapy, 163, 275

T
Taenia solium, 199
Tectorial membrane, 10, 12, 22, 121, 122,
244
Temporal bone, 3, 4, 6, 18, 84, 86, 89, 160,
184, 186, 224, 226, 260
Temporal lobe, 4, 15
Tensor tympani, 6, 7, 19

Teratogen, 29, 260
Tinnitus, 120, 149, 158, 160, 166, 194, 222,
229, 242, 249, 250, 253
Tobramycin, 243
Togavirus, 95
Toxins
endo-, 187, 188
exo-, 179
Toxocara canis, 199
Toxoplasma gondii, 143, 144, 145
Toxoplasmosis
clinical features, 146
congenital, 146, 149–50
acquired, 148–9
diagnosis, laboratory, 147, 262
epidemiology, 144, 150
hearing, effect on, 149–50
immune response to, 150
properties, 145
therapy, 147–8
Treponema pallidum, 155–161, 264
Trigeminal nerve (Vth cranial nerve)
Tuberculosis, 42, 196–7, 201, 247, 268
Tympanosclerosis, 173
Tympanic Membrane, 1, 4, 5, 6, 7, 18, 19,
167, 179, 233
perforation, 172, 173, 225
Tympanostomy, 174, 175, 176
Tympanum, 19
Typhoid Fever, 224–5
Typhus, 221–223

U
Utricle, 13, 14, 20, 122, 245

V
Vaccination/Vaccine
cytomegalovirus, 90–1
Haemophilus influenzae, 190, 212
meningococcal, 190
MMR, 102–6, 110, 28, 271–2
pneumococcal, 273
Vancomycin, 205, 253–4
Varicella zoster virus, 166, 200, 264, 267
Vestibular system, 13–15, 84, 86, 243, 245,
246, 249
Vestibular ganglia, 23, 89, 125
Vestibule, 7, 19

Vestibulotoxicity, 239, 243, 254
Viomycin, 254
Viraemia, 97, 117, 118, 119
Vogt-Koyanagi-Harada Syndrome, 201

W
West Nile virus, 201
World Health Organisation, 31, 33
    Survey, 33, 34, 40, 43, 46–7

Y
Yellow fever, 219
YLD, 31, 40, 44
YLL, 31, 40–43

Z
Zoster oticus, 166–7